Controversy in Anesthesiology

Edited by

JAMES E. ECKENHOFF, M.D.

Dean and Professor of Anesthesia
Northwestern University Medical School
Chicago, Illinois

W. B. SAUNDERS COMPANY   Philadelphia   London   Toronto

W. B. Saunders Company: West Washington Square
Philadelphia, PA 19105

1 St. Anne's Road
Eastbourne, East Sussex BN21 3UN, England

1 Goldthorne Avenue
Toronto, Ontario M8Z 5T9, Canada

Library of Congress Cataloging in Publication Data

Main entry under title:

Controversy in anesthesiology.

1. Anesthesia — Complications and sequelae.   2. Anesthetics
  — Toxicology.   I. Eckenhoff, James E. [DNLM:
  1. Anesthesia.   2. Anesthetics. W0200.3 C764]

RD82.5.C66   617'.96   79–3918

ISBN 0–7216–3322–6

Controversy in Anesthesiology   ISBN 0-7216-3322-6

Last digit is the print number: 9   8   7   6   5   4   3   2

CONTROVERSY

"There is no learned man but will confess he hath much profited by reading controversies; his senses awakened, his judgment sharpened, and the truth which he holds more firmly established. In logic they teach that controversies laid together more evidently appear; and controversy being permitted, falsehood will appear more false, and truth more true."

JOHN MILTON

CONTRIBUTORS

ROBERT H. BARTLETT, M.D., Professor of Surgery, University of California at Irvine; Chief, General Surgery Division, University of California at Irvine Medical Center.
IPPB SHOULD NOT BE ROUTINE PULMONARY PROPHYLAXIS

JOHN M. BEAL, M.D., Edward S. Elcock Professor of Surgery and Chairman, Department of Surgery, Northwestern University Medical School; Chairman, Department of Surgery, Northwestern Memorial Hospital, Chicago, Illinois.
SURGEONS AND THE "CAPTAIN OF THE SHIP" DOCTRINE

JOHN J. BONICA, M.D., D.Sc., F.F.A.R.C.S., Professor of Anesthesiology; Director, Pain Center, University of Washington School of Medicine, Seattle, Washington; Attending Anesthesiologist, University of Washington affiliated hospitals, Seattle, Washington.
ACUPUNCTURE ANALGESIA AND ANESTHESIA

BURNELL R. BROWN, JR., M.D., Ph.D., Professor and Head, Department of Anesthesiology, University of Arizona College of Medicine, Tucson, Arizona.
HALOTHANE HEPATITIS IS A REASONABLY WELL PROVED CLINICAL ENTITY

DAVID L. BRUCE, M.D., Professor of Anesthesiology, University of California at Irvine; Chief, Anesthesiology Service, Long Beach Veterans Administration Medical Center, Long Beach, California.
HALOTHANE AND HEPATITIS: A DIRECT RELATIONSHIP IS UNPROVED

ELLIS N. COHEN, M.D., Professor of Anesthesia, Stanford University Medical Center, Stanford, California.
INHALATIONAL ANESTHETICS MAY CAUSE GENETIC DEFECTS, ABORTIONS, AND MISCARRIAGES IN OPERATING ROOM PERSONNEL

JAY S. DEVORE, M.D., Assistant Professor of Anesthesiology and Obstetrics and Gynecology, University of California at Irvine; Director of Obstetric Anesthesia, University of California at Irvine

Medical Center; Attending Anesthesiologist, Long Beach Veterans Administration Medical Center, Long Beach, California.

ALL PARTURIENTS RECEIVING GENERAL ANESTHESIA SHOULD HAVE TRACHEAL INTUBATION

JOHN W. DITZLER, M.D., Former Professor of Anesthesia, Northwestern Medical School, Chicago, Illinois; Director of Resources, Veterans Administration, Washington, D.C.

NURSE ANESTHETISTS SHOULD BE TRAINED AND SUPERVISED BY ANESTHESIOLOGISTS

GALE E. DRYDEN, M.D., Assistant Professor of Anesthesiology, Indiana University School of Medicine; Chief of Anesthesiology, Wishard Memorial Hospital, Indianapolis, Indiana.

INHALATION ANESTHESIA EQUIPMENT SHOULD BE ASEPTIC FOR EACH USE

JAMES E. ECKENHOFF, M.D., Dean and Professor of Anesthesia, Northwestern University Medical School, Chicago, Illinois; Senior Attending Anesthesiologist, Northwestern Memorial Hospital; Consultant in Anesthesiology, Children's Memorial Hospital and the Veterans Administration Lakeside Medical Center, Chicago, Illinois.

DELIBERATE HYPOTENSION—A DEVIL'S ADVOCATE ANALYSIS

THOMAS W. FEELEY, M.D., Assistant Professor, Stanford University School of Medicine, Stanford, California; Associate Medical Director of Intensive Care, Stanford University Medical Center.

A NEED FOR ASEPTIC INHALATION ANESTHESIA EQUIPMENT FOR EACH CASE IS UNPROVEN

LOUIS L. FERSTANDIG, Ph.D., Vice President and Technical Director, Halocarbon Laboratories, Incorporated, Hackensack, New Jersey.

TRACE CONCENTRATIONS OF ANESTHETICS ARE NOT PROVED HEALTH HAZARDS

NICHOLAS G. GEORGIADE, M.D., P.D.S., Professor of Surgery and Chairman, Division of Plastic, Maxillofacial, and Oral Surgery, Duke University School of Medicine, Durham, North Carolina; Attending Surgeon, Duke University Hospital.

DELIBERATE HYPOTENSION—EDITORIAL COMMENT

AKE GRENVIK, M.D., Ph.D., Professor of Anesthesiology and Director, Division of Critical Care Medicine, University of Pittsburgh School of Medicine and Health Center Hospitals, Pittsburgh, Pennsylvania.

INTENSIVE CARE UNIT PATIENT CARE: A RESPONSIBILITY OF CRITICAL CARE MEDICINE PHYSICIANS

IRA P. GUNN, M.L.N., C.R.N.A., Educational Consultant, Council on Accreditation of Nurse Anesthesia Education Programs/Schools; American Association of Nurse Anesthetists, Council on Certification of Nurse Anesthetists.

NURSE ANESTHETISTS SHOULD CONTROL THE TEACHING AND PRACTICE OF THEIR PROFESSION

WILLIAM K. HAMILTON, M.D., Professor and Chairman, Department of Anesthesia, University of California at San Francisco School of Medicine; Attending in Anesthesia, University of California at San Francisco Hospitals, Moffitt Hospital, San Francisco General Hospital, and Veterans Administration Medical Center.

A NEED FOR ASEPTIC INHALATION ANESTHESIA EQUIPMENT FOR EACH CASE IS UNPROVEN

JOHN HEDLEY-WHYTE, M.D., David S. Sheridan Professor of Anesthesia and Respiratory Therapy, Harvard Medical School, Boston, Massachusetts; Anesthetist-in-Chief, Beth Israel Hospital, Boston, Massachusetts.

INTRA-ARTERIAL MONITORING: A ROUTINE AND SAFE PROCEDURE

JAY JACOBY, M.D., Ph.D., Professor and Chairman, Department of Anesthesiology, Jefferson Medical College, Philadelphia, Pennsylvania; Director, Department of Anesthesiology, Thomas Jefferson University Hospital.

INTRA-ARTERIAL MONITORING IS NOT A ROUTINE PROCEDURE

M. T. JENKINS, M.D., McDermott Professor and Chairman, Department of Anesthesiology, University of Texas Southwestern Medical School, Dallas, Texas; Chief of Anesthesiology, Parkland Memorial Hospital, Children's Medical Center, Dallas Veterans Administration Medical Center, and Texas Scottish Rite Hospital for Crippled Children.

NURSE ANESTHETISTS SHOULD NOT ADMINISTER REGIONAL ANESTHESIA

ANNE E. P. JONES, M.B.B.S., F.F.A.R.C.S., Assistant Professor-in-Residence of Anesthesia, University of California at Irvine; Attending Anesthesiologist, University of California at Irvine Medical Center.

TRACHEAL INTUBATION IS NOT MANDATORY IN INFANTS LESS THAN ONE YEAR OF AGE

A. ERCUMENT KOPMAN, M.D., Assistant Professor of Anesthesiology, Washington University School of Medicine, St. Louis, Missouri; Assistant Anesthesiologist, Barnes Hospital and St. Louis Children's Hospital.

BALANCED ANESTHESIA USING MORPHINE, NEUROMUSCULAR BLOCKERS, AND NITROUS OXIDE IS THE TECHNIQUE OF CHOICE

MICHAEL LESCH, M.D., Magerstadt Professor of Medicine, Northwestern University Medical School, Chicago, Illinois; Chief, Section of Cardiology, Northwestern Memorial Hospital; Attending Staff, Northwestern Memorial Hospital.

DELIBERATE HYPOTENSION – A DEVIL'S ADVOCATE ANALYSIS

MARY JEANETTE MANNINO, C.R.N.A., B.S., Clinical Instructor, Department of Anesthesiology, University of California at Irvine and California College of Medicine; C.R.N.A. Coordinator, University of California at Irvine Medical Center, Orange, California.

NURSE ANESTHETISTS SHOULD ADMINISTER REGIONAL ANESTHESIA

JOSEPH H. MARCY, M.D., Professor of Anesthesiology, University of Pittsburgh School of Medicine, Pittsburgh, Pennsylvania; Anesthesiologist, Children's Hospital of Pittsburgh.

ENDOTRACHEAL ANESTHESIA SHOULD BE USED IN ALL ANESTHETIZED INFANTS LESS THAN ONE YEAR OF AGE

LAWRENCE L. MICHAELIS, M.D., Associate Professor of Surgery, Northwestern University Medical School, Chicago, Illinois; Chief of Division of Cardiothoracic Surgery, Northwestern University Medical School.

THE ATTENDING SURGEON SHOULD RETAIN CONTROL OF SURGICAL PATIENTS IN THE INTENSIVE CARE UNIT

MALCOLM G. MILLER, M.B., Ch.B., Assistant Professor-in-Residence, University of California at Irvine; Attending Staff, Department of Anesthesiology, University of California at Irvine Medical Center.

INTRA-ARTERIAL MONITORING: A ROUTINE AND SAFE PROCEDURE

OTTO C. PHILLIPS, M.D., Clinical Professor of Anesthesiology, University of Pittsburgh School of Medicine, Pittsburgh, Pennsylvania; Chairman, Department of Anesthesiology, Western Pennsylvania Hospital, Pittsburgh, Pennsylvania.

AN ENDOTRACHEAL TUBE IS NOT MANDATORY WHEN GENERAL ANESTHESIA IS GIVEN TO A PARTURIENT

STEPHEN J. PREVOZNIK, M.D., Professor of Anesthesia, University of Pennsylvania, Philadelphia, Pennsylvania; Physician Anesthetist, Hospital of the University of Pennsylvania.

FLAMMABLE ANESTHETICS ARE OUTMODED

MAX SAMUEL SADOVE, M.D., Professor and Chairman, Department of Anesthesia, Rush, Presbyterian-St. Lukes Medical Center, Chicago, Illinois; Director of Pain Center, Rush, Presbyterian-St. Lukes Medical Center.

ACUPUNCTURE IS USEFUL IN PAIN MANAGEMENT

PETER SAFAR, M.D., Director of Resuscitation Research Center; and Anesthesiologist and Past Chairman, Department of Anesthesiology and Critical Care Medicine Health Center Hospitals, University of Pittsburgh, Pittsburgh, Pennsylvania.

INTENSIVE CARE UNIT PATIENT CARE: A RESPONSIBILITY OF CRITICAL CARE MEDICINE PHYSICIANS

M. RAMEZ SALEM, M.D., Professor and Assistant Chairman, Department of Anesthesiology, Loyola University Stritch School of Medicine, Maywood, Illinois.

DELIBERATE HYPOTENSION IS A SAFE AND ACCEPTED ANESTHETIC TECHNIQUE

BARRY ALAN SHAPIRO, M.D., Associate Professor of Clinical Anesthesia, Northwestern University Medical School, Chicago, Illinois; Medical Director, Department of Respiratory Therapy, Northwestern Memorial Hospital, Chicago, Illinois.

IPPB THERAPY IS INDICATED PREOPERATIVELY AND POSTOPERATIVELY IN SOME PATIENTS WITH PULMONARY DISEASE

C. R. STEPHEN, M.D., Professor of Anesthesiology, Washington University School of Medicine, St. Louis, Missouri; Anesthesiologist-in-Chief, Barnes Hospital, St. Louis Children's Hospital.

BALANCED ANESTHESIA USING MORPHINE, NEUROMUSCULAR BLOCKERS, AND NITROUS OXIDE IS THE TREATMENT OF CHOICE

LEROY D. VANDAM, M.D., Professor of Anesthesia, Harvard Medical School, Boston, Massachusetts; Anesthesiologist-in-Chief, Peter Bent Brigham Hospital, Boston, Massachusetts.

SPINAL ANESTHESIA – ACCEPTED

GLENN R. WEYGANDT, M.D., Associate Professor of Anesthesiology, Washington University School of Medicine, St. Louis, Missouri; Associate Anesthesiologist, Barnes Hospital, St. Louis Children's Hospital.

BALANCED ANESTHESIA USING MORPHINE, NEUROMUSCULAR BLOCKERS, AND NITROUS OXIDE IS THE TREATMENT OF CHOICE

CAROLYN J. WILKINSON, M.D., Assistant Professor, Department of Anesthesia, Northwestern University Medical School, Chicago, Illinois; Attending Staff, Northwestern Memorial Hospital, Chicago, Illinois.

HALOTHANE ANESTHESIA IS PREFERABLE TO MORPHINE

FOREWORD

This excellent volume reviews in depth a number of important topics of great interest to surgeons, anesthesiologists, and nurse anesthetists. The principle of the Captain of the Ship; How much responsibility can and should be given to nurse anesthetists; Who should be in charge of the Surgical ICU bring to mind earlier problems with which present generations are unfamiliar because increasingly close cooperation between surgeon and anesthesiologist has resolved them.

However, I cannot resist trying to put these problems into focus by recalling briefly my own personal experiences in the field of anesthesia. I was introduced to the use of ether anesthesia in 1931 at what was then known as the Womens' Free Hospital in Boston. Because of a lack of nurse anesthetists, second year medical students were regularly invited to act as anesthetists. Ordinarily, one of our classmates who had already given a few anesthesias was supposed to introduce us to the art. Unfortunately, the day that I arrived my "instructor" was ill; I was simply told by the circulating nurse to go ahead. She handed me a can of ether and a mask and said, "Don't let her pupils get too big." About the time the patient was entering the second stage of anesthesia, the operating table was seized by orderlies and, with me frantically hanging on, pushed into the operating room. The surgeon, Dr. Pemberton, who was a master surgical technician, said to me, "Son, pour it on," which I did. Within seconds the abdomen was draped, the incision made, and, even before I could get the patient deep enough to be any kind of a worry, Dr. Pemberton had the uterus out and was closing. The entire procedure required 25 minutes! Needless to say, I was back the next day as an accomplished anesthetist.

I must admit that that early experience gave me a sense of timing for the use of ether anesthesia that stood me very well over many years. As junior house officers at the Peter Bent Brigham Hospital we all gave anesthetics, inducing anesthesia with nitrous oxide and then shifting to ether. The introduction of tribromoethanol (Avertin) later was a boon to the emotional state of the patient, although it probably did not add much more.

At this period of time, the late 1930's, there were few places in the United States providing what might be called competent or sophisticated anesthesia. The University of Wisconsin, The Mayo Clinic, The Cleveland Clinic, and The Lahey Clinic were the leaders. I first became aware of modern anesthesiology while a Fellow at The Lahey Clinic in

1940 and during World War II, when Ralph Tovell was the Consultant in Anesthesiology for the European Theater of Operations and Paul Searles was assigned to the Harvard General Hospital Unit. Once having experienced the advantages of having a top flight anesthesiologist in charge of the patient I never wanted to return to the old days.

Despite the enormous advantages introduced by physicians as anesthesiologists, one must not forget the extraordinary competence of most of the nurse anesthetists in those days. Closure of patent ductus, coarctation of the aorta, mitral valvulotomy, pericardectomy, portocaval shunts, and countless other major advances in surgery were first performed successfully with experienced nurse anesthetists in charge. At one time spinal anesthesia was always administered by the surgeon and the use of adjuncts, such as tribromoethanol (Avertin) and thiopental (Pentothal), was also for the most part surgeon controlled. The responsibilities in today's operating theaters bear no resemblance to that era.

It is hoped that these reflections will encourage the reader to pursue this interesting and important historical review in depth to realize the changes that have occurred and the new problems and questions that are facing the specialty of anesthesiology. The book is very worthwhile.

J. ENGELBERT DUNPHY, M.D.
Professor of Surgery Emeritus
Consultant in Surgery
University of California, San Francisco

PREFACE

The editor acknowledges with thanks the participation and cooperation of the contributors to "Controversy in Anesthesiology." This group's acceptance of the request to write was prompt, manuscripts were in on time, recommendations for editorial changes were graciously accepted, and galleys were quickly returned. Authors for opposing positions were not always immediately found, however, some with known opinions on a controversy not wishing to put them in print alongside an opposite opinion. For instance, as noted later, obtaining a champion of deliberate hypotension was easy, but no one was willing to take the opposite side, hence, to the probable surprise of some, the editor wrote it along with an associate. Until the book is published, no author will have seen what was written by his or her counterpart. The purpose of the volume is to stimulate thought, in some instances to lay aside unwarranted acceptance of supposed fact and in others to call for the accumulation of data. In the editor's opinion, the authors have fulfilled their charge.

JAMES E. ECKENHOFF

CONTENTS

Part 1

NO LONGER AN ISSUE OF DEBATE

EDITORIAL COMMENT

by JOHN M. BEAL

Northwestern University Medical School

SURGEONS AND THE "CAPTAIN OF THE SHIP" DOCTRINE

The designation "Captain of the ship" is an outmoded phrase and indeed may be unfamiliar to recent medical graduates and residents both in anesthesia and in surgery. In fact, this designation of the surgeon should be relegated to its place in history and discarded as a concept now and in the future.

The Captain of the Ship concept is a rather amusing one, rarely held up in courts of law according to recent decisions and one which seems to be held dear to the surgeon only if the seas are calm. . . . Surgeons and anesthesiologists should consider each other members of the same team rather than adversaries, for only with a multidisciplinary approach and a free exchange of ideas can we continue to make medical progress (Lomanto, 1972).

The origin of the term "Captain of the ship" is uncertain but is interwoven with the relationships between surgery and anesthesia. Beginning in the middle of the 19th century, the advancements in surgery and anesthesia were linked closely. For centuries, the development of surgery had been impeded, not by the dexterity or ingenuity of surgeons but rather by the absence of anesthesia and the dangers of infection. The ability of ether to relieve pain during an operation was convincingly demonstrated in October 1846, by William Thomas Morton and John Collins Warren, and this agent was found to be an effective, safe general anesthetic. Another quarter of a century passed before a method to control the hazards of infection was available. The era of modern abdominal surgery did begin, however, little more than a decade after Joseph Lister ligated the external iliac artery for aneurysm under antiseptic conditions in 1868.

During the 18th century, many physicians in the United States received their medical education in the British Isles, and quite a few sought additional training there, whenever possible. By the end of the 19th century, things had changed, and surgeons in particular were attracted to Europe, especially France, Germany, and Austria. This was in large part due to the remarkable accomplishments of Billroth, von Langenbeck, Mikulicz, Kocher, and their followers. The European clinics offered an opportunity for the trainee to observe master

3

surgeons at work and to learn surgical techniques. The opportunities for surgical training in the United States were limited at this time, but, where available, surgeons were trained by the preceptor method. It is likely that, in addition to the medical knowledge obtained in the European clinics, attitudes formed there and perpetuated here led to the development of the "Captain of the ship" doctrine.

The chief of a European surgical clinic was indeed a powerful figure, often exercising dictatorial powers in the surgical suite. There is little doubt that many American surgeons attempted to emulate the imperious posture assumed by some European surgeons. At this same time, anesthesia was not developing very rapidly as a separate discipline. Chloroform, ether, and nitrous oxide were the available agents; of these, ether was the most reliable and safest, but chloroform was widely used in Europe. This limited supply of anesthetic agents did not seem to require the full-time attention of physicians. Indeed, for many years, anesthesia, most often administered as open drop ether, was given by nurses, medical students, interns, and sometimes orderlies. A few physicians acted as part-time anesthetists but devoted their principal medical practice to other areas. Anesthesia became a special area of nursing, and in hospitals, nurses were often urged to become anesthetists. Under these circumstances, the surgeon was responsible for the conduct of the operative procedure, including the entire operating team and the anesthetist. Nurses were employed by the hospital but in the operating room functioned under the direction of the surgeon. Legally, the surgeon was held liable for the entire surgical procedure, including fluid and blood therapy, as well as for anesthesia, in which he had had little or no training.

Physicians who limited their practice to anesthesia began to appear after the turn of the century, slowly increased in numbers, but received a strong impetus during World War II, when there were large numbers of injured who required anesthesia as well as surgical treatment to manage the war wounds. The introduction of cyclopropane, intravenous anesthesia, curare, and, in the 1950's, halogenated anesthetic agents was an impelling reason for specialization in anesthesia. The use of these agents in the anesthetic management of surgical patients required a greater knowledge of the pharmacologic action of anesthetic agents than the average physician or surgeon possessed. At the same time, the demand for anesthesiologists was increased by a boom in hospital construction; training programs in anesthesia expanded, and the role of the anesthesiologist became better defined.

The anesthesiologist is essentially a hospital-based physician who devotes more time to operating and recovery room activities than does any other physician. The anesthesiologist is in close contact with nursing personnel, and the availability of anesthetists has direct influence on surgical schedules and the smoothness with which they proceed. The anesthesiologist has become the trouble-shooter of the operating room; it is little wonder that anesthesiologists have been considered a threat to the dominance of the surgeon in the surgical theatre.

The expansion of the scope of the field of anesthesia into respiratory pathophysiology, applied pharmacology, fluid therapy, and intensive care has contributed significantly to both surgical and medical patient management. The courts have generally ruled that anesthesiologists have legal responsibility for their role in patient care and now, responsibility also for nurse anesthetists. In many institutions, anesthesiologists assume the role of director of the operating rooms and the recovery rooms.

The relationship between surgeons and anesthesiologists has evolved over the years from what was too often an adversary position to one of mutual respect and interdependence, although an occasional dying gasp reverberates from a proponent of the "Captain of the ship" doctrine. The nature of the professional sphere of activity of anesthesiologists indeed results in episodic patient care, whereas surgeons are responsible for continuing management of the surgical patient's problems. This difference in professional function leads to occasional conflicts, but the customary preoperative assessment of patients by anesthesiologists has done much to decrease this conflict, and the supportive role of anesthesiologists has provided better patient care in recovery rooms and intensive care units. Their participation in inhalation therapy and respiratory care sections has also enhanced patient treatment and, in addition, has done much to develop rapport between the disciplines. Mutual respect has also improved since surgeons have elected to operate upon the desperately ill and those at the extremes of life and to perform procedures with a degree of complexity that was only dreamed of 20 years ago. Without physicians equally well trained in anesthesiology as surgeons are in surgery, these endeavours would be doomed to failure.

The operating room is an area in which care is provided for patients who suffer from disease requiring operative intervention. Anesthesiologists contribute their skills in the selection and administration of anesthetic agents best suited to the patient's condition and monitor the patient in a manner that provides the safest environment for the patient and the surgeon. Surgeons devote their attention and skills to the eradication of the patient's disease or to the correction of the anatomic defect. Both work as parts of a team that also encompasses the nursing service and other supporting staff.

Without physician anesthesiologists, who would have developed the techniques essential for successful open heart operations and coronary artery operations? Who would have developed curare or endotracheal anesthesia? Who would dare experiment with promising new agents? And who would train the nurse-anesthetists and raise their educational experience and performance? Let us be dedicated professionals, get on with the job of giving the best possible care to the patient, and stop worrying who is more important or less important in the operating room where every member of the team has a significant and a vital role (Hoerr, 1971).

REFERENCES

Hoerr, S. O.: Anesthesiologist and surgeon. Surg. Gynecol. Obstet., 133:290, 1971.

Lomanto, C. Members of the Same Team. Surg. Gynecol. Obstet., 134:99, 1972.

by LEROY D. VANDAM

Harvard Medical School

SPINAL ANESTHESIA — ACCEPTED

DEVELOPMENT

Since its introduction, spinal anesthesia has provoked more continuous controversy than any other technique that comes to mind. Wanting professional anesthetists and faced by the mortality associated with the general anesthesia of the time, surgeons not only introduced the method but also continued to utilize it because of its certainty and the excellent muscle relaxation provided. To this day, surgeons and obstetricians give spinal anesthesia when trained anesthesia personnel are not available and then proceed with their surgical duties. Without the constant supervision of the patient we now know to be essential, undetected high levels of anesthesia may lead to arterial hypotension or respiratory paralysis, or both, with the inevitable hypoxemia. However, these were not the only problems. The local anesthetics first employed, cocaine then procaine, lacked the rigid standards for manufacture, sterilization, and storage mandated today. Furthermore, the need for an aseptic technique often must have been ignored. Thus, postanesthetic meningitis and a spectrum of neurologic deficits, in addition to the adverse physiologic effects noted, were common. Add to these phenomena the ubiquitous headache and high incidence of nausea and vomiting intraoperatively, and a dismal picture indeed emerges.

OPPOSITION

So far as the major complications were concerned, the clamor over the neurologic sequelae of spinal anesthesia reached a crescendo in the later 1940's, culminating with Thorsen's monograph on the subject (1947). Both he, by implication, and S. Foster Kennedy, a neurologist of New York, and his associates (1950) averred that paralysis was much too high a price to pay for the fine muscle relaxation afforded. Fortunately, at that time, the maturation of professional anesthesia in the United States (the British have never been addicted to regional anesthesia as in Germany and France), led to large scale studies of the method (Dripps and Vandam, 1954; Phillips et al., 1969), with resulting elucidation of the origins of the complications and the means for their prevention. Simultaneously, the matter of headache was squarely faced and the hypotension of sympathetic blockade more or less controlled via injection of sympathomimetic amines plus intravenous infusion of fluids to correct the disproportion between vascular volume and space.

CURRENT STATUS

The reader, if not already prejudiced, will soon learn that there are still pockets of resistance to the application of spinal anesthesia, mainly on the part of patients to be anesthetized. Some of the older surgeons cannot quite overlook the past, and others are dismayed if a patient is awake while teaching goes on in the operating room. In some areas of the country, anesthesiologists, although appreciative of the technique, refrain from its use because of a hostile medicolegal climate.

Spinal anesthesia does thrive in many a hospital, however, for the sale of manufactured spinal anesthesia kits approaches the hundreds of thousands annually. Nevertheless, from an analytic standpoint, even if spinal anesthesia were totally free of undesirable attributes, why perpetuate the technique? Peridural anesthesia is probably a safer method neurologically and the general anesthesia of today, with better agents and techniques, has reached a high degree of perfection, resulting in less morbidity and mortality in spite of the ever-increasing severity of operations performed and the physical status of subjects operated upon. The reply to this query is that no one method of anesthesia is acceptable under every circumstance. In comparison with general anesthesia, the mortality of spinal anesthesia is low (Beecher and Todd, 1954), although this statistic is tempered by the lesser severity of the operations for which spinal anesthesia is elected.

ALTERNATIVES

The use of balanced techniques is largely responsible for the improved current safety of general anesthesia, that is, utilization of a specific pharmacologic agent for each component of the anesthetic experience — unconsciousness, analgesia, and muscle relaxation. Even the new potent halogenated hydrocarbons, which incorporate all of these components, are used in balanced mode — essential practice to avert the circulatory depression associated with only slight increases in percentages of the inhaled mixtures. Although nonflammable, they are toxic in a way different from that of diethyl ether, more after the pattern of chloroform. Thus, halothane, fluroxene, and methoxyflurane, listed in order of their introduction, have been implicated in the development of postanesthetic hepatic necrosis. This occurrence probably relates to their metabolism to toxic by-products, evidence of a lack of inertness not suspected until the middle 1960's. Moreover, a metabolite of methoxyflurane, the fluorine molecule, causes tubular nephropathy resulting in renal failure. By reason of its chemical structure, the latest halogen, enflurane, may be less toxic, but the results of large scale clinical usage should be awaited before passing final judgment on its safety.

Nitrous oxide, because of its splendid analgetic properties the most commonly used inhalant, always raises the specter of hypoxia, since the inhaled mixtures do not allow high concentrations of oxygen. Delivery from faulty apparatus or inattention to flowmeter settings has resulted in many a hypoxic episode. Furthermore, nitrous oxide delivered in large volumes via partial rebreathing systems is an atmospheric contaminant, suspect of harming operating room personnel. A nonpharmacologic property of nitrous oxide that relates to its diffusion into gas pockets enhances intestinal distention, may disrupt closure in middle ear surgery, and is a potentially fatal hazard during air encephalography. Probably, the use of nitrous oxide has been largely responsible for the high incidence of symptomatic air embolism during intracranial operations.

The neuromuscular blockers that provide the relaxant component of balanced anesthesia require tracheal intubation for continuance of adequate alveolar ventilation; reversal of their paralytic effects at the end of operation not uncommonly leaves a patient at risk of respiratory insufficiency in the recovery period. In addition, the narcotic analgesics employed with nitrous oxide add to the problem through diminution in respiratory drive.

Thus, it seems apparent that general anesthesia entails formidable pharmacologic and physiologic trespass and the use of antidotes at the termination of anesthesia to counter the effects of the agents used. The actions of several of these agents are sometimes complicated by pharmacogenetic abnormalities, as in the syndrome of malignant hyperthermia, or prolongation of the action of succinylcholine by variants or diminution in amounts of circulating pseudocholinesterase.

PATIENTS AS ADVERSARIES IN THE CHOICE OF SPINAL ANESTHESIA

As mentioned earlier in this article, although some surgeons and even anesthesiologists are reluctant to accede to spinal anesthesia, the patient is the final arbiter of choice of anesthesia in this era of informed consent. More or less in order of frequency, these are the objections raised: A strong wish not to be aware of the happenings during operation — oblivion for the procedure; the lore based on decades of experience that headache is intimately associated with spinal anesthesia and that one must lie flat in bed without movement for some time postoperatively; the possibility that paralysis will be permanent; anxiety that the anesthetic will be ineffective or wear off prematurely; an aversion to "tinkering" with the spine, with backache as an outcome. These are formidable arguments often based on previous unsatisfactory experiences or knowledge of such complications in family or friend. However, the facts about these sequelae should be known to referring physician and patient alike. The discussion that follows considers well-known complications plus others not generally known to the public.

Oblivion

This is often an adamant stance on the part of the patient that is truly based on fear while other objections raised are also symbols of anxiety in adults reluctant to admit that they are simply frightened. No matter the theoretic or actual disadvantages of general anesthesia proffered, the patient is willing to take the chance, placing the onus on the anesthesiologist, rather than remain awake during operation.

Neurologic Sequelae

In his monograph on neurologic complications after spinal anesthesia, based on a questionnaire submitted to physicians in Scandinavia and a survey of the literature, Thorsen devised a useful classification of the problems encountered. Complications were classified as follows: (1) Those relating to physiologic changes — mainly the result of sympathetic nervous blockade; (2) incidents ascribed to the technique of lumbar puncture; and (3) those matters pertaining to injection of the local anesthetic.

Cerebral Complications

Brain. As in any form of anesthesia, cerebral damage can result from arterial hypotension or respiratory insufficiency, the hypoxemia in either case resulting in transient neurologic signs and symptoms or irreversible changes if hypoxemia is severe and when cardiac arrest ensues. Cerebrovascular accidents have occurred consequent to the hypotension derived from sympathetic blockade during spinal anesthesia and after an excessive hypertensive response to therapeutic injection of a vasopressor drug. Although the cerebral circulation normally adjusts to changes in systolic pressure within a range of 60 to 180 torr, the response is not immediate, and the autoregulative process may not be effective in the presence of cerebral arteriosclerosis or in the hypertensive individual. Bizarre symptoms, such as coma, memory loss, mental deterioration, confusion, and psychoses, probably are attributable to unrecognized or delayed treatment of hypoxemia in the majority of cases in the elderly. Cerebral anemia can be ameliorated by careful positioning of patients to avoid postural hypotension (accentuated by prior administration of a narcotic analgetic), by prophylactic intramuscular injection of a vasopressor drug or its intravenous infusion, and by expansion of the vascular space with lactated Ringer's solution. The latter is common practice prior to use of regional anesthesia for obstetric delivery — cesarian or vaginal — to avoid maternal hypotension and fetal distress secondary to diminished uterine blood flow. However, since there is a high incidence of urinary retention in patients given spinal anesthesia, excessive fluid administration only serves to accentuate the need for bladder catheterization postoperatively — not an innocuous procedure.

Headache (A component of the syndrome of decreased intracranial pressure). Headache of the postural kind, that is, aggravated by the erect position and relieved by recumbency, is surely attributable to lumbar puncture and leakage of cerebrospinal fluid (CSF). This contention is amply supported by experimental drainage of CSF in man, with relief of headache upon replacement of the fluid, and by prompt appearance of headache with withdrawal of CSF during pneumoencephalography. Supporting data come from the clinical observation that the occurrence of headache diminishes with use of progressively smaller gauge needles. The complaint approaches a 1 to 2 per cent frequency when a 26 gauge needle is employed, the headache less severe and of shorter duration.

Despite the fact that the leakage theory of lumbar puncture headache is tenable, surely there are modifying circumstances, in that not everyone with low CSF pressure develops a headache, headache is not always prevented by the small gauge needle, the incidence is higher in women (more so in the obstetric setting), and headache is progressively less with advancing age beyond the seventh decade (Vandam, 1956). These observations suggest that local factors modify the response, possibly through overlap of arachnoid and dura so that the puncture opening is sealed and the prevalence of fibrous elements in the meninges under different conditions, such as youth versus old age or alterations in tissue elasticity during pregnancy. In the aged, decreased intracranial, vascular distensibility and progressive loss of neural elements may account for the lesser incidence of headache.

On a theoretic basis, various measures have been employed to prevent headache: obviously, use of the smallest gauge needle, practically; puncture of the dura with the needle bevel parallel to the vertically arranged fibers, thereby avoiding a tear (not a proved remedy); puncture of the meninges at an acute angle so that the meningeal openings may overlap (fair experimental evidence but few supporting clinical data); and deliberate hydration intra- and postoperatively to promote formation of CSF. Hydration should be accomplished with saline solution for retention in the extracellular space, however; a purely aqueous solution such as dextrose in water does not serve the purpose since the free water is excreted upon metabolism of the dextrose.

Injuries Localized to the Spinal Cord and Its Coverings

Traumatic Lumbar Puncture. Repeated attempts at lumbar puncture may result in back pain, perforation of epidural veins, recovery of blood-stained CSF, and paresthesias in the lumbar distribution, while epidural hematoma formation is a threat in the presence of a defective clotting mechanism. Even in the most experienced hands, paresthesias may be encountered, a sign that a sensory nerve root in the cauda equina has been grazed by the needle. A persistent pares- thesia suggests impalement of the nerve root; in this circumstance, the needle should be withdrawn and redirected. Certainly the local anes- thetic should not be injected, since irreversible damage will result (vide infra). Even a transient paresthesia results in increased cellular- ity and protein content of CSF, suggesting a break in the CSF–neural barrier. On the experimental side, injection of blood or several of its degradation products causes a sterile tissue response manifested by arachnoiditis.

To avoid or minimize the possibility of traumatic puncture, the patient should be optimally positioned, the spine maximally flexed, with an assistant maintaining the pose. Preanesthetic detection of dis- torted spinal anatomy or pathology, such as scoliosis and arthritis, should suggest the sitting position for lumbar puncture, for which the spine is straightened and flexed under the gravity influence of the patient's body mass. An x-ray of the back is useful when bony pathol- ogy is suspect, and spinal anesthesia is deemed to be the method of choice. In any case, the entry site is carefully chosen — above the in- tercrestal line and at, or below, the third lumbar interspace. Finally, an anesthesiologist should be versatile enough to perform a midline, lateral, or sacral (Taylor method) approach to the lumbar subarach- noid space, when necessary.

Meningitis and Epidural Abscess.   Bacterial or chemical meningitis was once a well-known complication of diagnostic or spinal anesthetic lumbar puncture. Meningitis has, however, virtually disappeared under the persuasive influence of aseptic technique and the availabili- ty of prepackaged, sterile lumbar puncture and spinal anesthetic kits. Surely, the skin of the back should be carefully prepared with a col- ored antiseptic solution several times over, and spinal anesthesia should perhaps be avoided when there is a possibility of contamina- tion, as with ileostomy drainage, and dermal infection or when septice- mia is present.

Neurologic Complications Related to Injection of Local Anes- thetic

Two major complications of spinal anesthesia *not encountered in surveys of the method over the last 25 years* deserve mention for the dis- tressing and disabling illness that results: the cauda equina syndrome and chronic progressive adhesive arachnoiditis.

The Cauda Equina Syndrome.   This syndrome is so designated be- cause signs and symptoms are localized to the lumbar and sacral seg- ments of the cord. In any kind of chemical neurologic injury, in the present context related to injection of local anesthetic into the suba- rachnoid space, nerve fibers of smallest diameter are preferentially damaged. Thus, a patient with the syndrome presents with autonomic nervous disability, bladder and bowel dysfunction, disturbance in sweating and temperature regulation, as well as altered sensation to pinprick, all in the lumbosacral dermatomes. Mention was made previously of the possibility of inducing a partial cauda equina syndrome with traumatic lumbar puncture alone, but a more complete picture is seen when an intraneural or intraspinal injection of local anesthetic is made. Here, the anesthetic solution spreads along the nerve root to its origin in the spinal cord, thereby causing physical dissolution and ischemia of cells. When neither trauma nor intraneural injection can be implicated in causation of the syndrome, it is assumed that a toxic substance must have been injected, possibly a detergent used in cleaning apparatus or contamination of the local anesthetic with antiseptic solution. In the early days, when drugs were sterilized by storage in phenol solutions, it was possible for the caustic substance to seep into the anesthetic through an undetected crack in the glass ampule. Such an occurrence was implicated as the cause of major neurologic damage in a now famous British medicolegal decision.

Adhesive Arachnoiditis. Arachnoiditis is a more or less stereotyped kind of pathologic reaction in the central nervous system that was found at postmortem examination long before spinal anesthesia was first employed (Mackay, 1939). Occurring in patchy or diffuse distribution, this sterile, organizing inflammatory process may be idiopathic or may represent a response to trauma (as in intervertebral disc surgery), a reaction to a chemical irritant, or an infectious process. The subarachnoid space becomes obliterated by dense adhesions between meninges and cord, so that at laminectomy the structures cannot be separated (Fig. 1). The blood supply to the cord is enmeshed in an organizing inflammatory reaction, with resultant ischemia, destruction of cells and tracts, and a spectrum of neurologic deficits. On microscopic examination, the blood vessels are found to be obliterated by a vasculitis or organizing endarteritis.

Confusing Minor Neurologic Deficits. In one large scale comprehensive survey of delayed spinal anesthetic complications (Vandam, 1955), minor subjective phenomena sometimes associated with altered sensation in the lumbar and sacral dermatomes were discovered in a small percentage of patients. Similar complaints were not unearthed in a control group of subjects given general anesthesia for operation. Numbness and tingling were described along with objective numbness in some instances, not progressive and of relatively little concern to the patients thus afflicted. As traumatic lumbar puncture was not involved, it was assumed that the local anesthetic was responsible, possibly because the osmolality of the solutions injected differed considerably from that of CSF. No evidence was found to implicate the epinephrine used in the anesthetic mixture to prolong anesthesia, although ischemia of the cord caused by vasoconstriction would have been a plausible explanation. Finally, the syndrome of meralgia paresthetica might have been present in some, a not uncommon ailment, with numbness and dysesthesia in the distribution of the lateral femoral cutaneous nerve (Schneck, 1947). This complaint has been associated with arthritis of the spine, abdominal obesity, pregnancy, the wearing of cartridge belts by military personnel, and other mis-

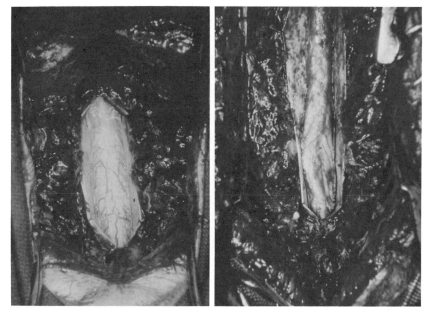

Figure 1. (*Left*) Normal spinal cord at laminectomy. The dura has been opened, and the arachnoid is still intact. Note the transparency of the latter and the delicate anastomosing network of blood vessels on the surface of the cord. (*Right*) A case of adhesive arachnoiditis shown at laminectomy. In contrast to the figure opposite, the dura has been opened and stripped, only with difficulty, from the underlying arachnoidal membrane. The latter is opaque, thickened, vascularized, and adherent to the underlying spinal cord which cannot be seen. The subarachnoid space is obliterated. (Reproduced with permission from: Vandam, L. D.: Spinal anesthesia. *In* Anesthesiology, Hale, D. E., Editor, Philadelphia, F. A. Davis Company, 1963.)

cellanea. Treatment entails local anesthetic injection of the nerve or surgical sectioning.

Antecedent Disease and Development of Neurologic Sequelae

In a high percentage of neurologic complications of spinal anesthesia, exacerbation of a previously present neurologic ailment, or its primary appearance, has been detected by both neurologists and anesthesiologists surveying the problem. Thus, Dripps and Vandam (Vandam and Dripps, 1956), as well as others, discovered the first symptoms and signs of spinal cord tumor after anesthesia, probably the result of CSF displacement or loss, with engorgement of blood vessels in the tumor mass. Other conditons that came to light for the first time, or were belatedly recalled by patients, included herpes zoster, hitherto quiescent encephalitis, vascular disease of brain or spinal cord, combined sclerosis, spinal column metastases from prostatic carcinoma (foot drop), protruding intervertebral disc, diabetic neuropathy, and development of bacterial meningitis in a patient with subacute otitis media.

These occurrences emphasize the importance of thorough history-taking and neurologic examination before electing spinal anesthesia. Even so, characteristically, some patients do not recall a neurologic problem until exacerbation occurs. Unfortunately, no matter the cause, spinal anesthesia is indicted, often by physicians uninformed or unwilling to tell a patient the truth about a potentially fatal disease. In a report by Marinacci and Courville (1958) of 482 patients whose complaints were attributed to spinal anesthesia, 478 were found to have unrelated neurologic conditions, mainly infectious neuritis or peripheral neuropathy.

ADDITIONAL PROBLEMS OF SPINAL ANESTHESIA

Regional Circulation

In the introductory paragraphs of this article, the problem of intracranial vascular hypotension resulting from sympathetic blockade was given prominence, but the circulation to other viscera is also affected via the same mechanism, in a more benign manner. Thus, the coronary circulation is to a large extent dependent on the level of the mean aortic diastolic pressure. With pooling of blood in the capacitance vessels, as well as peripheral vasodilation, the mean pressure falls during sympathetic blockade. The coronary circulation has the capacity to dilate rapidly, however, more so than the cerebral vessels within approximately the same pressure range, unless coronary arteriosclerosis is present. On the other hand, as heart rate decreases and afterload is lessened, both diminishing heart work, the need for oxygen is less under these circumstances. Toleration of a lesser perfusion pressure is thereby implied, but not necessarily so if the decline is much below the accustomed pressure for the individual.

Both splanchnic and renal blood flow decline during the decrease in mean arterial blood pressure, but, within a reasonable range, perfusion remains adequate without signs of anaerobic metabolism. Urine formation usually ceases when systolic pressure falls below 60 torr, but the parenchyma may still be well-perfused. In so far as postoperative alterations in hepatic function are concerned, there is little to choose between spinal and general anesthesia. The conduct of anesthesia and the magnitude of operation performed are probably more influential in the alterations in liver function tests found postoperatively. Moreover, vasodilation in the splanchnic circulation and kidney is considered beneficial in prevention and treatment of impending irreversible hemorrhagic or septicemic shock.

Respiratory Inadequacy

If the level of spinal anesthesia ascends to the point where all intercostal muscle activity ceases, respiration continues to be adequate under the influence of diaphragmatic contraction alone, unless its movement is impeded by placement of abdominal retractors or packs during abdominal operation. Lower intercostal paralysis is concomitant with relaxation of the abdominal wall muscles, so useful for the surgeon during laparotomy. If anesthesia ascends as far as the origins of the phrenic nerve roots at C3, C4, and C5, however, all respiratory action ceases and the patient is unable to talk and may lose consciousness even before hypoxemia develops. Thus, the need to observe the ascent of anesthesia from minute to minute during the phase before fixation of the local anesthetic to neural elements occurs by testing both sensory and motor levels.

Bowel and Urinary Tract

Interruption of sympathetic nervous outflow to the bowel results in unopposed parasympathetic activity, with smooth muscle contraction, hyperactive peristalsis, and sphincter relaxation. These happenings must be known in order to prevent spillage of intestinal contents during bowel anastomoses. Premedicants, however, such as the narcotic analgesics, and possibly large doses of atropine oppose the parasympathetic effect, preventing the contracted bowel that is responsible for the good operating conditions in abdominal surgery.

Spinal anesthesia has always been associated with a high incidence of urinary retention postoperatively and a consequent need for bladder catheterization. Surgeons and experienced patients are aware of the problem. As both sympathetics and the parasympathetics of the sacral division are blocked, bladder detrusor activity and reflex sphincter relaxation are impaired. The autonomic paralysis outlasts somatic sensory and motor block by far. Inability to empty the bladder is exaggerated by overdistension of the bladder secondary to zealous fluid administration during operation.

Nausea and Vomiting

When spinal anesthesia is given for abdominal operation, nausea and vomiting may be expected in at least 15 per cent and as high as 42 per cent of procedures, according to published reports dating back to the first decade of this century. These uncomfortable symptoms may appear as a result of hypotension and cerebral anemia but are usually in response to traction on abdominal viscera. Afferent pathways to the vomiting center in the medulla via splanchnic, phrenic, and vagal nerves are unblocked most of the time. Other explanations offered for the gastrointestinal distresss include the psychogenic, reflux of bile into the stomach or stimulation of the hindbrain when vasopressors with amphetamine-like properties are given.

UNUSUAL RESPONSES TO SPINAL ANESTHESIA

Failure of the Method

The large majority of partial or outright anesthetic failures probably can be ascribed to error in adding drugs to the spinal anesthetic mixture or when the mixture, after initial appearance of CSF, is injected partially or outside of the subarachnoid compartment, usually the subdural space. Hence, the wisdom of routine identification of all drugs added to the anesthetic solution and of advancing the bevel of the lumbar puncture needle well into the subarachnoid space and the need to aspirate CSF before and after injection and to position the patient properly according to the baricity of the solution employed should be recognized. If the anesthetic fails to take after a reasonable length of time, a second injection can be done, provided the operation is not unduly delayed. Otherwise, general anesthesia is the resort.

Tourniquet Pain

When a pneumatic tourniquet is inflated on leg or thigh for the purpose of a bloodless surgical field, a patient may experience a dull pain after 15 minutes or so that progresses to the unbearable as time passes by. Some would ascribe the pain to ascent of impulses over unblocked pathways in the paravertebral sympathetic chain as ischemia sets in. Others invoke the Gateway Theory of Pain Perception, noting that paralysis by tourniquet pressure of afferent fibers of large diameter permits the entry of pain impulses over the smaller fibers unblocked by the arrival of impulses that usually close the gate to the spinothalamic tract. In any case, afferent pathways are unblocked and the remedy would seem to lie in a high (T8-6) anesthetic block of afferent sensation when a tourniquet is used on the thigh, although this is not always successful.

Phantom Sensations

In the lower limb amputee, a hitherto dormant painful phantom may reappear briefly during the onset of spinal anesthesia, again suggesting that the gateway mechanism is temporarily inadequate. In another situation, a patient permitted to lie with knees flexed as spinal blockade approaches completion will claim that the legs are still bent even though now straightened. As the cerebral interpretation of body position can only rely upon afferent input, it would seem that the last interpretation of the position of the extremity is centrally retained, still a reality so far as the subject is concerned.

IS THE RESURGENCE OF PERIDURAL ANESTHESIA A THREAT TO THE SURVIVAL OF SPINAL ANESTHESIA?

The answer to this question lies both in the theoretic and practical realm. By the very nature of the site of placement of anesthetic in the peridural space, one should anticipate fewer neurologic sequelae with this method, certainly no headache unless inadvertent dural puncture occurs. In that case, the headache is usually severe, owing to the larger gauge needle employed in the peridural technique. Several retrospective studies of peridural anesthesia have uncovered none of the common neurologic sequelae hitherto ascribed to spinal anesthesia, even though the local anesthetic does diffuse into the subarachnoid space. Peridural anesthesia is enjoying a renaissance at a time when the lessons of spinal anesthesia are clearly in mind, i.e., the need for an aseptic technique and employment of reputable local anesthetics. Further, the newer anesthetics — lidocaine, mepivacaine, and bupivacaine — are used with more thorough prior study of their properties than the cocaine, procaine, and tetracaine of yore, the latter still the overwhelming choice in spinal anesthesia.

With minor differences, physiologic responses to spinal and epidural anesthesia are about the same. The main reasons for the continued popularity of spinal anesthesia however, lie in the lesser complexity of its administration, the greater certainty of obtaining effective anesthesia, the shorter time to onset, and the lack of influence of such variables as age and obesity, which dictate the dosage in peridural anesthesia. Furthermore, the large mass of local anesthetic (volume times concentration) used in peridural anesthesia, unlike the relatively miniscule amounts effective in spinal anesthesia, is to a degree absorbed into the systemic circulation, there likely to cause direct cardiovascular depression or central nervous system toxic effects. Unfortunately, because of the technical simplicity of spinal anesthetic administration, the method is often used by the inexperienced, with a resulting higher morbidity and mortality.

SUMMARY AND CONCLUSIONS

All but a few of the traditional sequelae of spinal anesthesia, those inherent in the technique of lumbar puncture and the introduction of a foreign substance into the subarachnoid space, are now infrequent occurrences. Accordingly, most physicians and surgeons abide by the anesthesiologist's choice of the method, often accepting the procedure for themselves when undergoing operation. Patients however, are still wary of the technique, for the reasons presented, and perhaps another generation or so must pass before the bad reputation of spinal anesthesia is forgotten, if ever. The technique, for all the advantages it has to offer, is an invaluable part of anesthetic methodology and is apparently here to stay.

REFERENCES

Beecher, H.K., and Todd, D.: A study of the deaths associated with anesthesia and surgery. Ann. Surg., 140:2, 1954.

DiGiovanni, A.J.: "Chemical Meningitis" tied to cleaning fluid bacteria. J.A.M.A., 214:2129, 1970.

DiGiovanni, A.J., and Dunbar, B.S.:

Epidural injections of autologous blood for post-lumbar puncture headache. Anesth. Analg., *49*:268, 1970.

Dripps, R.D., and Vandam, L.D.: Long-term followup of patients who received 10,098 spinal anesthetics: I. Failure to discover major neurological sequelae. J.A.M.A., *156*:1486, 1954.

Hurst, E.W.: Adhesive arachnoiditis and vascular blockage caused by detergents and other chemical irritants: An experimental study. J. Pathol. Bacteriol., *70*:167, 1955.

Kennedy, S.F., Effron, A.S., and Perry, G.: The grave spinal cord paralyses caused by spinal anesthesia. Surg. Gynecol. Obstet., *91*:385, 1950.

Mackay, R.P.: Chronic adhesive arachnoiditis. A clinical and pathological study. J.A.M.A., *112*:802, 1939.

Marinacci, A.A., and Courville, C.B.: Electromyogram in evaluation of neurological complications of spinal anesthesia. J.A.M.A., *168*:1337, 1958.

Marx, G.F., Saifer, A., and Orkin, L.R.: Cerebrospinal fluid cells and proteins following spinal anesthesia. Anesthesiology, *24*:305, 1963.

Phillips, O.C., Ebner, H., Nelson, A.T., and Black, M.H.: Neurologic complications following spinal anesthesia with lidocaine. Anesthesiology, *30*:284, 1969.

Schneck, J.M.: Meralgia paresthetica. J. Nerv. Ment. Dis., *105*:77, 1947.

Thorsen, G.: Neurological complications after spinal anesthesia. Acta Chir. Scand. [Suppl.] *95*:121, 1947.

Vandam, L.D., and Dripps, R.D.: A long-term follow-up of patients who recived 10,098 spinal anesthetics. II. Incidence and analyses of minor sensory neurological defects. Surgery, *38*:463, 1955.

Vandam, L.D., and Dripps, R.D.: Long-term follow-up of patients who received 10,098 spinal anesthetics. III. Syndrome of decreased intracranial pressure (headache and ocular and auditory difficulties). J.A.M.A., *161*:586 1956.

Vandam, L.D., and Dripps, R.D.: Exacerbation of pre-existing neurologic disease after spinal anesthesia. N. Engl. J. Med., *225*:843, 1956.

by STEPHEN J. PREVOZNIK

Hospital of the University of Pennsylvania

FLAMMABLE ANESTHETICS ARE OUTMODED

The Era of Flammable Anesthetics is, for all practical purposes, at an end. This ending has not come with the "bang" that many had forecast, for although explosions were a constant hazard, the actual number reported was small. Instead, the flammable agents have been steadily pushed aside by a "new order." Newer, better, and more predictable intravenous agents from tranquilizers and hypnotics to analgesics and muscle relaxants have appeared, with the result that a smooth, rapid, and safe level of anesthesia can be achieved without threat of explosion and fire. Likewise, the development of nonexplosive inhalation agents has added to this demise. If a *coup d'etat* could be singled out, it would have to be the twin blows of science and technology. The art of anesthesiology has been overtaken by the science of anesthesiology.

ADVANCES IN TECHNOLOGY

Many flammable agents have appeared on the anesthesia scene and then disappeared — ethylene, ethyl chloride, divinyl ether, and ethyl vinyl ether. Fluroxene, introduced in 1953, was originally thought to be nonflammable, but in higher concentration, this was not found to be true. The low potency of fluroxene resulted in a need for these higher concentrations, and its usefulness was thus curtailed. Despite a brief spurt of enthusiasm, fluroxene was withdrawn from the market less than 20 years after its introduction. Through all of this, ether and cyclopropane remained the mainstays of the anesthesiologist, but they were not without problems. Aside from the fire and explosion hazard, they caused many difficulties for patient and physician alike. Long, stormy inductions that gave real meaning to the "excitement" stage of anesthesia were commonplace. Maintenance of anesthesia was often precarious and consisted of hills and valleys of vascular stability and muscle relaxation. The arrhythmias seen with

19

cyclopropane, along with the sensitization of the myocardium to catecholamine activity, made many an anesthetic an exercise in terror.
Nausea and vomiting, lasting well into the postoperative period, was
an expected event and contributed greatly to a slow recovery from
anesthesia. The memory of smells, nausea, vomiting, and debilitation
made for poor patient acceptance.

It was no wonder that help in the form of new agents was eagerly
sought. The first real relief occurred in the early 1940's with the introduction of thiopental, followed in a few years by *d*-tubocurarine.
The introduction of these two agents signaled the decline of the flammable agents.

Advanced technology led to the development of the new and potent nonflammable halogenated hydrocarbons. The introduction of
halothane in 1956 gave the anesthesiologist an inhalation agent that
allowed for a relatively fast induction, ready control of anesthetic
depth, and prompt recovery (Johnstone, 1956). Absent were many of
the problems inherent in the administration of the flammable agents,
and compared to ether and cyclopropane, it was an "easy" anesthetic
to administer. The precision vaporizer (Feldman and Morris, 1958)
made it, and the other halogenated hydrocarbons to follow, easy to
administer; the amount of anesthetic agent meted out to the patient
was no longer an educated (or noneducated) guess. Precise concentrations of anesthetic agents could now be delivered and anesthetic depth
could be more readily controlled. Coupled with the concept of minimum alveolar concentration, it was now possible to avoid the potential
harmful effects of anesthetic agents at deep anesthetic levels (Eger,
Saidman, and Brandstater, 1965). By combining intravenous agents
for the induction of anesthesia (thiopental) and muscle relaxation
(succinylcholine chloride, and *d*-tubocurarine) with the potent new
agents, a state of surgical anesthesia could be achieved swiftly and
smoothly — a level rivaling that produced only by deep cyclopropane
or ether anesthesia or a combination of the two. Unlike cyclopropane
or ether anesthesia, this anesthetic state could be reversed with relative speed and ease.

It is also interesting to note that when the halothane hepatitis
crisis arose in the early 1960's, there was no great return to flammable
agents. Instead, alternate methods of producing an anesthetic state
were sought and intravenous agents enjoyed a resurgence of popularity that remains today.

ELECTRONIC ADVANCES

Advanced surgical technology also helped to speed the passing of
flammable agents. New surgical techniques and ventures into hitherto
inaccessible areas demanded that anesthesiology keep pace. Heart
chambers were invaded, organs — natural and artificial — were being
transplanted, and no age was immune from surgical intervention. Patients once considered too sick to be subjected to an operative procedure were becoming frequent and common patrons of the operating

room, each bringing advanced disease and special problems. As the patient's risk increased and the surgery proposed became more complex, it became obvious that "a finger on the pulse and a hand on the bag" simply wasn't good enough. Not only must the anesthetic agents be carefully administered but there also must be much more awareness of the minute to minute physiologic changes occurring while the patient is anesthetized. Although, at one time, the build-up of static electricity was a main concern of the anesthesiologist, now myriad monitors demand an electrical energy source in close proximity to the anesthesia machine. In the past, anesthesiologists might veto the surgeon's request to use live cautery, or electrocautery, on the basis of need to use an explosive agent. Now the explosive agents are avoided on the basis of need by the anesthesiologist for better and more complete monitoring. At the same time, the electrocautery has become a more integral part of most surgical procedures. At long last the surgeons and anesthesiologists have accepted electricity, and with that acceptance explosive agents are moving into the history books and medical museums.

COSTS

Another, perhaps mundane but realistic, problem reared its head — the economics of using flammable agents. It was clear to everyone involved with anesthetic management that the use of flammable agents was expensive as well as hazardous. New facilities required special construction of anesthetic locations: conductive flooring, special electrical circuitry, equipment design, and compliance with fire and safety codes. Stringent new codes required expensive renovation of older facilities. Personnel had to be indoctrinated in the "do's and don'ts" of working in hazardous locations. Rules and regulations regarding footwear, clothing or operating room personnel, and linens used in operating rooms had to be developed and constantly surveyed. All equipment in the operating room had to be grounded. Special procedures and solutions were evolved for mopping of floors, for if done improperly, the conductivity of the floor could be impaired. In new construction, to make any anesthetizing location safe for the use of flammable anesthetic agents, the cost per location increased by several thousands of dollars. Added to this was the cost of supplying equipment and furniture that conformed to fire and safety codes and the costs of routine maintenance and monitoring. Despite the fact that ether and cyclopropane were relatively inexpensive, their clinical application had become very expensive.

MIXED FACILITIES

Initially, in an attempt to offset the increase in cost of continued use of flammable agents, some hospitals resorted to "mixed facilities," having several operating rooms designated as "flammable anesthetizing locations" and confining the use of flammable agents to these rooms. This arrangement afforded some degree of flexibility, allowing for the use of these agents if, in the opinion of the anesthesiologist, they were indicated. Practically speaking, this solution was not quite as simple as it appeared. Usually, operating rooms are assigned to surgical schedules long before a decision is made as to the anesthetic agent to be used. The management of a busy surgical schedule often requires much arranging and rearranging to meet the circumstances of any given day, and setting aside one or two operating rooms "just in case" an anesthesiologist would like to use a flammable agent is not only inefficient but also generally impossible. The restriction of the use of these flammable agents has resulted in fewer people receiving training in the administration of these agents, thus increasing the likelihood of human error (Ngai, 1955). Training and policing anesthesiologists, as well as others of the surgical team, in explosive precautions for a "sometime thing" has proved burdensome and frustrating.

NFPA SAFETY CODE

The safety code (NFPA Bulletin 56A, 1977) has just about nullified any possible advantage a "mixed facility" has to offer. Section 6141 states, "All equipment intended for use in both flammable and nonflammable anesthetizing locations shall meet the antistatic requirements of Section 46." Thus, equipment used in areas where nonflammable techniques are permissible must either be explosion-proof or fixed to that room. Portable X-ray and all electrical equipment being used in a mixed facility must comply with the same requirements as those approved for hazardous locations (Sections 6143, 6144, and 6146). Section 6142 states, "Equipment intended for use only in nonflammable anesthetizing locations shall be labeled . . . and shall not be introduced into flammable anesthetizing locations." With restrictions such as these, it is easy to understand why most institutions have given up, or are giving up, on mixed facilities.

CURRENT TRENDS

The frequency of use of flammable anesthetic agents has declined steadily since the introduction of halothane, with virtual elimination by the mid-1970's. A study of use in the state of Pennsylvania in 1972 indicated that at that time, 56 per cent of hospitals in the state used flammable agents, but this figure can be misleading (Brian-Smith, 1972). A case in point is the experience at the Hospital of the University of Pennsylvania. In 1960, approximately 40 per cent of all anesthetic procedures involved the use of flammable agents. By 1970, flammable agents were still being used, but the incidence of use had dropped below 6 per cent, and in 1977, the use was banned. A similar history is observed at the Columbia-Presbyterian Medical Center, where about 26 per cent of the anesthetics administered in 1964 involved the use of flammable agents, decreasing to less than 12 per cent in 1969, less than 1 per cent in 1973 (Ngai, 1975), and today no flammable agents are used.

At present, only a few companies still manufacture anesthetic ether and cyclopropane in the United States. Although ether sales are up, according to one manufacturer, it is the industrial ethers that dominate the market, whereas ether for anesthesia makes up a small fraction of the total. One company still manufacturing cyclopropane listed 41 regular "customers" in 1972, but in the year 1977 only 13 hospitals ordered at least one cylinder of cyclopropane; only two hospitals appeared to be regularly using the agent.

In this day of advertising saturation, it is interesting that advertisements for diethyl ether and cyclopropane have long since disappeared from our professional journals. This is especially noteworthy since the words ether and anesthesia were considered synonymous in the United States as recently as 1945. It is likely that the manufacture of these agents will soon be phased out altogether.

RELUCTANCE TO ABANDON FLAMMABLE AGENTS

Greene has suggested that prior to 1950 a major difference in the practice of anesthesia in the United States, as compared to Great Britain, might well be that the safer anesthetic, ether, was used in the United States while Great Britain elected the more potent and dangerous agent, chloroform. In making this choice, Great Britain realized that chloroform represented not only a danger but also a challenge, one that would attract the attention of outstanding investigators. The dangers of chloroform demanded careful administration by physicians. By selecting the safer anesthetic, the United States could, and did, relegate its administration to the lesser qualified: medical students, surgical clerks, interns, and nurses (Greene, 1971). As intriguing as such as assumption might be, it will be pursued no further except to point out that a rivally was begun and a nationalistic form of chauvinism developed. This chauvinistic attitude might be one of the reasons we have persisted in the use of flammable agents.

One of the more pragmatic reasons that anesthesia departments held to the use of cyclopropane so long was its unique ability to provide surgical anesthesia without depressing the blood pressure. Generations of anesthesiologists had learned to rely heavily on cyclopropane for the hypovolemic, vascularly unstable patient. With the advent of ketamine, an intravenous agent was introduced that would induce general anesthesia, provide analgesia, and also support the blood pressure (Corssen and Domino, 1966). The use of ketamine as an induction agent in selected cases has replaced any reliance that was previously placed on cyclopropane.

Perhaps another reason that flammable agents remained in use as long as they did is the ego of some anesthesiologists. Banning these agents was seen as an infringement on the freedom of anesthesiologists to prescribe or to limit the choice of agents and techniques. Paradoxically, the anesthesiologist has never had so much choice among agents and techniques as is possible today. Some recall with fondness a mastery of cyclopropane and ether — an ability to induce and maintain anesthesia smoothly. Dimmed, however, are the memories of prolonged inductions complicated by excess salivation, vomiting, cyanosis, and cardiac irregularities. The prolonged emergence and the protracted postoperative nausea and vomiting are all but forgotten. Most forgotten are the time and number of procedures it took to attain the "mastery" so fondly remembered — an exposure and experience impossible to achieve in today's practice of anesthesia. Although reluctant to forgo flammable agents, the experience to gain expertise was denied, and now the matter is a *fait accompli*.

POSITION OF FLAMMABLE AGENTS TODAY

The actual frequency with which flammable agents are used today is difficult to document. An informal survey by the author into the use of flammable agents among the major medical centers in the United States revealed only one institution with anything resembling regular use. A small number of anesthesia departments claim to use the agents but admit the frequency of use is low. Without frequent use, it is impossible to train residents in the administration of the agents. A generation of anesthesiologists exists today with little, if any, experience in the use of cyclopropane. Greene refers to cyclopropane as a paleoanesthetic — "something of interest to historians ... but having little or no immediate practical value" (Greene, 1974). There is little doubt that the same could be said for diethyl ether.

Cyclopropane is still used, to a degree, in the investigator's laboratory because it has a unique effect: its ability to produce surgical anesthesia without depressing the blood pressure. In investigating this one action of cyclopropane, we have learned much about the state of anesthesia itself. Even here the use of cyclopropane as an investigative tool has declined greatly, easily discernible by thumbing through the Index Medicus for the past few years.

SUMMARY

The use of flammable anesthetic agents has been in steady decline for over 35 years. The beginning of this decline actually started in the early 1940's with the introduction of thiopental and d-tubocurarine and was greatly accelerated in the 1950's with the development of the potent, nonflammable, halogenated hydrocarbons. There is an extensive range of new agents — inhalational and intravenous — that, because of exhaustive prerelease testing, are understood reasonably well and are more controllable. They are safer, surer, and more patient-acceptable. Flammable agents are inferior to halogenated agents now available and therefore are no longer needed.

The increased use of electrical equipment in the operating room precludes the use of flammable agents, and the costs of new hospital construction, or renovation, to make anesthetizing locations safe for the use of flammable agents are prohibitive, considering any advantage gained.

Each year fewer anesthesiologists are being exposed to the use of flammable agents, suggesting that training in administration and the policing of explosive precautions by operating room personnel has become an episode in history.

Flammable anesthetic agents are in the final throes of a lingering death after a long and useful life. The time has come to "pull the plug!"

REFERENCES

Brian-Smith, R.: Use of explosive anesthetic agents. P. Med., 75:55–56, 1972.

Corssen, G., and Domino, E.F.: Dissociative anesthesia: Further pharmacologic studies and first clinical experience with the phencyclidine derivative CI-581. Anesth. Analg. (Cleve.), 45:29–40, 1966.

Eger, E.I., II, Saidman, L.J., and Brandstater, B.: Minimum alveolar anesthetic concentration: A standard of anesthetic potency. Anesthesiology, 26:756–763, 1965.

Feldman, S.A., and Morris, L.E.: Vaporization of halothane and ether in the copper kettle. Anesthesiology, 19:650–655, 1958.

Greene, N.M.: Consideration of the factors involved in the discovery of anesthesia and their effect on subsequent development of anesthesia. Anesthesiology, 35:515–522, 1971.

Greene, N.M.: Thoughts on a paleoanesthetic — editorial views. Anesthesiology, 40:320–322, 1974.

Johnstone, M.: Human cardiovascular response to fluothane anesthesia. Br. J. Anaesth., 28:392, 1956.

National Fire Protection Association (NFPA): Code for the Use of the Flammable Anesthetics, NFPA Bulletin 56A, 1977.

Ngai, S.H.: Explosive agents — are they needed? Surg. Clin. North Am., 55:975–985, 1975.

NO LONGER AN ISSUE OF DEBATE

EDITORIAL COMMENT

The existence of the controversies discussed in the preceding three articles may come as some surprise to anesthetists who began practice in the last 10 years. Nonetheless, to those of us who practiced in the 1940's and 1950's, the problems were very real and subjects of much debate, often heated and emotional. It is interesting that the solutions have not come about overnight or by mandate but rather by evolution.

Anesthesia went through stormy times in the three decades beginning with the 1930's. Few surgeons were willing to relinquish their control of either anesthesia or the operating room. This editor came up in an era when the operating room was dominated by the chief surgeon, whose word was law on anything, including scheduling and operating room rules and who would brook no intrusion into his authority. He wanted unsupplemented spinal anesthesia for cholecystectomies or gastrectomies, and we gave it, not always unsupplemented and sometimes with a little ventriloquism when he asked "Mrs. Finkelstein, how are you?" We learned things about spinal anesthesia under conditions we could not repeat today. Slowly, but surely, we taught him that we knew more about anesthesia than he did. We were convinced time would take care of the problem and attempted to prevent confrontation. The introduction of new potent anesthetics, the lack of depth of training for surgeons in anesthesia, some court rulings, and societal pressure for greater efficiency in the use of surgical facilities have all helped in settling the controversy. The increasing activities of anesthesiologists outside the operating room has also done much to dispel imaginary boundaries.

The assault on spinal anesthesia came principally through the courts and by some neurologists who believed the introduction of a local anesthetic into the subarachnoid space unacceptable. Because of unfavorable reports in the medical literature and court decisions in favor of plantiffs who developed complications after spinal anesthesia, the use of the technique nearly ceased in some states. It took many years to overcome this stigma. Here again, the establishment of a rigid aseptic technique and use of high quality agents along with the accumulation and publication of data from thousands of cases proved spinal anesthesia no more hazardous than any other anesthetic technique. Perhaps the accumulation of data by the University of Pennsylvania group, published by Dripps and Vandam, did as much as any one factor in establishing spinal as an acceptable technique. The medical profession and the courts now had positive evidence of acceptability. Today one chooses spinal on its merits from among all techniques available without undue fear of legal reprisal.

Although the first two controversies were between anesthesiologists and other specialists or the courts, the third was principally within anesthesiology and among anesthetists. Prevoznik develops the story well. With the introduction of new potent nonflammable agents, permitting smooth induction and rapid uneventful recovery, and the requirement of better monitoring devices, the use of flammable agents diminished. Cost awareness questions the need to build and maintain expensive facilities required when flammable agents are used. Many experienced in the use of ether and cyclopropane were reluctant to give them up, citing real and fancied advantages. The conclusion has been reached by obtaining data on what techniques were being taught and being used by anesthetists and what agents are being sold by manufacturers. The answer is in: flammable techniques are neither taught nor used to any significant extent nor is the sale of the agents appreciable. Anesthetists have practically demonstrated that nonflammable agents are superior and that flammable ones are no longer needed.

A study of anesthesia history is valuable for anesthetists to understand their origins and the development of the characteristics of their daily life and to be aware of ways to deal with the present. It is said that "time heals all." Well, maybe time plus something else. These three chapters suggest time plus demonstration of competency, time plus developing data of acceptability, and time plus acquiring statistics of daily habits.

Part 2

HALOTHANE AND HEPATITIS

THE PROPOSITION:

A relationship between halothane and post halothane hepatitis is proved.

ALTERNATIVE POINTS OF VIEW:

By Burnell R. Brown, Jr.
By David L. Bruce

EDITORIAL COMMENT

by BURNELL R. BROWN, JR.

University of Arizona College of Medicine

HALOTHANE HEPATITIS IS A REASONABLY WELL PROVED CLINICAL ENTITY

Many halide alkyl compounds classify as direct hepatic toxins, including the anesthetic chloroform. Recognizing this precedent, during the initial pharmacologic investigation of Suckling's newly synthesized anesthetic, halothane ($CF_3CHClBr$), Ráventos (1956) examined liver cellular changes in 30 rats, 3 dogs, and 5 monkeys after exposure to the anesthetic. He reported only "minor changes." Halothane was released for general clinical use in the United States early in 1959. Within several years, a plethora of articles reporting unexplained jaundice and massive hepatic necrosis and implicating halothane as a vector were published (Virtue and Payne, 1958; Brody and Sweet, 1963; Lindenbaum and Leifer, 1963). These cases created a great deal of controversy, much of which generated more heat than light. Anesthesia was in a state of change, and halothane was the drug spearheading the metamorphosis. This potent, nonflammable anesthetic possessed many desirable features and allowed the use of sophisticated electronic monitors that could not be used during the era of diethyl ether and cyclopropane. Pleasant rapid induction, delivery of high oxygen concentrations, and quick, predictable awakening were a few of the virtues of this substantial breakthrough in inhalation anesthetics. The users of the anesthetic were convinced of the overall admirable qualities of the drug; hepatologists, not intimately concerned with anesthetic administration, saw only the rare, yet often fatal complication of postoperative hepatic necrosis. Many of them considered the anesthetic anathema. An additional, and most cogent, problem was that the sobriquet "halothane hepatitis" constituted a diagnosis of exclusion. Histologic and liver enzyme changes in cases attributed to this adverse reaction were nonspecific and could not be differentiated from viral hepatitis. Thus, strong polarization occurred between those who believed halothane was a panacea and those who ubiquitously

31

attributed all postoperative jaundice to the anesthetic. Unfortunately, the zeal of many hepatologists who labeled every case of a patient turning yellow postoperatively as being anesthetic-induced led to many incorrect diagnoses. The author is aware of patients with jaundice following spinal anesthesia, patients in the incubation phase of viral hepatitis prior to anesthesia, patients with Weil's disease, and patients with severe sepsis — all diagnosed as "halothane hepatitis." Such incorrect diagnoses of the cause of hepatic necrosis following halogenated anesthetics, although classic negative reports, have been published (Douglas et al., 1976).

The flurry of case reports implicating halothane led to the National Halothane Study (Bunker, 1965). This large-scale epidemiologic effort was commendable but suffered in two respects: it was distinctly biased, since several participating hospitals had already published case reports indicting halothane, and it was retrospective in nature. It did bring out several salient features on the subject, however. Halothane appeared to have an excellent overall safety record as an anesthetic, and the entity "unexplained jaundice" following use of halothane did occur. Unexplained does not *de facto* pinpoint halothane as the cause but rather places it in the possible cause category. Another interesting facet brought out was the association of unexplained jaundice and repeated administrations of halothane. Other authors reported that there was a high liver injury attack rate in patients who had had more than one halothane anesthetic. Little (1968) reported that 49 per cent of his series had received two or more administrations of halothane prior to developing hepatic damage, and Klatskin (1968) noted that 68 per cent of his series had more than one anesthetic with the drug. A recent report by Trowell and associates demonstrated that British women given halothane anesthesia for radium therapy of carcinoma of the cervix had gross elevations of serum glutamic pyruvic transaminase (SGPT) levels with multiple administrations, although none of the 39 patients in this series developed overt liver necrosis (Trowell, Peto, and Crampton-Smith, 1975).

The high degree of association of multiple administration and jaundice following anesthesia with halothane and the inability to produce significant liver damage in laboratory animals with the drug led to the speculation that the entity, if it existed at all, was a drug-induced allergy. Substantiation of this theory was reinforced by the findings of Paronetto and Popper, in which incorporation of tritiated thymidine in the harvested lymphocytes of "halothane hepatitis" patients was enhanced by halothane (Paronetto and Popper, 1970). Two reports were published in which anesthetists suspected of being sensitized to halothane were administered a challenge test with a short exposure to subanesthetic concentrations of the anesthetic. Deterioration of liver function followed shortly thereafter, leading to the conclusion that the individuals were allergic to the anesthetic (Belfrage, Ahlgren, and Axelson, 1966; Klatskin and Kimberg, 1969). The result of this activity was that halothane hepatitis became entrenched in the literature as a drug allergy specific to man and classified as a true entity. Reports of eosinophilia, skin rashes, and arthralgias coincident with halothane hepatitis appeared confirmatory. Based on this thesis, it was stated that halothane should not be repeated within 3 to 12 months, a statement predicated on inductive reasoning, *not fact*.

The controversy continued as new investigations were published and new thoughts came to light. Many cases of unexplained jaundice occurred following a single administration. How could this be an allergy if the patient had not had previous exposure to the allergen? Gronert and associates reported a retrospective series of multiple halothane anesthetics in a large burn center; there were no data to indict halothane as a hepatic sensitizing agent (Gronert, Schaner, and Gunther, 1968). Numerous attempts were made in the laboratory to produce centrolobular hepatic necrosis in animals, based upon halothane allergy, but to no avail (Reeves and McCracken, 1976; Mathieu et al., 1975). The positive lymphocyte transformation test of Paronetto and Popper was discredited by Walton and coworkers (Walton et al., 1973) and by Moult and associates (Moult et al. 1975). It was held (by absence of cited cases) that newborns were not susceptible to the complication. A series of South African women with carcinoma of the cervix were given multiple halothane anesthetics without rises in liver enzymes (Allen and Downing, 1977), in contrast to the findings of Trowell and his collaborators (Trowell, Peto, and Crampton-Smith, 1975). It was not the intent of these articles to discredit the fact that jaundice could be attributed to halothane, but rather they reported futile attempts to search for a mechanism. The hypothesis (but not the fact) of the heralded challenge test as proof of halothane allergy was enough to make an Aristotelian syllogist despair. Although there may be a cause and effect relationship between administration of a drug and an adverse reaction, in no way does this explain mechanism. It is difficult, in view of the multitude of case reports and the similarity in structural formula of halothane and known halogenated hepatic toxins, to discredit the problem. In the main, it is surely overdiagnosed, which lends fuel to the support of opponents of the concept.

A well-done retrospective analysis of halothane-induced liver damage was recently reported from Sweden (Böttinger, Dalen, and Hallen, 1976). Several interesting points accrue from this study. First, 82 per cent of the affected patients had multiple exposures. Second, the demographic composition of the halothane hepatitis victims, when contrasted to medical ward cases of viral hepatitis, was different. Liver injury following halothane is common in middle-aged, obese females. Viral hepatitis is a disease of youth. Third, the incidence of halothane hepatitis or unexplained jaundice following halothane anesthesia is increasing in Sweden. The widespread use of halothane when coupled with such retrospective reviews does not prove halothane is the offending agent, however. Wright and co-authors demonstrated in a prospective study that repeated halothane anesthetics produce elevations of liver enzymes, although none in this series developed liver necrosis (Wright et al., 1975). Such prospective studies are difficult to discredit, but without an acceptable mechanism, strictly phenomenologic reports lack substance.

A synthesis of several unrelated observations have directed the search for a cause of halothane hepatitis toward a mechanism other than allergy. Slater (1966), Recknagel and Ghoshal (1966), Castro and associates (1968), and others espoused the theory that active metabolites of halogenated liver toxins, rather than the parent molecules, are responsible for hepatic necrosis. In animal studies, this theory has been found to be correct. Van Dyke, Chenoweth, and Van Poznak (1964) and Stier and coworkers (1964, 1967) demonstrated that halothane is biotransformed to a considerable extent in both man and animals. The metabolites of halothane found in these initial studies were innocuous. Brown and Vandam speculated, however, that the syndrome of halothane hepatitis might lie in altered biotransformation of the anesthetic (Brown and Vandam, 1971). Biotransformation of a drug is an extremely complex set of reactions. Variables may alter both qualitative and quantitative biotransformation of most drugs, including inhalation anesthetics. Age, sex, amount of body fat, liver blood flow, genetic predisposition, and microsomal enzyme induction due to prior exposure to a drug are among the endogenous and exogenous factors that must be taken into account when exploring the overall metabolism of any given drug.

Cohen and collaborators performed a detailed analysis of urinary metabolites of man following halothane anesthesia (Cohen et al., 1975). They determined the presence of two metabolites that were probably of sufficient degree of reactivity to adversely interact with liver macromolecules. The amount of these metabolites was too small to predict that they could produce overt liver damage, however. Although the biotransformation of halothane had previously been held to be oxidative, these reactive metabolites could have been produced by reduction. In this regard, Uehleke and coworkers demonstrated *in vitro* that with reduced oxygen concentrations, halothane produced far more covalent binding to liver constituents than in the presence of excess oxygen (Uehleke, Hellmer, and Tabarelli-Poplawski, 1973). Covalent binding signifies that reactive intermediate metabolites have interacted with functional protein and lipid complexes to denature them. Widger and associates substantiated increased binding, increased inorganic fluoride release, and histologic damage with hypoxic oxygen concentrations during halothane anesthesia (Widger, Gandolfi, and Van Dyke, 1976). Thus, there was evidence that changing halothane biotransformation qualitatively to a reduction reaction could lead to intermediates capable of interacting with the liver and perhaps damaging it.

The author and his co-investigators have succeeded in routinely producing centrolobular necrosis of the liver in animals by changing biotransformation towards a reductive one (qualitative change) that is induced (quantitative change) (McLain, Brown, and Sipes; Sipes and Brown, 1976). In Model I (Table I), Arochlor is a potent agent that

Table 1. Animal Models of Centrolobular Hepatic Necrosis After
1 Per Cent Halothane Anesthesia for One Hour

Model I
  A. Animals pretreated with a single dose of Arochlor 1254 (a mixture of
     polychlorobiphenyls) 300 mg./kg. 5 days before anesthesia.
  B. Anesthesia: 1 per cent halothane, 99 per cent oxygen.

Model II
  A. Animals pretreated with phenobarbital for 5 days prior to anethesia
     (1 mg./ml. drinking water).
  B. Anesthesia: 1 per cent halothane, 14 per cent oxygen, 85 per cent nitrogen.

induces reductive pathways to a far greater extent than does phenobarbital. Model II is predicated on reduced oxygen availability to microsomal enzymes so that reductive metabolism is forced. Two reduced metabolites of halothane have been found in the plasma of
these models: CF_2CClBr and CF_3CH_2Cl. The latter metabolite was
speculated to be a product of halothane biotransformation and is hepatotoxic to animals in small quantities (Brown and Vandam, 1971).
Cohen's group has found that this volatile metabolite is produced in
man. The total amount so produced was quite low, however — too low
in fact to produce liver damage in his small series of volunteers. It is
interesting to speculate that if biotransformation of halothane were
altered by environmental or genetic factors, this metabolite could be
formed in quantities sufficient to result in liver damage. Suffice it to
say that Koch's postulates have been realized with halothane; it is possible to juggle biotransformation in laboratory animals such that classic centrolobular necrosis is produced by clinical concentrations of the
anesthetic.

DISCUSSION AND SUMMARY

The evidence appears to be overwhelming that the pathologic
state termed halothane hepatitis exists. It is a rare phenomenon that
cannot be predicted at this time. A rare, sporadic event is not unusual
for a drug reaction. This unfortunate side effect should not ban the
use of an otherwise safe, highly versatile anesthetic. The finding that
halothane anesthesia can produce centrolobular necrosis given the
correct, although ill-defined, set of variables is an important one. The
theory of biotransformation to reactive intermediates is consonant
with information concerning hepatotoxicity of other halogenated compounds, such as chloroform, carbon tetrachloride, and fluroxene.
Obviously, the middle-aged, obese individual is at high risk, because
this group implies more varied metabolism than neonates. The obese
person is known to biotransform more anesthetic for any given dose
than the svelte person, owing to the fat storage capacity of lipophilic
inhalation anesthetics. The hazard produced by repeated halothane

anesthetics could represent additional covalent binding, with the result that liver enzymes are increased, or, in the catastrophic case with necrosis, an environmental change (drugs or pollutants) between administrations. The individual who is genetically and environmentally at high risk would suffer liver damage on first administration. The challenge tests previously alluded to might represent such individuals who are responding in a dose-related manner to altered biotransformation of the anesthetic.

In summary, the salient features implicating halothane hepatitis as a true entity, in order of importance, are as follows:

1. There are a large number of anecdotal case reports of unexplained jaundice following halothane administration, even when serologic tests for hepatitis A and B are employed.
2. Halothane is chemically related to other alkyl halides known to produce liver damage.
3. Individuals at risk, when challenged with subanesthetic concentrations of halothane, have responded with liver damage in a dose-related fashion.
4. Animal models of halothane hepatitis are now easily produced in the laboratory. Thus, if animals can respond with centrolobular necrosis following halothane, it is quite possible man can.
5. The reactive metabolites thought to be responsible for the liver injury following halothane in animals can be detected in man. If the levels of these metabolite intermediates were increased, there is reason to believe necrosis would result.

REFERENCES

Allen, P.J., and Downing, J.W.: A prospective study of hepatocellular function after repeated exposures to halothane or enflurane in women undergoing radium therapy for cervical cancer. Br. J. Anaesth., 49:1035–1039, 1977.

Belfrage, S., Ahlgren, I., and Axelson, S.: Halothane hepatitis in an anesthetist. Lancet, 2:1466–1467, 1966.

Böttinger, L.E., Dalen, E., and Hallen, B.: Halothane induced liver damage: An analysis of the material reported to the Swedish adverse drug reaction committee, 1966–1973. Acta Anaesth. Scand., 20:40–46, 1976.

Brody, G.L., and Sweet, R.B.: Halothane anesthesia as a possible cause of massive hepatic necrosis. Anesthesiology, 24:29–37, 1963.

Brown, B.R., Jr., Sipes, I.G., and Baker, R.K.: Halothane hepatotoxi-city and the related derivative 1,1,1-trifluoro-2-chloroethane. Environ. Health Perspect., 21:185–188, 1971.

Brown, B.R., Jr., and Vandam, L.D.: A review of current advances in metabolism of inhalation anesthetics. Ann. N.H. Acad. Sci., 179:235–243, 1971.

Bunker, J.P., Forest, W.H., Jr., Mostell, F., et al. (eds.): The National Halothane Study. A study of the possible association between halothane anesthesia and postoperative hepatic necrosis. Bethesda, Maryland, NIGMS, 1965.

Castro, J.A., Sasame, H.A., Sussman, H., et al.: Diverse effects of SKF 525-A and antioxidants on carbon tetrachloride induced changes in liver P-450 content and ethylmorphine metabolism. Life Sci., 1:129–136, 1968.

Cohen, E.N., Trudell, J.R., Edmunds, N.H., et al.: Urinary metabolites of halothane in man. Anesthesiology, *28*:392–399, 1976.

Cohen, E.N.: Unpublished observations.

Douglas, J.H., Eger, E.I., II, Biava, C.G., et al.: Hepatic necrosis associated with viral infection after enflurane anesthesia. N. Engl. J. Med., *296*:552–555, 1977.

Gronert, G.A., Schaner, P.J., and Gunther, R.C.: Multiple halothane anesthesia in the burn patient. J.A.M.A., *205*:878–880, 1968.

Klatskin, G.: Mechanisms of toxic and drug induced hepatic injury. *In* Fink, B.R. (ed.): Toxicity of Anesthetics. Baltimore, Williams and Wilkins, 1968.

Klatskin, G., and Kimberg, D.V.: Recurrent hepatitis attributable to halothane sensitization in an anesthetist. N. Engl. J. Med., *280*:515, 522, 1969.

Lindenbaum, J., and Leifer, E.: Hepatic necrosis associated with halothane anesthesia. N. Engl. J. Med., *268*:525–530, 1963.

Little, D.M.: Effects of halothane on hepatic function. *In* Greene, N.M. (ed.): Halothane. Philadelphia, F.A. Davis, 1968.

Mathieu, A., DiPadua, D., Kahan, B., et al.: Humoral immunity to metabolites of halothane, fluroxene, and isoflurane. Anesthesiology, *42*:612–616, 1975.

McLain, G.E., Jr., Brown, B.R., Jr., and Sipes, I.G.: Unpublished observations.

Moult, P.J.A., Adjukiewicz, A.B., Gaylarde, P.M., et al.: Lymphocyte transformation in halothane-related hepatitis. Br. Med. J., *2*:69–70, 1975.

Paronetto, F., and Popper, H.: Lymphocyte stimulation induced by halothane in patients with hepatitis following exposure to halothane. N. Engl. J. Med., *283*:277–289, 1970.

Ráventos, J.: The action of fluothane — a new volatile anesthetic. Br. J. Pharmacol. Chemother., *11*:394–410, 1956.

Recknagel, R., and Ghoshal, A.: Lipoperoxidation as a vector in carbon tetrachloride hepatotoxicity. Lab. Invest., *15*:132–146, 1966.

Reeves, J.G., and McCracken, L.E.,

Jr.: Failure to induce hepatic pathology in animals sensitized to a halothane metabolite and subsequently challenged with halothane. Anesth. Analg., *55*:235–242, 1976.

Rehder, K., Forbes, J., Alter, H., et al.: Halothane biotransformation in man: A quantitative study. Anesthesiology, *28*:711–715, 1967.

Sipes, I.G., and Brown, B.R., Jr.: An animal model of hepatotoxicity associated with halothane anesthesia. Anesthesiology, *45*:622–628, 1976.

Slater, T.F.: Necrogenic action of carbon tetrachloride in the rat: A speculative mechanism based on activation. Nature, *209*:36–40, 1966.

Stier, A., Alter, H., Hessler, O., et al.: Urinary excretion of bromide in halothane anesthesia. Anesth. Analg. *43*:723–728, 1964.

Trowell, J., Peto, R., and Crampton-Smith, A.: Controlled trial of repeated halothane anaesthetics in patients with carcinoma of the uterine cervix treated with radium. Lancet, *1*:821–824, 1975.

Uehleke, H., Hellmer, K.H., and Tabarelli-Poplawski, S.: Metabolic activation of halothane and its covalent binding in liver endoplasmic proteins *in vitro*. Arch. Pharmacol. *279*:39–44, 1973.

Van Dyke, R.A., Chenoweth, M.B., and Van Poznak, A.: Metabolism of volatile anesthetics. I. Conversion in vivo of several anesthetics to $^{14}CO_2$ and chloride. Biochem. Pharmacol., *13*:1239–1248, 1964.

Virtue, R.W., and Payne, K.W.: Postoperative death after fluothane. Anesthesiology, *19*:562–563, 1958.

Walton, B., Dumond, D.C., Williams, C., et al.: Lymphocyte transformation: Absence of increased responses in alleged halothane jaundice. J.A.M.A., *225*:494–498, 1973.

Widger, L.A., Gandolfi, A.J., and Van Dyke, R.A.: Hypoxia and halothane metabolism *in vivo*: Release of inorganic fluoride and halothane metabolites binding to cellular constituents. Anesthesiology, *44*:197–201, 1976.

Wright, R., Chisholm, M., Lloyd, B., et al.: Controlled prospective study of the liver function of multiple exposures to halothane. Lancet, *1*:791–821, 1975.

by DAVID L. BRUCE

University of California, Irvine

HALOTHANE AND HEPATITIS: A DIRECT RELATIONSHIP IS UNPROVED

Halothane does not cause human hepatitis. No data exist to prove that it does. To be sure, *post hoc ergo propter hoc* reports abound in the literature, but these only suggest that a problem exists without giving any basis for either its cause or its solution. Currently, visions of contingency fees dance in the heads of litigious lawyers, and this fact alone requires that we examine seriously any evidence for "halothane hepatitis."

Even without this self-protecting motivation, however, we have an ethical obligation to do no harm to our patients. People *have* died of liver failure following halothane anesthesia. It is obviously important to know whether halothane itself caused these catastrophes or a combination of anesthesia, operation, and other stressful factors somehow tipped the scale toward progression of pathologic processes either potential or already extant but asymptomatic.

Halothane came into general clinical use in the United States in 1958. That same year, two cases of fatal hepatic necrosis were reported in the American literature to follow halothane anesthesias (Burnap, Galla, and Vandam, 1958; Virtue and Payne, 1958), but in both instances, severe cardiovascular depression had been present intraoperatively and this tempered any judgments against the anesthetic agent itself. In 1960, a French report (Vourc'h et al., 1960) of fatal hepatic necrosis after an uncomplicated inguinal herniorrhaphy went unnoticed in the United States. Not so easily overlooked was a group of reports (Temple, Cote, and Gorens, 1962; Brody and Sweet, 1963; Tornetta and Tamaki, 1963; Lindenbaum and Heifer, 1963; Bunker and Blumenfeld, 1963) appearing from mid-1962 to 1963. In May 1963, a warning was issued by the manufacturer of halothane, stating that "the administration of halothane to patients with known liver or biliary tract disease is not recommended." A month later, the National Halothane Study was begun.

That study sought to determine the incidence of fatal massive hepatic necrosis and of overall mortality within six weeks of the administration of halothane or other general anesthetic agents. Data accrued by 34 institutions between 1959 and 1962 were analyzed retrospectively by a panel of anesthesiologists, internists, pathologists, statisticians, and surgeons. Their findings were published in a 418 page report (Bunker et al., 1969). Despite the fact that the results of 856,500 operations were scrutinized, the study team could not conclude more than "The possible rare occurrence of halothane-induced hepatic necrosis after single or multiple administration could not be ruled out." That was nine years ago. How much farther has our factual data base extended since then?

The same year that the National Halothane Study appeared, Klatskin and Kimberg published a case report (Klatskin and Kimberg, 1969) that caused Combes to declare editorially in the New England Journal of Medicine that "The current status of halothane liver damage has gone beyond the point of whether such an entity exists" (Combes, 1969). To this day, that single case convinces many that halothane is, indeed, a "sensitizing" agent capable of causing liver damage when administered to patients, particularly if given repeatedly. Therefore, in taking a position denying a direct relationship between halothane and hepatitis it will be necessary to examine the facts of that case in some detail.

The patient was a physician in his mid-40's who practiced anesthesiology. At age 21, he had undergone desensitization to ragweed, thought to be the basis of his allergic asthma and hay fever. Other than that, he was healthy until he developed hepatitis after almost one year of daily use of halothane as a resident in anesthesiology. This was initially diagnosed as viral hepatitis. When he resumed work two months later, he had a relapse. This pattern repeated itself several times until steroid therapy was started. When taking prednisone he worked without relapse and finished his training. For the next two years he practiced anesthesiology "but was exposed to halothane only occasionally." Midway through this two-year period, he had a physical examination that "gave no clinical or biochemical evidence of hepatic disease." Later, he had a relapse thought to represent recurrent hepatitis and was treated successfully with prednisone. Liver biopsy showed posthepatitic cirrhosis. Thereafter, he could work without illness only if he continued taking steroids. Repeat liver biopsies showed progression of liver damage but could not differentiate recurrent viral hepatitis from drug sensitization, by now regarded as suspect. During a time when his hepatitis was inactive and he was not receiving medications, he was challenged by the inhalation of 0.1 to 0.2 per cent halothane in oxygen for five minutes. Within four hours he had myalgia, and six hours later his temperature and pulse reached 102.8 F. and 108, respectively. Over the next two days his serum glutamic oxaloacetic transaminase (SGOT) level rose from 41 to 700 international units. He recovered, but the conclusion drawn from this challenge was that he was specifically sensitive to halothane.

This report is dramatic and indeed does suggest sensitization to halothane. There are obstacles, however, to accepting that conclusion. It seems unlikely that a year of "almost daily" exposure to an agent would be required to sensitize a subject, particularly one prone to allergy. While at home, convalescing from his second relapse, the patient noted signs and symptoms of recurrent hepatitis when he increased his physical activity, and the levels of his liver enzymes increased again, even though he had not returned to work and had not been re-exposed to halothane. When he *did* resume his residency, he was apparently well for two weeks before a third relapse occurred. This, plus the later history of two years of uneventful practice punctuated by occasional exposure to halothane, suggests that his "sensitization" was not of such severity that exposure to halothane always led to exacerbation of his hepatitis. He began to treat himself with steroids whenever he felt ill. A flight to Europe caused him to start such self-medication. Before submitting to the halothane challenge, he was advised that this might represent a serious risk to him. Although the report does not discuss his emotional state on the day of that test, he may, with good reason, have been a bit apprehensive, to put it mildly. Would it not have been at least as stressful as a flight to Europe? In point of fact, this patient cannot with absolute certainty be excluded as having had chronic, relapsing viral hepatitis, with exacerbations brought on by physical and emotional stress.

Simpson and colleagues commented on these "anomalies" in the history of that now famous, anonymous anesthesiologist and reviewed the evidence for the existence of "halothane hepatitis" that had accrued by 1972 (Simpson, Strunin, and Walton, 1973). They concluded that a cause and effect relationship between halothane exposure and postoperative jaundice could not be supported but added that it was equally impossible to deny categorically such a possibility. Dykes and associates in a scholarly survey of the epidemiologic, immunologic, and metabolic aspects of the relationship of halothane to the liver concluded, "We believe that the only truly compelling evidence for the existence of 'halothane hepatitis' remains the two anesthetists who demonstrated a true positive halothane challenge" (Dykes et al., 1972). One of those two anesthetists was the anesthesiologist whose history I have just reviewed. The other has not been commented upon because of the paucity of information offered therein. It is interesting, and typical of the literature on this topic, that two reviews written within a year of each other drew different conclusions about how "compelling" the evidence offered by the reports of the sensitized anesthetists was.

Perhaps these people disagreed, but in a review of the complication of postoperative jaundice, a section was devoted to "halothane hepatotoxicity" (LaMont and Isselbacher, 1973). In the mind of the medical public, the role of halothane as a hepatotoxin was no longer putative. Attention had turned to the definition of a "safe" interval between halothane exposures (Bruce, 1972). While this occupied the attention of clinicians, laboratory work continued to seek the reason(s) for a relationship between halothane and hepatic complications. Reports too numerous to review gave results of metabolic and immunologic studies, *in vivo* and *in vitro*, and the consensus was that if a relationship existed, it was through a metabolite of halothane, perhaps a free radical impossible to identify with existing techniques, rather than the unchanged, parent molecule.

If one accepts this thesis, it would follow that patients whose rate of drug metabolism is accelerated by their chronic use of enzyme-inducing drugs would be at greater risk for "halothane hepatitis" than those taking no medications would be. Greene's survey suggested that this is not the case (Greene, 1973), but the trouble with all attempts to survey this complication is its rarity. An event, in this case "halothane hepatitis," alleged to occur once in 10,000 cases is unlikely to show significantly different incidences in comparisons of groups numbering in the 100's. Since the metabolites of halothane under consideration are thought to be either hepatotoxic or immunogenic, they must be atypical rather than routine breakdown products. This hypothesis is attractive, since it is compatible with the relative frequencies of enzyme abnormalities, pseudocholinesterase deficiency being an example. It is not unreasonable to believe that 1 in 10,000 patients has an enzyme system that produces toxic or immunogenic products from halothane. Now, is there any evidence that such a thing is even possible?

There is. Burnell Brown and colleagues have convincingly shown that the rat, by suitable treatment, may be made to metabolize halothane *via* a reductive, rather than oxidative, pathway and that an unidentified reductive metabolite is uniformly hepatotoxic in that model system (Sipes and Brown, 1976). Even though these animals had to be pretreated with chemicals, anesthetized, and subjected to hypoxia, a principle was established in these experiments. Halothane metabolism could be manipulated to produce hepatotoxic effects in the rat. If this phenomenon can be caused in rats, it *may* occur in man. We have no way now of knowing if it does. In time, we will.

In the meantime, we can conclude that if liver toxicity can follow the use of halothane, it is the result of atypical, and completely unpredictable, metabolism of that drug. That is where the problem lies, not with the drug itself. Halothane does not cause hepatitis. Admonitions against administering halothane to patients with known liver disease and against repeat administrations within six months and these sorts of quasi–common sense approaches to the use of this valuable anesthetic agent are totally without foundation in fact. So are most medical malpractice cases based on violations of these irrational rules.

We are left with the probability that a rare and *a priori* unidentifiable patient may reduce, rather than oxidize, halothane. The only time we would know if this could happen would be after the fact of halothane administration. The first such anesthesia should probably be allowed to show signs of resultant liver dysfunction, which would be evident in significantly elevated enzymes within 10 days or so, before repeat anesthesias are given with this agent. Other than that, our best course is to follow the old saw of the consultant, to "avoid hypoxia." *Plus ça change, plus c'est la même chose.*

REFERENCES

Brody, G.L., and Sweet, R.B.: Halothane anesthesia as a possible cause of massive hepatic necrosis. Anesthesiology, *24*:29–37, 1963.

Bruce, D.L.: What is a "safe" interval between halothane exposures? J.A.M.A., *221*:1140–1143, 1972.

Bunker, J.P., and Blumenfeld, C.M.: Liver necrosis after halothane anesthesia. Cause or coincidence? N. Engl. J. Med., *268*:531–534, 1963.

Bunker, J.P., Forrest, W.H., Jr., Mosteller, F., and Vandam, L.D. (eds.): The National Halothane Study. A study of the possible association between halothane anesthesia and postoperative hepatic necrosis. Bethesda, Md., National Institutes of Health, National Institute of General Medical Sciences, 1969.

Burnap, T.K., Galla, S.J., and Vandam, L.D.: Anesthetic, circulatory and respiratory effects of Fluothane. Anesthesiology, *19*:307–320, 1958.

Combes, B.: Halothane-induced liver damage — an entity. N. Engl. J. Med., *280*:558–559, 1969.

Dykes, M.H.M., Gilbert, J.P., Schur, P.H., et al.: Halothane and the liver: A review of the epidemiologic, immunologic and metabolic aspects of the relationship. Can. J. Surg., *15*:1–22, 1972.

Greene, N.M.: Halothane anesthesia and hepatitis in a high-risk population. N. Engl. J. Med., *289*:304–307, 1973.

Klatskin, G., and Kimberg, D.V.: Recurrent hepatitis attributable to halothane sensitization in an anesthetist. N. Engl. J. Med., *280*:515–522, 1969.

LaMont, J.T., and Isselbacher, K.J.: Medical intelligence, postoperative jaundice. N. Engl. J. Med., *288*:305–308, 1973.

Lindenbaum, J., and Leifer, E.: Hepatic necrosis associated with halothane anesthesia. N. Engl. J. Med., *268*:525–530, 1963.

Simpson, B.R., Strunin, L., and Walton, B.: Halothane hepatitis: Fact or fallacy. Bull. N.Y. Acad. Med., *49*:708–721, 1973.

Sipes, I.G., and Brown, B.R., Jr.: An animal model of hepatotoxicity associated with halothane anesthesia. Anesthesiology, *45*:622–628, 1976.

Temple, R.L., Cote, R.A., and Gorens, S.W.: Massive hepatic necrosis following general anesthesia. Anesth. Analg., *41*:586–592, 1962.

Tornetta, F.J., and Tamaki, H.T.: Halothane jaundice and hepatotoxicity. J.A.M.A., *184*:658–660, 1963.

Virtue, R.W., and Payne, K.W.: Postoperative death after Fluothane. Anesthesiology, *19*:562–563, 1958.

Vourc'h, G., Schnoebelen, E., Buck, F., et al.: Hépatonéphrite aiguë mortelle après anesthésie comportant de l'halothane (Fluothane). Anesth. Analg. (Paris), *17*:466–475, 1960.

HALOTHANE AND HEPATITIS

EDITORIAL COMMENT

For the past 15 years, anesthetists have been concerned over the relationship of halothane anesthesia and the appearance of hepatitis in the postoperative period. Few equate haltohane and hepatitis in the same fashion as chloroform and hepatitis. Many have established guidelines for use or exclusion of the agent, nearly all of which, both Brown and Bruce point out, are without a basis in fact. Others have continued a fairly liberal use of halothane in the absence of conclusive evidence of a relationship and rarity of a complication. Considering the unwarranted medicolegal accusations and the attention given hepatitis, the continued popularity of the agent is surprising, bespeaking its overall superiority for general anesthesia.

Bruce has taken the position that a relationship between halothane and hepatitis is unproved except if a patient has an unsuspected and undetectable abnormality of metabolic pathways leading to production of a hepatotoxic metabolite. He therefore lays the blame for hepatitis after halothane not on the anesthetic but on the factors that altered metabolic pathways, be they genetic or drug-induced. He points as proof that Brown by suitable pretreatment can change oxidative metabolism to reductive metabolism, thereby producing a hepatotoxic metabolite.

On the other hand, Brown is more swayed by the anecdotal reports and available data and considers a relationship of hepatitis to halothane reasonably proved. By manipulation of metabolic pathways in laboratory animals and by exposing the animals to halothane, he can reliably produce hepatitis. He couples halothane and hepatitis, whereas Bruce couples deranged metabolic pathways and hepatitis. Perhaps the difference in interpretation is immaterial.

Both authors are clear on the fact that the agent is a superior one, that the complication is rare, that a toxic metabolite must be produced through abnormal metabolic pathways, and that these pathways cannot be predicted except through the prior appearance of hepatitis following halothane exposure.

Part 3

ANESTHETIC EFFECTS UPON REPRODUCTION

THE PROPOSITION:

Inhalation anesthetics cause genetic defects, abortions, and miscarriages in operating room personnel.

ALTERNATIVE POINTS OF VIEW:

By Ellis N. Cohen
By Louis L. Ferstandig

EDITORIAL COMMENT

by ELLIS N. COHEN
Stanford University Medical Center

INHALATIONAL ANESTHETICS MAY CAUSE GENETIC DEFECTS, ABORTIONS, AND MISCARRIAGES IN OPERATING ROOM PERSONNEL

An awareness that waste anesthetic gases were contaminants of the operating room environment undoubtedly coincided with the introduction of inhalation anesthesia into clinical practice. This had to be so, since the earliest techniques for administration of chloroform and ether consisted of vaporizing the liquid anesthetic onto several layers of gauze placed over the patient's nose and mouth. One's sense of smell was thus sufficient to detect significant anesthetic contamination. Although recognized, this pollution did not generate serious concern, and only sporadic efforts were made to reduce the waste anesthetic concentration because of occasional side effects in sensitive individuals.

The first suggestion of concern associated with waste anesthetic gas pollution followed publication of a study investigating the working conditions of Russian anesthetists (Vaisman, 1967). Of some 354 anesthetists surveyed, many reported multiple complaints, including itching (8 per cent), headaches (78 per cent), and fatigue (85 per cent). Unfortunately, the study was uncontrolled, and in the light of vague polysymptomatology, it was tempting to dismiss the findings entirely. What commanded attention was the observation indicating that 18 of 31 pregnancies among these anesthetists ended in spontaneous abortion and that only seven of the pregnancies were without complication. This did generate concern, and the subsequent 10 years have resulted in numerous experimental studies, as well as in large epidemiologic surveys (212 citations by 1977). Although most of these investigations have supported Vaisman's original observations, clear experimental evidence establishing a direct association between the trace anesthetic gases and health risks associated with the operating room has not appeared. Nonetheless, a large body of evidence confirms the presence of an occupational hazard and strongly suggests an association with trace anesthetics present in the operating room.

DATA OBTAINED AT CLINICAL ANESTHETIC CONCENTRATIONS

Although concentrations of trace anesthetics customarily measured in an unscavenged operating room average 500 ppm. nitrous oxide and 10 ppm. halothane, these concentrations represent only 0.1 to 0.2 per cent of that breathed by a patient during clinical anesthesia. On the other hand, occupational exposure for the anesthetist and operating room attendants is essentially continuous throughout their active professional life. Since the lipid soluble inhalation anesthetics are eliminated relatively slowly, the amount of trace anesthetics retained in the body during a given year may exceed that of several clinically administered anesthetics. These calculations make no allowance for the phenomenon of enzyme induction or for the proportionate increase in anesthetic metabolism also occurring at low anesthetic concentrations. Both of these factors enhance the amount of anesthetic metabolism and possibly associated toxicity.

In Vitro Studies

An early demonstration that prolonged administration of nitrous oxide resulted in depression of the bone marrow (Lassen et al., 1956) led to trials of this anesthetic for the treatment of leukemia (Eastwood et al., 1963), as well as to numerous studies confirming a depressant effect of anesthetics on cell growth and cell division. The ability of inhalation anesthetics in concentrations used clinically to inhibit cell division has been known for some time, a phenomenon intensively studied in plants, animals, and cell cultures (Fink and Kenny, 1968; Jackson, 1972; Sturrock and Nunn, 1975). Of considerable interest is evidence that halothane inhibits DNA synthesis in the rat hepatoma cell (Jackson, 1968) and inhibits RNA synthesis in the cultured lymphocyte preparation (Bruce, 1975). Exposure of Chinese hamster fibroblasts to this anesthetic results in the formation of abnormal multinucleated cells (Sturrock and Nunn, 1975). There is thus significant evidence that concentrations of inhalation anesthetics used clinically influence cell multiplication and normal cell growth.

Many *in vitro* studies have been carried out exposing various microbial systems to the inhalation anesthetics in an attempt to investigate possible mutagenic effects. Studies with halothane, methoxyflurane, enflurane, trichloroethylene, and isoflurane examined over a wide range of concentrations have failed to produce mutagenicity in histidine-dependent strains of *Salmonella typhimurium.* In contrast, fluroxene was followed by a sixfold increase in mutant colonies beginning at vapor concentrations of 1 per cent (Baden et al., 1977). Although mutagenesis in this system has not been reported following the use of halothane, its urinary metabolites have been implicated, an observation remaining to be confirmed (McCoy et al., 1977).

In Vivo Animal Studies

An embryolethal and fetal-toxic effect of inhalation anesthetics administered in concentrations used clinically has been demonstrated in both mammalian and avian species (Smith, Gaub, and Moya, 1965; Fink, Shepard, and Blandau, 1967; Basford and Fink, 1968). Toxicity is manifested as an increase in fetal death rates and in incidence of congenital defects, the responses being most pronounced during the first trimester. Toxicity increased with prolonged exposure to the anesthetics. Whether these effects are solely dependent on the anesthetic is unknown. At least one group failed to demonstrate anesthetic toxicity in rats and rabbits exposed at clinical anesthetic concentration (Kennedy et al., 1976).

Studies of the effect of anesthetics on spermatogenesis are of interest. Rats administered subanesthetic concentrations of nitrous oxide (20 per cent) exhibit damage to the seminiferous tubules. Spermatozoa count is reduced, and abnormal multinucleated cells appear in the testis within 14 days (Kripke et al., 1976). In more sensitive animals, these responses were noted as early as the second day. All animals recovered normal spermatogenesis within three days after return to room air.

Human Studies

Although an estimated 50,000 women in the United States annually undergo a surgical procedure and anesthesia during gestation, limited data exist to define the associated risk to pregnancy and fetus. A single study reported by Shnider and Wester examined 9073 pregnant women (Shnider and Wester, 1965), 1.6 per cent of whom underwent operation and anesthesia during pregnancy. Upon eventual delivery, there was a birth defect rate of 5.44 per cent, essentially the same as that of the unoperated control group. Further data are needed.

Inhalation anesthetics are associated with an effect on the immune response; concentrations used clinically depress phagocytic action in man (Lofstrom and Schildt, 1974) as well as reduce susceptibility to infection with murine hepatic virus (Moudgil, 1973). Depression of lymphocyte transformation also follows major surgery and anesthesia, although this likely relates to degree of surgical trauma rather than to the depressant effects of inhalation anesthetics (Cullen and van Belle, 1975).

DATA OBTAINED AT TRACE ANESTHETIC CONCENTRATION

Although inhalation anesthetics administered at concentrations used clinically are generally recognized to produce toxic responses in the fetus, we have become concerned with a potential hazard associated with exposure to trace concentrations of anesthetics. At first glance, the amount of anesthetic agent present in the operating room atmosphere would seem insignificant, since it is measurable in parts per million. On the other hand, occupational exposure of physicians, nurses, and dental personnel to trace concentrations is continuous and may be long-term, and under these circumstances, measurable physiologic responses occur (Cascorbi, Blake, and Helrich, 1970; Evers and Racz, 1974; Ghonheim et al., 1975). Similar factors likely participate in the increased spontaneous abortion and congenital abnormality rates in infants of exposed operating room personnel and possibly in other health hazards as well. Although a direct causal relationship between these responses and trace anesthetic gases has not been proved, there are approximately 214,000 operating room personnel in the United States exposed to waste anesthetics, and the issue of their health is a matter of national concern.

In Vitro Studies

Despite the large numbers of experimental studies conducted at anesthetic concentrations used clinically that document an effect on cell cultures and microbial systems, similar investigations are not available for trace concentrations of anesthetics.

In Vivo Animal Studies

Although one study indicated the absence of any effect on reproduction in mice repeatedly exposed to 16 ppm. halothane (Bruce, 1973), a subsequent study with nitrous oxide demonstrated a definite toxic response at low trace anesthetic concentration (Corbett et al., 1973). Rats exposed to 1000 and 15,000 ppm. of nitrous oxide showed significant increases in fetal death rates (spontaneous resorption) at both dose levels. Diurnal variation in response was also observed. In contrast, a recent study has failed to demonstrate fetal toxicity in rats following chronic exposure to a range of trace concentrations of halothane, methoxyflurane and nitrous oxide (Pope et al., 1978). It has also been reported, however, that rats less than 60 days old chronically exposed to 10 ppm. halothane manifest lasting behavioral deficits and ultrastructural central nervous system damage, effects less apparent in older groups (Quimby et al., 1974).

Recent studies indicate chromosomal changes in spermatogonial and bone marrow cells of the rat at two trace-dose levels of halothane and nitrous oxide (Coate, Kapp, and Lewis, 1979). Male rats were exposed for 52 weeks (7 hours per day, 5 days per week) to 50 ppm. nitrous oxide and 1 ppm. halothane and to 500 ppm. nitrous oxide and 10 ppm. halothane. The latter dose level resulted in cellular aberrations consistent with marked genetic damage, including chromatid gaps, chromosomal breaks, and chromosomal markers such as exchange figures, rings, and miscellaneous marker chromosomes. Although similar findings were noted at the lower concentrations, they were not as marked. These data have serious implication in view of the reports enumerated in the paragraphs to follow.

Human Studies

The most significant data concerning possible effects of trace anesthetics are those resulting from epidemiologic investigations. Although most of these studies are retrospective and necessarily suffer from the limitations of this approach, a large body of data has accumulated suggesting an association between working in an anesthetic-contaminated environment and an increased incidence of spontaneous miscarriage and congenital abnormalities in offspring. A direct relationship between these hazards and levels of trace anesthetic gases and the duration of anesthetic exposure is more difficult to document, although some data are available. Additional information is required, and alternate etiologic factors must also be excluded. The latter include severe occupational stress, exposure to chemicals used in the operating room, and presence of oncotic viruses. Few studies have been undertaken in these areas, and data are limited.

As an outgrowth of the survey by Vaisman (Vaisman, 1967), small scale epidemiologic studies were conducted in Denmark and in the United States. The Danish study surveyed 578 nurses and 174 female and male anesthetists, and the incidence of spontaneous abortion was compared before and after employment in the anesthesia department (Askrog and Harvald, 1970). Miscarriage rates were increased (17 per cent versus 10.7 per cent) during the period of employment of the women in the anesthesia department. It was also reported that wives of exposed male anesthetists showed an increased rate of spontaneous miscarriage. Unfortunately, both this study and that by Vaisman lacked adequate statistical control. The United States study (Cohen, Bellville, and Brown, 1971) however, did not suffer from this deficiency. Spontaneous miscarriage rates in 67 female operating room nurses and 92 female anesthesiologists were surveyed, with controls provided by comparable groups of general duty nurses and nonanesthetist female physicians. Spontaneous miscarriage rates among operating room nurses were increased to 29.7 per cent and those in anesthesiologists to 37.8 per cent, approximately a threefold increase over control groups (8.6 to 10.3 per cent). The differences were statistically significant.

The first large-scale epidemiologic survey was reported in 1972 from the United Kingdom and examined anesthetic practice and pregnancy outcome in a large population of female anesthetists (Knill-Jones, Moir, and Rodriques, 1972). A questionnaire was sent to 1241 female anesthetists and to 1670 female physicians not associated with anesthesia. The frequency of spontaneous abortion was significantly higher in anesthetists (18.2 per cent) compared to the control group (14.7 per cent). It was also noted that anesthetists working during pregnancy delivered children with a significantly higher incidence of congenital abnormalities (6.5 per cent) compared to those not at work during pregnancy (2.5 per cent). The rate of miscarriage in the non-anesthetist control group was higher (4.9 per cent) than that in the nonworking anesthetists, an insignificant statistical difference. Involuntary infertility among the exposed anesthetists was noted twice as frequently (12 per cent versus 6 per cent) as in the control group.

This disturbing report led to an evaluation of the incidence of birth defects among offspring of Michigan female nurse anesthetists (Corbett et al., 1974). The results of a mail survey of 621 female nurse anesthetists indicated that children born to mothers who worked during pregnancy had an 8.8 per cent incidence of birth defects compared to 3.8 per cent among children whose mothers did not work during pregnancy — statistically significant differences.

The United Kingdom survey also led to a study of the incidence of spontaneous abortion among 300 married Finnish nurses (Rosenberg and Kirves, 1973). The rate among scrub nurses was 21.5 per cent, among intensive care unit nurses 16.7 per cent, among anesthesia nurses 15 per cent, and among casualty department nurses 8.3 per cent. The incidence of miscarriage among anesthesia and intensive care unit nurses was comparable. If one grouped anesthesia and scrub nurses and compared them to women working outside the operating room (intensive care and casualty department nurses), however, the mean spontaneous abortion rate was 19.5 per cent for the former and 11.4 per cent for the latter. These findings are significantly different. The pre-employment spontaneous miscarriage rates of the two groups were 13.9 per cent and 12.5 per cent, respectively.

The largest epidemiologic survey to date is that conducted by a committee of the American Society of Anesthesiologists (Cohen et al., 1974). This national survey included all anesthesiologists, nurse anesthetists, and operating room nurses and technicians in the United States. Some 49,585 exposed personnel were surveyed, as was a control group of 23,911 pediatricians and general duty nurses. The study indicated that female anesthesiologists, nurse anesthetists and operating room nurses and technicians were subject to a statistically significant increased risk of spontaneous abortion, approximately 1.3 to 2 times that of the unexposed control group. There was an increased risk of congenital abnormalities among live-born babies of exposed female physicians and nurse anesthetists compared to control; the incidence of abnormalities, skin defects excluded, was approximately twice that of control for female physician anesthetists and increased 26 per cent for nurse anesthetists compared to their controls. An intragroup analysis of exposed female anesthesiologists, compared with unexposed physicians who had been away from the operating room at least one year prior to pregnancy, further substantiated these results. The congenital abnormality rate calculated for children of the exposed anesthesiologists was 5.9 per cent and 3.4 per cent for those of the unexposed female physicians. Similar data derived from nurse anesthetists indicated a rate of 9.6 per cent congenital abnormalities for the exposed group and 5.9 per cent for the unexposed. There were no significant differences in congenital abnormality rates between exposed and unexposed operating room nurses and technicians.

A particularly interesting and unexpected finding was the increased congenital abnormality rate noted in children of exposed male anesthesiologists, even though their wives had not been exposed to the operating room; the increase approximated 25 per cent, and was statistically significant. This suggests mutagenic damage within the male reproductive system. The data for children born to wives of male nurse anesthetists and male operating room nurse technicians reveal a similar trend, but the data base was small, and the difference was statistically insignificant.

A third large retrospective study of male anesthetists in the United Kingdom similarly analyzed anesthetic practice and pregnancy (Knill-Jones, Newman, and Spence, 1975). Some 7949 male physicians were surveyed, including an anesthetist group and a control group of nonanesthetist physicians. Although paternal operating room exposure had no influence on the frequency of spontaneous abortion among the nonexposed wives, maternal exposure was associated with an abortion rate of 15.5 per cent, compared to 10.9 per cent when neither the women nor their husbands were exposed. The frequency of congenital abnormalities was 4.5 per cent for children of exposed male anesthetists and 3.6 per cent for the nonexposed male physicians. For female physicians, the rate of congenital abnormalities in their offspring was 5.5 per cent for exposed women versus 3.6 per cent for the unexposed female physicians. Matching pregnancies of the exposed and nonexposed groups for maternal smoking, birth order, and maternal age at the time of birth further emphasized the significantly increased differences in spontaneous abortion and congenital abnormality rates.

Recently, a comparative analysis has been made of data from the three large retrospective surveys conducted in the United States and the United Kingdom. The analysis indicates close agreement with respect to the apparent association between anesthetic practice and obstetric mishap in both countries (Spence, Cohen, and Brown, 1977). In these analyses (Table 1), the adjusted combined data for female

Table 1. Adjusted and Combined Rates From United States
and United Kingdom Surveys

	Age (in years)	Preg-nancies	Miscar-riages/ Pregnan-cies, %	Live-Born Children	Congenital Abnormalities/ Live-Born Children, %
Exposed female anesthetists					
United States	41.6	596	15.7 ± 1.5	494	5.5 ± 1.0
United Kingdom	39.3	737	17.5 ± 1.4	599	5.5 ± 0.7
Combined data			16.7 ± 1.0*		5.5 ± 0.7**
Control female physicians					
United States	47.2	355	9.6 ± 1.6	313	2.8 ± 1.9
United Kingdom	41.8	2150	14.0 ± 0.8	1817	4.2 ± 0.4
Combined data	—		13.3 ± 0.7		4.0 ± 0.4
Exposed male anesthetists					
United States	45.2	4143	12.1 ± 0.5	3597	5.3 ± 0.4
United Kingdom	39.8	1382	13.9 ± 0.9	1180	4.2 ± 0.7
Combined data	—		12.6 ± 0.5†		5.0 ± 0.3*
Control male physicians					
United States	51.8	2261	12.0 ± 0.7	1970	3.9 ± 0.4
United Kingdom	41.6	2493	11.5 ± 0.6	2174	3.6 ± 0.4
Combined data	—		11.7 ± 0.5		3.7 ± 0.3

(Modified from Spence, A. A., Cohen, E. N., and Brown, B. W.: Occupational hazards for operating room–based physicians. J.A.M.A., 238:955–959. 1977.)

  *p > 0.01: exposed compared to controls
 **p = 0.04: exposed compared to controls
 †p = 0.10: exposed compared to controls

anesthetists yields a spontaneous abortion rate of 16.7 per cent versus 13.3 per cent for control, a highly significant difference statistically. The adjusted combined congenital abnormality rate for children of exposed female physicians is 5.5 per cent versus 4.0 per cent for control, also statistically significant. For exposed male anesthetists, the combined adjusted rates for spontaneous miscarriage in their wives was 12.6 per cent and 11.7 per cent for wives of nonexposed physicians, a difference that is not significant. The adjusted combined data for congenital abnormalities in children of exposed male anesthetists (5.0 per cent) indicate a highly statistically significant difference compared to children born to wives of the unexposed physicians (3.7 per cent). It would appear that, despite many differences in methods of survey and in statistical analysis, there is corroboration in the conclusions drawn from three independent studies.

A small-scale survey has also been undertaken of anesthetic health practices among dentists (Cohen et al., 1975). Analysis of data from 4797 general dental practitioners and 2642 oral surgeons indicates that 20.2 per cent of the former and 74.8 per cent of the latter were exposed to inhalation anesthetics in the dental operatory a minimum of three hours per week. When the dentists exposed to anesthetic were combined into one group and compared to unexposed dentists, there was a significant increase in the incidence of spontaneous abortion (16.0 per cent) among spouses of those exposed compared to wives of those unexposed (9.0 per cent). Data on congenital abnormalities of children born to wives of exposed dentists suggest an increase (4.7 per cent versus 4.1 per cent) when compared to wives of unexposed dentists, but the data base is small and statistically insignificant.

A finding of related interest in the dental survey was the approximate 2½-fold increase in liver disease among exposed versus unexposed male dentists. There are also data in the dental study that support a specific relationship between the incidence of these health problems and exposure to waste anesthetic gases. General dentists and oral surgeons provide similar dental care to their patients under similar operative and stress conditions, whether local or inhalation anesthetics are used. Separation of the dentists into two groups, those exposed to anesthetic gases and those not exposed, reveals significant differences in disease rates. The presumption that anesthetic gas exposure is the only known operating variable makes the case for association of a health hazard and anesthetic exposure in the dentist stronger than that available for operating room personnel, for whom many variables exist, and a similar control group is unavailable. The dental study provides data from which one can reasonably associate exposure to the waste anesthetic gases and resultant obstetric health hazards.

Data from operating room–exposed anesthetists also indicate the presence of enzyme induction associated with this exposure, which might contribute to increased toxicity following accelerated metabolism of the trace anesthetic gases. There are, however, insufficient data at present to define this problem. Although there is little question as to the increased health hazard to individuals working in the operating room, this conclusion must be advanced cautiously. As the American Society of Anesthesiologists Ad Hoc Committee carefully reported, "the epidemiologic studies were retrospective in nature, obtained by mail, and involve data that are subject to misinterpretation, misrecollection and variation due to the experience and education of the respondent" (Cohen et al., 1975). It is hoped a resolution of the question of health hazards in operating room personnel will be obtained from the results of a repeat survey to be conducted in the near future. If the extensive application of gas scavenging techniques during the intervening period results in a decrease in the incidence of spontaneous abortion and congenital abnormalities in children of operating room–based physicians and nurses, one could then speak of a direct cause and effect relationship with greater confidence. In the meantime, the available data suggest the likelihood of such an association and obligate us as responsible individuals to do everything possible to reduce the levels of waste anesthetic gases through careful operating room monitoring and efficient gas scavenging techniques.

REFERENCES

Askog, V., and Harvald, B.: Teratogenic effect of inhalation anesthetics. Nord. Med., *83*:498–504, 1970.

Baden, J. M., Kelley, M., Wharton, R. S., et al.: Mutagenicity of halogenated ether anesthetics. Anesthesiology, *46*:346–350, 1977.

Basford, A., and Fink, B. R.: Teratogenic activity of halothane in rats. Anesthesiology, *29*:1167–1173, 1968.

Bruce, D. L.: Halothane inhibition of RNA and protein synthesis of PHA-treated human lymphocytes. Anesthesiology, *42*:11–14, 1975.

Bruce, D. L.: Murine fertility unaffected by traces of halothane. Anesthesiology, *38*:473–477, 1973.

Cascorbi, H. F., Blake, D. A., and Helrich, M.: Differences in the biotransformation of halothane in man. Anesthesiology, *32*:119–123, 1970.

Coate, W. B., Kapp, R. W., and Lewis, T. R.: Chronic low-level halothane-nitrous oxide exposure. Reproduction and cytogenetic effects in rats. Anesthesiology (In press).

Cohen, E. N., Bellville, J. W., and Brown, B. W.: Anesthesia, pregnancy, and miscarriage. A study of operating room nurses and anesthetists. Anesthesiology, *35*:343–347, 1971.

Cohen, E. N., Brown, B. W., Bruce, D. L., et al.: Occupational disease among operating room personnel. A national study. Anesthesiology, *41*:321–340, 1974.

Cohen, E. N., Brown, B. W., Bruce, D. L., et al.: A survey of anesthetic health hazards among dentists. J.A.D.A., *90*:1291–1296, 1975.

Corbett, T. H., Cornell, R. G., Endres, J. L., et al.: Effects of low concentrations of nitrous oxide on rat pregnancy. Anesthesiology, *39*:299–301, 1973.

Corbett, T. H., Cornell, R. G., Endres, J. L., et al.: Birth defects among children of nurse anesthetists. Anesthesiology, *41*:341–344, 1974.

Cullen, B. F., and van Belle, G.: Lymphocyte transformation and changes in leukocyte count. Effects of anesthesia and operation. Anesthesiology, *43*:563–569, 1975.

Eastwood, D. W., Green, C. D., Lamdin, M. A., et al.: Effect of nitrous oxide on the white cell count in leukemia. N. Engl. J. Med., *268*:197–299, 1963.

Evers, W., and Racz, G. B.: Occupational hazards in anesthesia. Survey of blood enzymes, morphology and serum proteins in anesthesia residents. Anaesthe. Resusc. Intensive Ther., *2*:179–181, 1974.

Fink, B. R., and Kenny, G. E.: Metabolic effects of volatile anesthetics in cell culture. Anesthesiology, *29*:505–516, 1968.

Fink, B. R., Shepard T. H., and Blandau, R. J.: Teratogenic activity of nitrous oxide. Nature, *214*:146–148, 1967.

Ghonheim, M. M., Delle, M., Wilson, W. R., et al.: Alteration of warfarin kinetics in man associated with exposure to an operating room environment. Anesthesiology, *43*:333–336, 1975.

Jackson, S. H.: The metabolic effect of halothane on mammalian hepatoma cells in vitro. I. Inhibition of cell replication. Anesthesiology, *37*:489–492, 1972.

Jackson, S. H.: The metabolic effect of halothane on mammalian hepatoma cells in vitro. II. Inhibition of DNA synthesis. Anesthesiology, *39*:405–409, 1973.

Kennedy, G. L., Smith, S. H., Keplinger, M. L., et al.: Reproductive and teratologic studies with halothane. Toxicol. Appl. Pharmacol., *35*:467–474, 1976.

Knill-Jones, R. P., Moir, D. D., Rodrigues, L. V., et al.: Anesthetic practice and pregnancy. Controlled survey of women anaesthetists in the United Kingdom. Lancet, *1*:1326–1328, 1972.

Knill-Jones, R. P., Newman, B. J., and Spence, A. A.: Anaesthetic practice and pregnancy. Controlled survey of male anaesthetists in the United Kingdom. Lancet, *2*:807–809, 1975.

Kripke, B. J., Kelman, A. D., Shah,

N. K., et al.: Testicular reaction to prolonged exposure to nitrous oxide. Anesthesiology, *44*:104–113, 1976.

Lassen, H. C. A., Henrickson, E., Neukirch, F., et al.: Treatment of tetanus: Severe bone marrow depression after prolonged nitrous oxide anaesthesia. Lancet, *1*:527–530, 1956.

Lofstrom, B., and Schildt, B.: Reticuloendothelial function under general anesthesia. Acta Anaesthesiol. Scand., *18*:34–40, 1974.

McCoy, E. E., Hankel, R., Robbing, K., et al.: Presence of mutagenic substances in the urine of anesthesiologists. Abstracts of Environmental Mutagen Society, Eighth Annual Meeting, Colorado Springs, 1977, p. 34.

Moudgil, G. C.: Influence of halothane on mortality from murine hepatitis virus (MHV$_3$). Br. J. Anaesth., *45*:1236, 1973.

Pope, W. D. B., Halsey, M. J., Lansdown, A. B. G., et al.: Fetotoxicity in rats following chronic exposure to halothane, nitrous oxide or methoxyflurane. Anesthesiology, *48*:11–16, 1978.

Quimby, K. L., Aschkenase, L. J.,

Bowman, R. E., et al.: Enduring learning deficits and cerebral synaptic malformation from exposure to 10 parts of halothane per million. Science, *185*:625–627, 1974.

Rosenberg, P., and Kirves, A.: Miscarriage among operating theatre staff. Acta. Anaesth. Scand. (Suppl.), *53*:37–42, 1973.

Shnider, S. M., and Wester, G. M.: Maternal and fetal hazards of surgery during pregnancy. Am. J. Obstet. Gynecol., *92*:891–900, 1965.

Smith, B. E., Gaub, M. L., and Moya, F.: Investigation into the teratogenic effects of anesthetic agents: The fluorinated agents. Anesthesiology, *26*:260–261, 1965.

Spence, A. A., Cohen, E. N., and Brown, B. W.: Occupational hazards for operating room–based physicians. J.A.M.A., *238*:955–959, 1977.

Sturrock, J. E., and Nunn, J. F.: Mitosis in mammalian cells during exposure to anesthetics. Anesthesiology, *43*:21–23, 1975.

Vaisman, A. I.: Working conditions in surgery and their effect on the health of anesthesiologists. Eksp. Khir. Anesteziol., *3*:44–49, 1967.

by LOUIS L. FERSTANDIG

Halocarbon Laboratories, Inc.

TRACE CONCENTRATIONS OF ANESTHETICS ARE NOT PROVED HEALTH HAZARDS

The anesthesia literature contains many articles implicating trace concentrations of anesthetics as health hazards to operating room personnel. Spontaneous abortion, abnormalities among offspring, infertility, and cancer have been attributed to chronic exposure to traces of anesthetics. Several epidemiologic studies and many laboratory studies on animals have dealt with abortion and abnormalities among offspring. These will be reviewed and certain conclusions will be drawn.

EPIDEMIOLOGIC STUDIES

Pitfalls of Epidemiologic Studies

These studies are valuable tools, the use of which will continue to add to preventive medicine. They are fraught with problems, however (MacMahon and Pugh, 1970). I believe that the epidemiologic studies that have been published to date on a relationship between anesthetics and disease have had flaws, some of which are discussed below.

The choice of cohort or control group is of critical importance to the validity of the conclusions to be drawn. The first study of health hazards among operating room personnel (Vaisman, 1967) lacked a cohort. Drawing reliable conclusions, therefore, depends on guesswork. Another serious failing of epidemiologic studies is the use of improper cohorts. For example, I believe that the choice of pediatricians as cohorts for anesthesiologists (Cohen et al., 1974) is questionable because the two groups have considerably different published mortality rates (Goodman, 1975). Also, to use cohorts of different ages may lead to invalid conclusions (Askrog and Harvald, 1970).

58

Cohorts may have other equally important but unrecognized differences from the study group. For this reason, low values for p are essential. The value of $p < 0.05$, used in many epidemiologic studies as the statistically significant level, has been called too high (Walts, Forsythe, and Moore, 1975), and a suggestion has been made that even a level of 0.01 may be risky for such studies.

The use of personal questionnaires to obtain medical information raises doubts of the validity of the conclusions. For example, questions using terms such as "abortion" and "abnormality" can lead to a variety of answers. Medical records are preferred to questionnaires, although here, too, variability of accuracy among observers and institutions exists. All reported studies of health hazards in the operating room are of the unsupported questionnaire type.

Retrospective studies are inferior to prospective studies. The former depend upon memory or records written without knowledge that the findings would be reviewed. In prospective studies, specific information is requested in advance of compilation of the record, so that the records are more likely to be complete and appropriate tests done. None of the reported studies on operating room health hazards were prospective.

No published study was designed to test the hypothesis that a cause and effect relationship exists between exposure to trace concentrations of anesthetics and certain diseases. The at-risk groups studied have all been operating room personnel and the stress of the surgical environment is a possible cause of disease. Fink and Cullen (1976) discuss one small study that suggests that stress, not trace concentrations of anesthetics, causes increased abortion among some nurses. Recently, Pope and coworkers (1978) reported that animals that were thought to be stressed by experimental handling had a dramatically higher fetal loss. However difficult, the design of epidemiologic studies among operating room personnel must exclude causes of gestational defects other than exposure to anesthetics for meaningful conclusions to be drawn.

Epidemiologic data are unacceptable when authors point to an increased rate of disease for the study group compared to cohorts if the results are not statistically significant. That is precisely what statistics teaches us to avoid: the increased rate is *not meaningful* if not statistically significant.

Operating Room Studies

In 1967, Vaisman discussed the working conditions of Russian anesthesiologists. Using a questionnaire technique, 354 physicians specializing in anesthesia were queried; 303 responded, 110 of whom were female. Despite the fact that the questionnaire was not published, the responses suggest that the questions were general in nature. The following were the complaints, with percentage of affirmative responses: headaches, 78.5 per cent; increased irritability, 49.0

per cent; increased fatigability, 84.8 per cent; frequent upper respiratory inflammation, 60.4 per cent; angina, 20.6 per cent; and poor surgical unit layout, 75.0 per cent. Among 31 pregnant women, 18 miscarriages were reported; three had more than one miscarriage each. Vaisman concluded that many working conditions contributed to the complaints noted: chronic inhalation of anesthetic vapors, a high degree of stress, irregular work and rest schedules, excessive workload, and the prolonged strain of concentrated attention. The small size of the study and the lack of controls have been commented upon, but the paper is widely quoted in the literature because of its historic importance.

Askrog and Harvald (1970) are also frequently quoted, and, although the study used controls, the same subjects at a younger age were used as controls for their experiences when older. This is a recognized error in epidemiology. In fact, the data within the paper illustrate the error; the year-by-year trend in abortion rate grew during the three years of data collection. For this reason, this report is suspect.

Another frequently quoted study (Cohen, Bellville, and Brown, 1971) was based on data from 67 operating room nurses and 50 female anesthesiologists who had 10 and 14 miscarriages in their respective groups. There is no quarrel with what was reported, but it is of interest that of the 50 anesthesiologists polled, 20 reported one or more pregnancies and those 20 had 14 miscarriages. Two respondents accounted for eight miscarriages; in one woman, two occurred at age 39 and two at age 40. Excluding the two habitual aborters, the rate of miscarriage did not differ significantly from the rate in the control group. The other participants in the study reported normal live births similar in rate to that of the control group.*

Knill-Jones and her associates (1972) evaluated pregnancy and anesthetic practice in 563 married women anesthesiologists and in 828 women doctor controls. Three groups were compared: anesthesiologists at work and two sets of controls: nonworking anesthesiologists and other physicians. The data show that children of anesthesiologists working during pregnancy had a higher frequency of congenital abnormality than did those of nonworking anesthesiologists but *not* significantly different from those of other women physicians. Spontaneous abortion was significantly higher for the working anesthesiologists than for the other doctor group but *not* significantly different from nonworking anesthesiologists. The lack of coincidence of the two control groups and the reversal of effects between the control groups suggests to me that there is no relationship between anesthetics and abortion or miscarriage. Even the authors state, "No such association can be derived from our survey. . . ."

Later work by the same group (Knill-Jones, Newman, and Spence, 1975) failed to support the earlier report of increased congenital abnormalities following maternal exposure to the operating

---

*Data supplied by Dr. J. W. Bellville.

room environment. Knill-Jones and Spence, two of the original authors of the last two studies, are co-authors of another paper (Spence, Knill-Jones, and Newman, 1974) and write, "Although it was tempting to identify a triad of abortion, infertility and congenital abnormality which might all be ascribed to an abnormality of embryo development perhaps induced by anaesthetics, there was no direct evidence for such a suggestion and several pointers to the contrary." These points were as follows: mean maturity to abortion was the same for anesthetists and controls; there was no specific system involvement to explain the increase in congenital abnormality; and the women anesthetists who conceived after a period of involuntary infertility were almost all working in the operating room during early pregnancy.

The most comprehensive epidemiologic study was reported by Cohen and associates (1974). The salient points made about gestational problems are that some women on operating room teams are prone to spontaneous abortion and to the occurrence of congenital abnormalities in their children. Similarly, unexposed wives of male operating room personnel are also reported to have an increased risk of congenital abnormalities in their children.

This study has been criticized by Walts, Forsythe, and Moore (1975), generally by Fink and Cullen (1976), and in detail in a review (Ferstandig, 1978). Walts, Forsythe, and Moore objected to the method of data collection, the use of $p < 0.05$ as a level of statistical significance, and the logic used in deriving conclusions. Fink and Cullen, after considering all available data on operating room health hazards, including this study, state that ". . . the present evidence is wholly inclusive." The review article points out flaws in the data and conclusions. Since these publications are readily available, only some new comments seem appropriate.

The data in the national study are internally inconsistent. The $p < 0.05$ significance level indicates a lack of agreement in health hazards between anesthesiologists and nurse anesthetists; wherever one group is reportedly at risk, the other is not.

Probably the most significant finding in the survey was that neither anesthesiologists nor nurse anesthetists were found to have an increased risk of abortion when compared to unexposed members of their own respective societies.

The points in these last two paragraphs present a dilemma. We have two sets of data in the same survey that disagree:

1. Significant findings of gestational defects for female anesthesiologists (compared to female pediatricians) are *always* accompanied by nonsignificant findings for female nurse anesthetists (compared to female nurses) and vice versa, a fact pointed out by the authors.
2. Four of six findings for all female operating room personnel are nonsignificant when compared to unexposed members of their respective societies.

If we choose pediatricians and nurses as cohorts, we arrive at conflicting data for equally exposed groups. If we choose unexposed members of the study group professional societies as cohorts (seemingly a better choice), we derive more consistent data. Logic clearly dictates that, for greater consistency, unexposed members of one's own professional society be used as cohorts; although a sufficient number of such a cohort in the appropriate age group might be hard to find.

For a more meaningful understanding of the epidemiologic studies, the results of the national study, the two studies by Knill-Jones and her coworkers (1972 and 1975), and a study among dentists (Cohen et al., 1975) are assembled in Table 1. It shows at a level of $p < 0.05$, the significant findings as pluses and the nonsignificant as minuses. If all of the findings in the table were pluses or minuses, the conclusions would be obvious, but the results are mixed, and, therefore, I would like to do my own logical analysis. The table shows the following:

1. Significant findings for ASA members never correspond to the significant findings for AANA members in *any* comparison.
2. Nowhere in the table is there a group that has a significant increase in both abortions and congenital abnormalities.
3. There are three places where the least exposed group in the national study, AORN/T, has significant findings and the more exposed groups (AANA and ASA) do not.
4. There are three reports in which a significant finding changes to a nonsignificant one when another plausible cohort is used (ASA vs. AAP to ASA vs. unexposed ASA, and twice for female anesthesiologists vs. nonworking female anesthesiologists to female anesthesiologists vs. other female physicians.)
5. The data from dentists' wives disagree with those from anesthesiologists' wives.
6. The data from wives of British physician anesthetists differ from those of wives of American anesthesiologists with respect to major congenital anomalies.

Logical analysis provides two alternatives: we can accept the data as predicting a specific disease risk for given groups, e.g., female anesthesiologists experience more spontaneous abortions than do female nurse anesthetists, or we can reject all of the data because of illogical results among the different studies. I believe that logical analysis leaves only the second choice.

The most recent paper concerning occupational hazards in operating room personnel (Spence et al., 1977) is a compilation of three retrospective studies (Knill-Jones et al., 1972; Cohen et al., 1974; and Knill-Jones, Newman, and Spence, 1975), all of which have been cited. The authors believe that the surveys corroborate each other and that the combination of the three is stronger than each alone. In combining the papers, the authors have not considered the negative findings among nurse anesthetists (there aren't many in the United Kingdom) and the negative findings when the unexposed society members are cohorts. Furthermore, I doubt whether the combination of different age groups, practices, countries, and control groups

Table 1. Epidemiologic Surveys of Gestational Problems: Significant Findings (+), Nonsignificant Findings (−), and Level of Significance at 5 Per Cent

Study Group	Cohort	Spontaneous Abortion		Congenital Abnormality in Offspring	
		Exposed Females	Wives of Exposed Males	Exposed Mothers	Wives of Exposed Males
(Cohen et al., 1974)					
ASA*	AAP**	+	−	−	+
AANA†	ANA‡	−	−	+	−
AORN/T§	ANA	+	+	−	−
ASA	ASA Unexposed	−		−	
AANA	AANA Unexposed	−		+	
AORN/T	AORN/T Unexposed	+		−	
(Cohen et al., 1975)					
Exposed dentists	Unexposed dentists		+		−
(Knill-Jones et al., 1972)					
Female anesthesiologists	Other female physicians	+		−	
Female anesthesiologists	Nonworking female anesthesiologists	−		+	
(Knill-Jones et al., 1975)					
Male anesthesiologists	Other male physicians		−		−
Female anesthesiologists	Other female physicians	+		−	

*American Society of Anesthesiologists members
**American Academy of Pediatrics members
†American Association of Nurse Anesthetists members
‡American Nurses Association members
§Combined membership of Association of Operating Room Nurses and Association of Operating Room Technicians

is epidemiologically valid. The combinations do, however, produce lower p values because of the increased populations. The epidemiologic questions raised for each survey remain, however, and I believe new valid conclusions cannot be drawn from the combinations.

I believe that evidence from within the surveys and from external sources suggests that the choice of cohort is the major reason for illogical patterns and contradictions in data. In fact, these surveys present evidence of a lack of a health hazard from traces of anesthetics in operating room personnel.

LABORATORY GESTATION STUDIES

Reviewing animal studies on the relationship between anesthetics and gestational abnormalities is important for two reasons: (1) animals are reasonable substitutes for humans in experimental studies, and (2) the results of studies in animals have been referred to by authors of epidemiologic reports as evidence that trace concentrations of anesthetics in the operating room are responsible for health hazards. A concise review will be given here but details and references can be found elsewhere (Ferstandig, 1978).

Cellular Studies

Cell division and metabolism, important during gestation, may, by inference, predict gestational defects. A review of the effects of anesthetics on these functions follows.

The earliest observation that anesthetics affect growth appears to be in 1878, when a publication stated that it was well known among florists that high concentrations of ether inhibit plant growth and cell division. Since then, there have been many papers on the effects of anesthetics on the dividing cell. A review by Anderson (1966) after the thalidomide experience and a more recent one by Jackson (1975) describe in great detail the effects of anesthetics, sedatives, narcotics, and tranquilizers on cell division and growth. Most of these central nervous system depressants exhibit the same effect as colchicine, a potent agent that halts mitosis at metaphase.

At about 0.5 MAC halothane does not affect mouse heteroploid cell growth in five days and has small effect on mouse neuroblastoma cells; at 1 MAC, cell growth continues but at reduced rate. At levels well over 1 MAC, halothane reduces cell division in a ciliate protozoan, the root tip of the broad bean, hamster lung fibroblasts, rat hepatoma cells, and neuroblastoma cells. In fertilized sea urchin eggs, 2 per cent halothane causes the mitotic spindles (microtubules) to disappear within three minutes, and they reappear within three minutes of removal of the anesthetic. In the crayfish ventral nerve cord, clinical levels of halothane cause microtubules to disappear in one to three hours, and in neuroblastoma cells, 1.3 to 2.4 per cent halothane alters microtubules. The axopods of a heliozoon have microtubules that disappear at about 2 MAC of methoxyflurane, halothane, chloroform, divinyl ether, and cyclopropane. The tubules reappear within minutes of anesthetic removal. The phenomena reported required surgical levels of anesthetics and were reversible, but no long-term subanesthetic level studies have yet been reported.

Several studies have been designed to determine if anesthetic inhibition of cell division involved RNA and DNA. These studies showed that the extent of DNA synthesis and RNA synthesis, the time required for synthesis, and the DNA and RNA contents of certain cells were unaltered or only slightly changed even after prolonged clinical anesthetic doses. It is unlikely that the mechanism of anesthetic cell growth inhibition involves the fundamental building blocks — RNA and DNA.

There is an anesthetic dose–related reduction in respiration of rat liver mitochondria *in vitro,* shown by a reduction of oxygen uptake beginning just below 1 per cent halothane and continuing until a minimum of about 25 per cent of normal oxygen uptake is reached with halothane levels of 3 to 9 per cent. The respiratory depression is almost totally reversible below 3 per cent halothane. Halothane, methoxyflurane, enflurane, and ether all show this reversible depression below 2 to 2.5 MAC. The reversible depression of respiration of mitochondria coincides with the inhibition of cell growth, indicating that the effects are probably linked.

All anesthetics appear to interfere *in a reversible* manner with cell division in a variety of cells at middle to upper clinical levels. No report positively demonstrates a connection between this effect and neoplastic or teratogenic disease, however.

Animal Gestation Studies

The application of animal studies to human beings must be interpreted warily. Diet affects tumor susceptibility, stress affects reproductive abilities, hypoxia causes congenital malformations, and even 0.2 MAC anesthetic levels change sleeping behavior compared to controls. The use of large numbers of animals to achieve greater statistical significance does not eliminate these influences among the exposed groups, and because of the difficulty in controlling many variables, a certain skepticism is required before valid conclusions may be drawn.

The early testing of the teratogenic effects of anesthetics on animals was with chick embryos. Exposure to about 80 per cent nitrous oxide and 20 per cent oxygen failed to significantly increase teratogenicity or lethality compared to controls, but 90 per cent nitrous oxide and 10 per cent oxygen resulted in a greater lethal effect than 90 per cent nitrogen and 10 per cent oxygen did, but teratogenicity was not significantly elevated.

Concentrations of 13 to 30 per cent ether for six hours caused a large increase in chick embryo deaths and anomalies over controls.

Cyclopropane also showed toxic and teratogenic effects after six hours at 20 to 40 per cent.

In a multilevel study of chick embryos using several fluorinated anesthetics, neither lethal nor teratogenic effects were noted at about 0.5 to 1.5 MAC after six hours of exposure. Death rates increased above 2 per cent halothane (not significantly) and 0.5 per cent methoxyflurane (significantly), however.

All the anesthetics studied (ether, cyclopropane, nitrous oxide, halothane, methoxyflurane, and fluroxene) showed effects on chick embryos, but only at high clinical or above clinical concentrations. The similarity of results following administration of these anesthetics and the fact that they do not have metabolites in common suggest that death and teratogenicity could be due to general anesthesia rather than to a specific metabolite. One possible explanation is that hypoxia associated with deep anesthesia causes the observed response, for it is known that hypoxia alone has lethal and teratogenic effects in chick embryos and certainly can cause death and possibly teratogenicity in humans. Other explanations could be reduced cellular metabolism and cell division caused by deep anesthesia, as observed in tissue studies.

In 1967, Fink and his associates for the first time demonstrated the toxic effects of anesthetics on pregnant rats. Pregnant rats exposed to 45 to 50 per cent nitrous oxide for two, four, or six days starting on day 8 of gestation resulted in a significant incidence of fetal resorptions and abnormalities of fetal vertebrae and ribs. Similar results were obtained after one-day exposures to 70 per cent nitrous oxide, most evident with exposure on day 9. The authors noted that the skeletal defects were reminiscent of responses of fetuses of pregnant mice subjected to hypoxia.

Pregnant rats were exposed to 0.8 per cent halothane for 12 hours during one day or one night of pregnancy. After "blind" examination, the number of lumbar rib anomalies was found to be highly significant following exposure at day 8, 9.5, or 10 but not at day 8.5 or 9. Vertebral anomalies and resorptions were similarly scattered. Regardless of the lack of statistical significance in the results, the authors (Basford and Fink, 1968) noted that the abnormalities were strikingly similar, both in kind and frequency, to those following nitrous oxide.

Pregnant hamsters exposed to 60 per cent nitrous oxide plus 0.6 per cent halothane for three hours on day 9, 10, or 11 of gestation responded with an increase in fetal resorptions for day 11 only ($p<0.05$) (Bussard et al., 1974). The weight of the fetuses also declined compared to controls after exposure on days 10 and 11.

In an effort to determine if halothane induces reproductive abnormalities in rats or rabbits, Kennedy and coworkers (1976) subjected female rats to 1.4 per cent halothane for one hour per day on postinsemination days 1 to 5, 6 to 10, or 11 to 15, and rabbits were exposed to 2.1 to 2.3 per cent halothane for one hour per day for days 6 to 9, 10 to 14, or 15 to 18. Neither adverse reproductive nor teratologic effects were observed.

In a very careful study, Pope and associates (1978) exposed rats to 0.16 to 0.32 per cent halothane, 1 to 50 per cent nitrous oxide, 10 per cent nitrous oxide plus 0.16 per cent halothane, or 0.01 to 0.08 per cent methoxyflurane for eight hours per day throughout 21 days of gestation. The principal finding was a reduction in fetal weights for the higher subanesthetic concentrations. There was no increase in fetal loss or fetal abnormalities compared to controls. During this study, any animal exhibiting stressful behavior during the necessary handling was removed and labeled as a member of a "stress group." The animals in this group had the largest loss in fetal weight and a dramatic rise in fetal death (65 to 100 per cent) unrelated to their original exposure.

The most impressive animal study to date (Wharton et al., 1977) involved approximately 4000 mouse fetuses, almost equally divided between controls and experimental animals. Male and female mice were exposed daily to halothane for nine weeks prior to mating, and the mother's exposure was continued during pregnancy. Exposures up to 500 ppm. of halothane for two hours each day failed to lead to morphologic effects on fetuses. At 3000 ppm. (0.3 per cent) of halothane for four hours each day, some developmental variations occurred but no major abnormalities.

In summary, it appears that short exposure to even high concentrations of inhalation anesthetics either has no adverse gestational effects in animals or has statistically questionable effects. Prolonged exposure to levels of anesthetic greatly exceeding values reported for halothane in the operating room environment (about 10 ppm. in unscavenged operating rooms) did not lead to a morphologic effect. Therefore, contrary to assertions in epidemiologic reports, animal studies do not positively support a cause and effect relationship between anesthetics and health hazards associated with chronic operating room exposure and, in fact, suggest that we must exclude other factors (i.e., stress) before proving anesthetics an operating room environment health hazard.

Laboratory Studies on Fertility

There are few reports of the effects of anesthetics on fertility *per se*. Male and female mice exposed to 16 ppm. halothane for seven hours per day, five days per week for six weeks prior to mating showed no difference from controls in the number of pregnancies, implants, resorptions, or live fetuses (Bruce, 1973). A large study involving 168 female and 84 male mice showed that exposure to as high as 0.4 MAC halothane for four hours daily for 63 days prior to mating had no effect on the percentage of pregnancies, number of implants and live fetuses, fetal weight, or fetal length (Wharton et al., 1976). A study of rats exposed to 1.4 to 1.5 per cent halothane for one hour daily in days 1 to 5, 6 to 10, or 11 to 15 before mating showed no difference from controls in mating, fecundity, or fertility index (Kennedy et al., 1976).

Kripke and colleagues (1977) exposed male rats to 20 per cent nitrous oxide for either 8 or 24 hours daily for up to 35 days. Four to six rats from each group and from controls were sacrificed at 12 time periods during the 35 days. Dry testes weight data were given for only three groups without specifying whether daily exposure was 8 or 24 hours: I. (four rats) having 28 days of exposure; II. (five rats) having 32 days of exposure followed by three days in air before sacrifice; and III. (five rats) having 32 days of exposure followed by six days in air. Groups I and II had lowered dry testes weights than controls ($p<0.05$). I cannot determine how meaningful these data are. No other testes weights were given even though there were four groups with longer exposure than those used to determine the statistical significance. Detailed morphologic descriptions were reported but no statistical analysis was made of these findings.

Thus, there is no substantial evidence of damage to animal fertility and evidence of lack of damage due to traces of anesthetics or repeated exposure to concentrations of volatile anesthetics used clinically.

SUMMARY AND CONCLUSIONS

The epidemiologic studies on health hazards associated with working in the operating room are open to question because of flaws in design. Some entirely lack controls, most have inappropriate controls, and all, I believe, suffer from internal inconsistency. Several of the studies have contradictory findings. Although these studies predict increased risks for specific groups (e.g., spontaneous abortions in female anesthesiologists), they do not make such predictions for other equally exposed groups (e.g., spontaneous abortion in female nurse anesthetists). This inconsistency occurs so frequently that I believe the data in the surveys cannot be used to form valid conclusions. Evidence points to poor choice of cohorts as the major flaw.

Even if the epidemiologic data are accepted, none of the studies was designed to establish a cause and effect relationship between chronic exposure to trace concentrations of anesthetics and gestational changes. Some authors of epidemiologic reports claim that research on the effects of anesthetics on cells and animals supports this cause and effect relationship. Careful review of these reports proves to me that trace concentrations of anesthetics are *not* implicated in any disease alluded to in the epidemiologic studies.

When histotoxic effects are observed in gestational studies, clinical or near clinical levels were required and all anesthetics showed similar effects. However, since it is unrealistic to expect the widely different metabolites of all the anesthetics to have identical toxic effects, metabolites probably can be ruled out as the common cause. The most likely causes for the observed histotoxicities are the profound physiologic phenomena associated with anesthesia. Since trace concentrations have not been proved to produce these phenomena, the studies at clinical levels do not predict the effects at trace levels.

REFERENCES

Anderson, N. B.: The effect of CNS depressants on mitosis. Acta Anaesth. Scand., *10*:1, 1966.

Askrog, V., and Harvald, B.: Teratogenic effects of inhalation anesthetics. Nord. Med., *83*:498, 1970.

Basford, A. B., and Fink, B. R.: The teratogenicity of halothane in the rat. Anesthesiology, *29*:1167, 1968.

Bruce, D. L.: Murine fertility unaffected by traces of halothane. Anesthesiology, *38*:473, 1973.

Bussard, D. A., Stoelting, R. K., Peterson, C., and Ishaq, M.: Fetal changes in hamsters anesthetized with nitrous oxide and halothane. Anesthesiology, *41*:275, 1974.

Cohen, E. N., Bellville, J. W., and Brown, B. W., Jr.: Anesthesia, pregnancy, and miscarriage: A study of operating room nurses and anesthetists. Anesthesiology, *35*:343, 1971.

Cohen, E. N., Brown, B. W., Jr., Bruce, D. L., et al.: Occupational disease among operating room personnel: A national study. Anesthesiology, *41*:317, 1974.

Cohen, E. N., Brown, B. W., Jr., Bruce, D. L., et al.: A survey of anesthetic health hazards among dentists. J.A.D.A., *90*:1291, 1975.

Ferstandig, L. L.: Trace concentrations of anesthetic gases: A critical review of their disease potential. Anesth. Analg., *57*:328, 1978.

Fink, B. R., and Cullen, B. F.: Anesthetic pollution: What is happening to us? Anesthesiology, *45*:79, 1976.

Fink, B. R., Shepard, T. H., and Blandau, R. J.: Teratogenic activity of nitrous oxide. Nature, *214*:146, 1967.

Goodman, L. J.: The longevity and mortality of American physicians 1969–1973. Milbank Memorial Fund Quarterly, Summer 1975, p. 353.

Jackson, S. H.: Anesthetics and cell multiplication. Clin. Anesth., *11*:75, 1975.

Kennedy, G. L., Smith, S. H., Keplinger, M. L., and Calandra, J. C.: Reproductive and teratologic studies with halothane. Toxicol. Appl. Pharmacol., *35*:467, 1976.

Knill-Jones, R. P., Moir, D. D., Rodrigues, L. V., and Spence, A. A.: Anesthetic practice and pregnancy: Controlled survey of women anaesthetists in the United Kingdom. Lancet, *1*:1326, 1972.

Knill-Jones, R. P., Newman, B. J., and Spence, A. A.: Anaesthetic practice and pregnancy: Controlled survey of male anesthetists in the United Kingdom. Lancet, *2*:807, 1975.

Kripke, B. J., Kelman, A. D., Shah, N. K., et al.: Testicular reaction to prolonged exposure to nitrous oxide. Anesthesiology, *42*:104, 1976.

MacMahon, B., and Pugh, T. F.: Epidemiology Principles and Methods. Boston, Little, Brown and Company, 1970.

Pope, W. D. B., Halsey, M. J., Lansdown, A. B. G., et al.: Fetotoxicity in rats following chronic exposure to halothane, nitrous oxide, or methoxyflurane. Anesthesiology, *48*:11, 1978.

Spence, A. A., Knill-Jones, R. P., and Newman, B. J.: Studies of morbidity in anaesthetists with special reference to obstetric history. Proc. R. Soc. Med., *67*:989, 1974.

Spence, A. A., Cohen, E. N., Brown, B. W., Jr., et al.: Occupational hazards of operating room-based physicians. J.A.M.A., *238*:955, 1977.

Walts, L. F., Forsythe, A. B., and Moore, J. G.: Critique: Occupational disease among operating room personnel. Anesthesiology, *42*:608, 1975.

Wharton, R. S., Baden, J. M., Hitt, B. A., and Mazze, R. I.: Fertility and embryolethality in mice chronically exposed to halothane. Abstracts, ASA meeting, San Francisco, October 1976, p. 143.

Wharton, R. S., Wilson, A. I., Little, D., et al.: Fetal morphologic abnormalities in mice following chronic subanesthetic halothane exposure. Abstracts, ASA meeting, New Orleans, October 1977, p. 627.

Vaisman, A. L.: Working conditions in surgery and their effect on the health of anesthesiologists. Eksp. Khir. Anesteziol., *3*:44, 1967.

ANESTHETIC EFFECTS UPON REPRODUCTION

EDITORIAL COMMENT

A study of the two sides of this controversy should prove to be worthwhile to the discerning anesthetist, of interest to the epidemiologist, and invaluable to those who would become involved with research on some of the possible, but less well defined, effects of anesthetics that are difficult to assess.

If the result of my questioning is correct, most anesthetists, trained or in training, who have heard of or read about the possible effects of trace concentrations of anesthetic agents upon human reproduction are reasonably assured that a toxic effect has been demonstrated conclusively. If not, some have said, pointing to the scavenging systems in modern operating rooms, why all the effort and expense? Yet, perusal of Cohen's and Ferstandig's papers reveals that they both realize that incontrovertible evidence of trace concentrations of anesthetics causing reproductive effects does not exist. Cohen hedges in his title by writing "may cause" and Ferstandig by "are not proved." Cohen is sufficiently impressed with the published data to conclude, ". . .the available data suggest the likelihood of such an association and obligate us as responsible individuals to do everything possible to reduce the levels of waste anesthetic gases." In fairness to many of the authors of papers cited by Ferstandig, they have repeatedly pointed out the lack of definitive proof, but the possibility of the relationship warrants, in their opinion, the effort in scavenging operating rooms of anesthetic gases.

Ferstandig's paper could perhaps be used by a class in epidemiology. As well as any I have seen in the recent scientific literature, it points out pitfalls in epidemiologic research. I suppose an epidemiologist today does not have to turn to the scientific literature to demonstrate easy routes to false conclusions. Evidence appears daily in the newspapers and government pronouncements — the false and unwarranted conclusions most often being used for political gain. Unfortunately, in the newspaper, the reader rarely has the benefit of two sides of a controversy, or even the sources of the data upon which the conclusions are drawn.

Although perhaps beyond the scope of the two reports, it is interesting that neither author questions the source of operating room pollution and whether the whole problem could be abolished by eliminating the source. Some believe that changing from high flow systems of administering anesthetics to low flow or closed systems would do away with the problem, save as much as $100,000,000 annually, and prevent contamination of the atmosphere. There are those who view the latter as a major environmental health hazard. Anesthesiologists would do well to examine these beliefs carefully.

Part 4

STERILIZATION OF ANESTHETIC EQUIPMENT

THE PROPOSITION:

Inhalation anesthesia equipment should be either disposable or sterilized after each use.

ALTERNATIVE POINTS OF VIEW:

By Gale E. Dryden
By William K. Hamilton, Thomas W. Feeley

EDITORIAL COMMENT

by GALE E. DRYDEN
Indiana University School of Medicine

INHALATION ANESTHESIA EQUIPMENT SHOULD BE ASEPTIC FOR EACH USE

The members of all facets of the health care profession are obligated to provide drugs, equipment, and skills that deliver safe and effective patient care. In recent years, the profession and the federal government have initiated a review of the safety and effectiveness of current medical care. Many changes have resulted.

The principles of asepsis are fundamental in medical practice and should always be applied to the best of our ability. A single break in good aseptic practice may or may not result in morbidity or mortality, but this should not be used as an excuse to relax the application of accepted principles of good patient care. The application of these fundamentals should not be dictated by inconvenience, traditional work habits, or personal preferences. Judged by the rules for maintaining asepsis, some anesthesia practices and procedures fail to meet established standards; yet, there exists a controversy about the need to clean inhalation anesthesia equipment after each use. The bases for differences of opinion are usually philosphic attitudes, educational background, or data interpretation. Comments in each of these areas will be made in advocating the routine cleaning of all parts of inhalation anesthesia equipment.

PHILOSOPHIC ATTITUDE

A basic principle of medical practice is first to do no harm. To fulfill this goal, emphasis on preventive care must be maintained. For example, in order to appropriately manage the physiologic changes that occur during anesthesia, a minimun routine in monitoring is performed, even though direct benefits are not always measurable for

73

each patient. In like manner, the benefits of routine cleaning of anesthesia equipment cannot always be measured for each patient. To select the patient that might become infected from contaminated equipment would require complete knowledge of the flora in the equipment and each patient's susceptibility. These facts are not readily available. Therefore, routine preventive cleaning is ideal.

Tradition and familiarity often lead to the acceptance of a practice past due for re-evaluation. If patients and practitioners in the other medical fields were aware of the aseptic breaks common in anesthesia practice and equipment care, they would have reason to inquire why, since there are readily available and reasonable ways to sterilize or clean anesthesia systems. When applied, they measurably reduce the risk of cross-infection.

CONCEPTS OF DISEASE TRANSMISSION

The theory of disease transmission by germs, which include a broad spectrum of bacteria and viruses, is over 100 years old, but certain elements of the mechanics of transmission are still vague, a lack of knowledge recently demonstrated by the mysteries of Legionnaire's disease. The minimum infective amount and the incubation periods for infectious diseases varies, depending on the relationship between the organism (the seed) and the patient (the soil). For example, one million or more *Staphylococcus albus* microorganisms may be required to produce an abscess in unbroken skin. If there is a skin break, however, then a few organisms will produce an infection. Recent studes (Westood and Sattar, 1976) reveal that a single virus is sufficient for infection, and transmission of adenovirus infection in man can occur with one infective unit per 60,000 liters of air. Incubation times may vary from a few hours for some organisms to several weeks or months for tuberculosis and infectious hepatitis. The low infective doses, prolonged incubation periods, and lack of understanding of the mechanics of transmission often make it difficult to determine the source of infection.

The anesthesiologist manipulates and invades the respiratory tract and the vascular tree in nearly every phase of patient care. These systems are frequently the portals of entry and location for infection; therefore, attempts to prevent contamination during patient contact should be standard practice.

Infections of the upper respiratory tract are a common malady among our population, and more than 50 per cent originate from the viral spectrum. Since the common laboratory studies do not apply in viral identification, only minimal effort has been made to study viruses in anesthesia apparatus. Nevertheless, the virus hazards remain an important concern because of their wide distribution, the ease of their spread by extremely dilute infective units, and the difficulty of killing them. The insidiousness of their presence is marked by illnesses with unpredictable degress of morbidity and by dissemination by healthy asymptomatic carriers.

BODY DEFENSES

The normal defense mechanisms of the body are changed by a wide variety of influences, including the psychologic and physical stress and drugs associated with operation and anesthesia. The use of immunosuppressive drugs that lower the body's defenses is common in the management of many ailments. The increasing problems with opportunistic and antibiotic-resistant organisms, the changing role of pathogenic and nonpathogenic bacteria, the altered host organism, and symbiotic relationships further increase hazards of infection.

The effects of anesthetics on leukocytes, lymphocyte transformation, and phagocytosis have been studied, and alterations have been noted. The changes noted, however, were transient and not as profound as those associated with the combination of anesthesia and operation (Duncan and Cullen, 1976).

An increase in the incidence of influenzal pneumonia in mice following ether anesthesia has been shown, but clinical concentrations of currently used anesthetic agents offer no recognized bacteriostatic effects. The high incidence of pulmonary infections after general and local anesthesia is not fully understood but is thought to be partially due to reduced mucocilary function and bacterial clearance. Even in some healthy patients, the immunosuppresive effects and altered host resistance due to anesthesia and operation may be sufficient to allow infections to develop with challenges that would ordinarily be contained (McLean and Meakins, 1975.)

The presence of pre-existing pulmonary disease increases the risk for postoperative pulmonary complications. The normal defenses of the respiratory tract include the mucus membrane, which warms, moistens, and filters the air as it passes into the lungs. Tracheal intubation by-passes these protective areas, and nasotracheal intubation adds a 16 per cent risk of bacteremia. Shortly after birth, the upper respiratory tract becomes colonized with a changing variety of organisms that live in harmony, most of the time, with their host. If these organisms are introduced into other areas of the body or are transferred to other individuals, they may multiply and cause an infectious disease. During good health, the airway below the glottis is normally sterile. While the patient is awake, the glottis closes by reflex to prevent foreign bodies from entering the lung, a protection lost during anesthesia. The trachea and bronchi down to the respiratory bronchioles are lined by mucosa with ciliated epithelium that acts to trap and sweep upward out of the lung small particles that have passed the glottis. The cough reflex supports airway cleansing. These protective functions are reduced by the use of dry gases, topical anesthetic agents, anticholingerics, narcotics, and other depressants. The normal respiratory unit is dry and doesn't provide a place for bacteria to settle but when atelectasis, pulmonary vascular overload, or other conditions cause the alveolus to become moist or closed, bacteria may settle and find conditions favorable to their colonization.

ANESTHESIA EQUIPMENT CONTAMINATION AND PRACTICES

The results of many studes (Shiotoni et al., 1971; Tinne, Gordon, and Bair, 1967; Joseph, 1952; Dryden, 1969; Atik and Hanson, 1970; Lockwood and Tyler, 1971; Olds et al., 1972; Roberts, 1972; Walters, 1974) indicate that equipment used for general anesthesia and respiratory therapy is often grossly contaminated by organisms including cocci, bacilli, yeasts, molds, fungi, and viruses.

The fear of abscess and meningitis from contaminated equipment promotes the use of sterile spinal needles, epidural catheters, and syringes. These items are used by washed and gloved operators in a scrubbed and draped field.

The same high standard of aseptic care expected for regional anesthesia should, but frequently does not, continue when placing and manipulating needles and fluid lines in blood vessels. The skin is not always well-prepared, drapes are not used, and the operator often works without either washed or gloved hands.

There is even less concern about the management of equipment used for inhalation anesthesia. One hundred fifty-seven directors responded to a survey of all anesthesia residency programs in the United States. Eighty-two of these had bacteriologically investigated their inhalation anesthesia apparatus. Fifty-six found positive cultures, but only 44 made some, albeit incomplete, attempts at cleaning equipment between uses. A four year follow-up survey of those who first responded indicated an increased awareness and effort toward cleaning inhalation systems, but the absorber and ventilator remained unattended (Dryden, 1973). This relaxed attitude may be based on the fact that the air we breath and the upper airway itself are not sterile; therefore, there is no need to provide clean anesthesia apparatus, even though it is known that respiratory infections occur from air and contaminated equipment. Others mistakenly believe that soda lime will trap and kill bacteria in gases passing through the absorber.

SODA LIME NOT EFFECTIVE AS A FILTER OR BACTERICIDAL AGENT

Fresh soda lime is a U.S.P. product with a specific chemical and physical composition. The manufacturers do not claim that it is sterile or a germicidal product. Attempts to sterilize soda lime with ethylene oxide change the chemical composition and reduce the carbon dioxide uptake capacity. Steam sterilization may cause the granules to fragment and cause caking, which increases air flow resistance.

Carbon dioxide absorbent materials at one time were thought to act as bactericidal agents that prevent contamination of the absorber system. This concept has been repeatedly disputed and is refuted by the ineffective kill of *Mycobacterium tuberculosis* by Baralyme and soda lime (Dryden, 1969). Studies conducted by the Center for Disease Control isolated *Pseudomonas aeruginosa* many times from circle absorbers including soda lime granules.

Soda lime does kill certain organisms and acts as a mechnical trap that catches some organisms as they flow past the soda lime. These actions are inadequate for preventing organisms from moving with the air stream through intragranular spaces. Many parts of the absorber are not in contact with the soda lime; therefore, they are not subject to any of its chemical influences. Movement of bacteria through soda lime was demonstrated by challenging a firmly packed 450 gm. Waters to-and-fro absorber with a single 1000 ml. surge of air that had been seeded with *Serratia marcescens*. Culture of the cellulose filter on the opposite end of the absorber was positive.

THE ABSORBER AND VENTILATOR

Two major pieces of anesthesia equipment — the carbon dioxide absorber and the ventilator — are particularly difficult to clean in a routine manner. These pieces also form the center of most discussions about the proper cleaning of anesthesia equipment.

Most currently used carbon dioxide absorbers were designed and manufactured in such a way that they are heavy, difficult to remove, and made of materials that excluded heat sterilization. Cold sterilization requires 10 hours of contact exposure to 2 per cent alkaline glutaraldehyde to produce sterility. The many cavities in an absorber make it difficult to be certain that there are no air pockets preventing contact with the sterilizing solution. The initial cost and bulk of the large capacity, permanently mounted metal absorber prohibit economic ethylene oxide sterilization. As a consequence, the usual care of a permanently mounted carbon dioxide absorber is limited to changing the soda lime as it exhausts and periodically draining the accumulated condensation from the bottom of the absorber housing.

If an absorber has not been drained for a long time, a foul-smelling, scum-covered condensation is found in the bottom. Besides being unaesthetic and a bacterial reservoir, the use of such unclean equipment has been named as the cause of postoperative nausea.

The degree of contamination of equipment by the patient lessens by distance from the patient; however, all parts exposed to gases exchanged by the patient become contaminated to some degree. Shinotani and coworkers (1971) reported that healthy patients contaminate the absorber at an average rate of 35 organisms per minute. The kind and number of organisms that remain and act as a reservoir of risk to the next patient depend upon many variables, such as time, temperature, humidity, material available to act as media, and the type of organisms present. If left unused, further seeding from the air can occur and in time proliferate into a multiple organism reservoir (Fig. 1). It is evident that contamination is a problem with all inhalation equipment. Techniques for resolving these patient risks need to be developed and practiced.

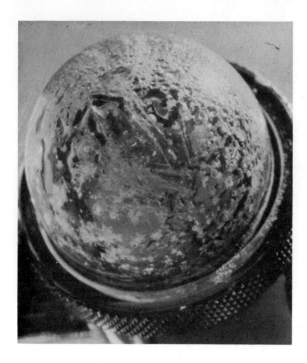

Figure 1. An in-use circle absorber valve cover, with an overgrowth of organisms. Culture revealed gram negative bacilli, yeast and mold.

CARE OF ABSORBERS

There is no way to simply and totally clean many of the large-capacity, permanently mounted, machined metal, carbon dioxide absorbers. If they cannot be revised to permit easy removal and complete cleansing, it would seem best to discontinue them as outdated equipment and select circle absorbers that will provide the needed patient protection through single-use units or those that permit easy disassembly and sterilization, such as that provided by Anesthesia Associates. The to-and-fro method of carbon dioxide absorption has functional limitations, but it offers an economic, easy to clean carbon dioxide absorption system.

CARE OF ANESTHESIA VENTILATORS

Anesthesia ventilators are a mechnical substitute for breathing bags. The ventilator bellows and parts exposed to respired gases become contaminated in a manner similar to that for breathing bags. Unfortunately, because of mechanical shielding, the ventilator bellows may be ignored for long periods, permiting accumulation of condensate, which acts as a nutrient for pathogenic organisms. In an exaggerated case of neglect, this author has seen a ventilator fail to function because of the excess volume and weight of condensate in the bellows.

Respiratory ventilators with humidifiers have been demonstrated to cause pneumonia owing to colonization of the humidifiers (Lockwood and Tyler, 1971; Reinarz, Pierce, and Benita, 1965). The condensate in the anesthesia circuit, absorber, and ventilator offers a similar situation for the development of a bacterial reservoir.

Proper management of anesthesia ventilators begins with selecting one that permits isolation of the patient circuit from the driving mechanism. The bellows and all other patient-exposed parts should be easy to remove and able to withstand steam sterilization. Several current models meet these requirements. Experience has shown that longevity of the Monahgan and Ohio bellows is one year when steam-sterilized after each use.

THE ANESTHESIA CIRCUIT

The anesthesia hoses, mask, and breathing bag become contaminated by the patient during use. If left uncleaned, the accumulated moisture allows organisms to survive, multiply and act as a reservoir for transmission to subsequent users. Living viruses have been identified on anesthesia masks three hours after use. Walter (1974) reported the transmission of cowpox from anesthesia masks.

The currently available rubber anesthesia breathing tubes, breathing bags, and masks lend themselves to recycling through pasteurization, steam, ethylene oxide, or glutaraldehyde soak. The light weight plastic versions will not withstand steam sterilization but will cycle through low-temperature sterilizing programs. In each case, however, they must first be thoroughly washed free of mucus that can shield organisms from the sterilizing agent.

NONREBREATHING SYSTEMS

The various modifications of nonrebreathing systems for anesthesia are smaller and simpler than circle absorber systems. These characteristics permit easier handling and simpler cleaning for recyling. Some nonrebreathing devices are available as single-use products modestly priced.

ANCILLARY EQUIPMENT

Endotracheal tubes should be sterile, since they enter a sterile area of the body. Although contamination from flora of a patient's upper airway may occur, the patient may have developed antibodies for these organisms. Trauma by the tube and the reduced defenses of the respiratory tract may allow even such organisms an opportunity to colonize and infect their host.

Cleaning of endotracheal tubes for reuse is difficult to assure both bacteriologic and chemical safety. As a consequence, there has been an increasing acceptance of endotracheal tubes as single-use items.

During use, stylets, laryngoscopes, and airways become grossly contaminated. Therefore, they must be thoroughly washed and prepared to prevent contamination of the next patient. These items are available as single-use products or in materials that will permit sterilization by steam or ethylene oxide.

Suction catheters are often necessary to remove secretions from the airway. It requires skill to guide the tip of the catheter into a tube without touching other areas that can contaminate the catheter and transform it into an inoculator of the lower airway. A sleeved catheter or gloves should be used to prevent finger contamination of the catheter as it is advanced into the endotracheal tube. Cleaning suction catheters for reuse is not recommended because of the difficulty associated with long narrow lumina.

THE ROLE OF BACTERIAL FILTERS

All bacterial filters for patient care have limitations, so their purposes need to be defined in order to make the best selection. Filters are designed to reduce the number of large organisms that can pass through; a lower challenge number results in fewer organisms passing the filter. Since filters are incapable of providing 100 per cent performance for the total spectrum of infective organisms, their use should be advocated when added protection is needed. For example, high-pressure filters in oxygen lines and low resistance filters in intake ports of respiratory therapy ventilators help reduce the environmental air contamination; however, ventilators still become contaminated owing to filter failure and retrograde bacterial movement (Roberts, 1972).

INCIDENCE AND DOCUMENTED INFECTIONS FROM ANESTHESIA EQUIPMENT

There are several reasons why the true incidence of bacterial contamination and of infections transmitted via anesthesia equipment cannot be documented. Many patients successfully meet the bacterial challenge with their own defense mechanisms. At other times, antibiotics are given postoperatively for symptoms unrelated to the anesthesia technique; these antibiotics simultaneously subdue potential pulmonary infection. Even if there are signs of respiratory infection, it often is treated and responds quickly, and the surgeon may fail to record the complication for coding that will permit identity for simple mechanical data retrieval.

Albrecht and Dryden (1974) investigated postoperative respiratory complications following general anesthesia before and after initiating a program providing each patient with a totally clean inhalation anesthesia system. Emphasis was placed on keeping contamination to a minimun during use. For example, if the endotracheal tube contacted a contaminated area outside the patient's mouth before insertion, it was discarded. The incidence of pulmonary complications dropped from 26 per cent to 3 per cent with these procedural changes.

There are hundreds of documented infections from anesthesia apparatus. There are undoubtedly many cases of unpublished infections and deaths for each of the published examples. Several authors have reported fatalities from contaminated anesthesia apparatus. They include: Six cases of gram-negative pneumonitis with four deaths, the organisms traced to operating room anesthesia devices by phage types (Atik and Hanson, 1970); seven cases, with three deaths, of *Pseudomonas aeruginosa* pneumonitis, with the causative organism isolated from anesthesia equipment (Tinne, Gordon, and Bain, 1967); an outbreak of respiratory infections with one death due to *P. aeruginosa* in a group of patients exposed to a contaminated anesthesia machine while undergoing cardiac surgery (Olds et al., 1972). These outbreaks stopped when the anesthesia apparatus was cleaned properly.

COSTS

The degree of effort exerted must be assessed in relationship to the benefits derived. The cost of providing clean medical devices is small when compared with the cost of antibiotics and increased hospital stays. I am aware of the death of a healthy 21-year-old from fulminating gram-negative pneumonitis that became evident the first postoperative day. Death occurred on the 15th postoperative day. The interval hospital, medical, surgical, and respiratory care costs exceeded $20,000.

The cost of cleaning the patient's inhalation system need not be excessive and may be kept low by recycling or by utilizing single-use equipment. Disposable equipment is practical when it provides cost savings and is more efficient and safer than recycling a similar product. The cost of single-use hoses, bag, and circle absorber for an inhalation anesthetic, including mask and endotracheal tube, is less than the charges for typing and crossmatching one unit of blood.

A cost analysis covering two years and 10,000 anesthetic procedures utilizing recycled polyethylene circuits and low-cost conductive rubber breathing bags sterilized with ethylene oxide indicated a maximal saving of 15 cents per unit when compared to using the same components only once. The inconvenience of detecting defects due to aging and recent reduction in the price of disposable circuits has made the single-use program the most desirable in our institution.

The national nosocomial infection rate is estimated to be 7 per cent with an average increased hospitalization of seven days. The extra cost exceeds $1,000 per patient. Although many postoperative nosocomial infections are not respiratory, the knowledge that patients do contaminate anesthesia circuits during use and the documentation of infections originating from anesthesia equipment are sufficient evidence for anesthetists to initiate routine precautions that will remove this potential source of harm.

The use of sterilized needles and syringes to prevent transmission of infectious hepatitis is an example of an accepted routine practice of preventive medicine based upon a low but positive incidence of transmission.

SUGGESTED GUIDELINES FOR ASEPTIC PRACTICE IN ANESTHESIA

There are no generally accepted guidelines that describe and direct the use and care of general anesthesia equipment so that it minimizes risk of equipment to patient contamination.

In 1977, the American Operating Room Nurses Association published a list of recommendations for the care of anesthesia apparatus, including the following: The entire inhalation anesthesia system must be terminally decontaminated, cleaned, and/or sterilized after each use; the exterior surfaces of equipment that do not come into direct contact with the respiratory circuit must also be routinely decontaminated; the equipment used in recovery rooms should be treated the same as operating room anesthesia equipment; frequent hand washing should be performed to reduce the bacterial count on the hands; all cleaning and sterilizing procedures should be done by trained, conscientious workers.

These standards are similar to those applied in other areas of medical care. Anesthesiologists should accept similar standards in principle and encourage their application as a part of the operating room clean-up regime. This would be a step forward in delivering better care for anesthetized patients.

REFERENCES

Albrecht, W.H., and Dryden, G.E.: Five year experience with the development of an individually clean anesthesia system. Anesth. Analg., 53:24–28, 1974.

Atik, M., and Hanson, B.: Gram-negative pneumonitis: a new postoperative menace. Am. Surg., 36:198–204, 1970.

Dryden, G.E.: Risk of contamination from the anesthesia circle absorber: an evaluation. Anesth. Analg., 48:939–943, 1969.

Dryden, G.E.: Anesthesia equipment sterility: repeat of a questionnaire. Anesth. Analg., 52:167–169, 1973.

Duncan, P.G., and Cullen, B.E.: Anesthesia and immunology. Anesthesiology, 45:522–536, 1976.

Joseph, J.M.: Disease transmission by inefficiently sanitized anesthetizing apparatus. J.A.M.A., 149:1196–1198, 1952.

Lockwood, W.R., and Tyler, M.: Inhalation therapy equipment as a reservoir of infectious agents. South. Med. J., 64:860–862, 1971.

MacLean, L.D., Meakins, J.L., Taguchi, K., et al.: Host resistance in sepsis and trauma. Ann. Surg., 182:207–216, 1975.

Olds, J.W., Kisch, A.L., Eberle, B.J.,

et al.: Pseudomonas aeruginosa respiratory tract infection acquired from a contaminated anesthesia machine. Ann. Rev. Resp. Dis., 105:628–632, 1972.

Reinarz, J.A., Pierce, A.K., and Benita, B.M.: The potential role of the inhalation therapy equipment in nosocomial pulmonary infection. J. Clin. Invest., 44:831–839, 1965.

Roberts, B.R.: Infections and sterilization problems. In International Anesthesiology Clinics. Vol. 10, No. 2. Boston, Little, Brown and Co., 1972.

Shiotani, G.M., Nichols, P., Ballinger, C.M., et al.: Prevention of contamination of the circle system and ventilators with a new disposable filter. Anesth. Analg., 50:844–855, 1971.

Tinne, J.E., Gordon, A.M., and Bain, W.H.: Cross infection by Pseudomonas aeruginosa as a hazard of intensive surgery. Br. Med. J., 4:313–315, 1967.

Walter, C.W.: Cross-infection and the anesthesiologist. Twelfth annual Baxter-Travenol Lecture. Anesth. Analg., 53:631–644, 1974.

Westwood, J.C.N., and Sattar, S.A.: The minimal infective dose. In Berg, G., Bodily, H., Lennette, E., Meinick, J., and Metcalf, T. (eds.): Viruses In Water. Washington, D.C., American Public Health Association, Inc., 1976.

by WILLIAM K. HAMILTON

THOMAS W. FEELEY
University of California, San Francisco

A NEED FOR ASEPTIC INHALATION ANESTHESIA EQUIPMENT FOR EACH CASE IS UNPROVEN

Infections following anesthesia and operation, be they in the wound, the urinary tract, the respiratory tract, or elsewhere, are a primary concern for all involved with surgical care. Prevention of infection is the object of much of the pre- and intraoperative care given by nurses, surgeons, and anesthetists. High cost in both morbidity and dollars justifies the surgeon's fear of infection and has resulted in a widely accepted code of aseptic practice. The anesthesia fraternity has not followed such a rigid discipline. We have been less careful than our surgical colleagues, and our behavior is often the cause of anguish and despair among nurses, surgeons, and more meticulous anesthesiologists.

Throughout the world of medicine, much is professed and practiced with little scientific foundation. Such practices are often the result of tradition or exist because of a paucity of scientific evidence for a more exact practice. Perhaps nowhere is this more evident than in the prevention of postoperative infection. This problem is replete with various whims and pet projects of the protagonists of an assortment of preventive procedures, many of which exist without the slightest evidence of clinical efficacy and with only fragmentary scientific basis. One need only recall the variety of "skin prep solutions" used over the years. There have been many mercurials and an infinite number of iodides, all praised as "the only way to go." The color of the surgical abdomen seems to have varied almost as much as fashions in dress. We also observe a variety of prophylactic practices in antibiotics, airflow generators, suture material, and surgical technique,

84

again argued without evidence that clinical benefit results. Often, these unproved practices are supported by what is attractively labeled as "common sense."

One cannot deny the value of and necessity for intuitive reasoning and "common sense" in practice. We are not likely to have solutions to all of our problems; in fact, the art of medicine probably will contribute as much or more to clinical practice as pure science will for many years to come. A danger exists, however, when the ideas basic to "common sense" are incomplete or misapplied. The danger is worsened when the *theory* is so attractive as to command emotional support strong enough to discourage meaningful evaluation of *results*. Establishment and acceptance of such theories may seriously delay progress. Claude Bernard is quoted as saying, "It is the things we do know that are the great hindrance to our learning the things that we do not." We must continue to consider alternative solutions to problems and admit controversy rather than rigidly defend even what appears to be the most attractive logic.

The controversy discussed here is the use of sterile inhalation anesthesia circuits for each anesthetic to prevent postanesthetic respiratory infections. Anesthesia circuits have been suspect as a source of transmission of infection from one patient to another since their introduction into anesthesia practice (Adriani and Rovenstine, 1941; duMoulin and Hedley-Whyte, 1977). It is understandable that breathing from someone else's equipment appears undesirable and dangerous. It is aesthetically attractive to use sterile or new inhalation equipment at each setting. An argument against such a procedure is hard to sell. One company that markets single-use equipment has recently circularized a toy balloon to emphasize the undesirability of breathing from a container previously used by another.

A review of the literature, however, establishes that a real doubt exists concerning need for sterile anesthetic circuits for each inhalation anesthetic (duMoulin and Hedley-Whyte, 1977; duMoulin and Saubermann, 1977; Stark, Green, and Pask, 1962; Pandit, Melita, and Agarwall, 1967). We find no substantial evidence, clinical or experimental, that anesthesia circuits are a source of postoperative infection and conclude that anesthesia equipment is not as culpable as it seems on first glance.

Despite the lack of evidence, pressure is increasing, largely on the part of purveyors of equipment and hospital committees behaving in traditional committee sytle. We are all besieged by sales representatives armed with

1. Quotations and incomplete excerpts from inconclusive and often unsound articles.

2. Threats of the medicolegal consequence of not using disposable products.

3. Assurance that expense is no problem because third party payers will cover the cost of disposable equipment — and in fact allow a reasonable profit.

4. Unproved claims of dollar savings that will result from decrease in cleaning time and personnel.

Until recently, little formal consideration was given to this problem. As of 1968, less than half of all anesthetics administered in hospitals having anesthesia training programs were given through sterile rubber goods. (Sterility was achieved either by use of ethylene oxide or buffered gluteraldehyde or by autoclaving.) Most anesthetics were administered through tubing and masks that were washed with soap and water between cases. Outbreaks of infection related to this practice were not substantial.

This controversy could be categorized as being of academic interest only and would perhaps be amusing were it not for the enormous cost generated by the use of disposable equipment or complex sterilizing procedures. As an additional problem, practices without scientific evidence often lead to restrictive standards imposed by those unwilling to examine the question thoroughly. The potential for such standards is exemplified in the June 1977 issue of AORN, the Journal of the Association of Operating Room Nurses, in which standards requiring sterilization of the entire anesthetic system were proposed, without evidence of either an existing problem or the efficacy of the suggested procedure (Standards, 1977). In addition to the cost and the unsatisfactory practice regulations that might ensue, one is faced with the significant problems of storage and disposal of an extravagant dissipation of our petroleum by-products.

Many hospitals and anesthesia departments have yielded to persuasion, and thus the costs of medical care are given another boost. A precise projection of costs resulting from general use of completely disposable inhalation anesthesia circuits cannot be made. In our 500-bed hospital, we estimate a cost increase of tens of thousands of dollars — exclusive of the cost of storage and disposal. Projected nationally, we believe the cost could exceed 10 million dollars annually. It is not surprising that industry finds this an attractive activity. Despite the manufacturers' claims, there is serious doubt that adopting disposable inhalation anesthesia equipment has actually reduced the number of cleaning personnel employed.

There are many reports that espouse the cause of sterilized and single-use equpment for inhalation anesthesia. Although it is possible to list these with comments as to why each is not appropriate or convincing, it is shorter to discuss them generally. These articles may be categorized as falling into one or more of the following categories:

First, there are reports that have discussed and sometimes even measured bacterial contamination of anesthesia circuitry (Joseph, 1962; Snow, Mangiaracine, and Anderson, 1962). Although no one doubts the accuracy of the measurements, this is certainly not the end point in which we are interested. We are concerned with the *clinical infection of patients*. Contamination of equipment is important only in so far as it can be shown to *cause* patient infection.

Second, there are anecdotal, or at least nonepidemic, incidents and case reports of transmitted infection (Atik and Hanson, 1970; Olds, Kisch, and Eberle, 1972; Tinne et al., 1967). These are not supported by bacteriologic data that satisfy cause and effect criteria. Most often, equipment cultures have been taken *after* infections occurred, and the anesthesia circuits used have not been "found guilty."

Third, there is one clinical series that reports an astounding reduction in the incidence of postoperative respiratory infection subsequent to the adoption of sterile anesthesia equipment (Albrecht and Dryden, 1974). The experimental design of this study appears to us to be grossly inadequate. The control series had an inordinately high incidence of postoperative respiratory infection that is not approached in most hospitals using unsterile equipment. The experimental group was tested at a different time period than the control group — in some instances separated by years. There is little discussion of what else may have changed during the time period involved, but a "vigorous campaign was instituted." The criteria for diagnosis of respiratory tract infection are incompletely described. One of the authors of this report is our adversary in this controversy and has been involved in manufacture and marketing disposable inhalation anesthesia equipment.

Fourth, there are a number of editorials and individual statements (such as this) that represent personal or group opinions without data (Editorial, 1952, 1964; Dryden, 1975).

Fifth, some reports render a guilt by association verdict in noting that since inhalation therapy and intensive care unit equipment have been found to transmit infection, anesthesia equipment must be equally at fault (Tinne et al, 1967). We cannot be certain of differences between these somewhat similar situations, but longer exposure time and prevalence of humidifiers with reservoirs in inhalation therapy and intensive care equipment may be partial explanations.

What about evidence that standard reusable equipment is safe? There are two recent publications (duMoulin, 1977) that call attention to the unlikeliness of anesthesia circuits as sources of nosocomial infections. One of these references quotes the proceedings of an international conference on nosocomial infections . . . "the paucity of positive evidence implicating anesthesia equipment as a source of infection is truly remarkable in view of the nonstandardized methods currently employed and the almost total neglect of routine decontamination in the past" (Hebert, 1970). DuMoulin states that the environment within the circle system is probably not conducive to bacterial survival because of a flow of cool dry gas, the bacteriostatic properties of rubber and metal, and the strongly alkaline condensate in the absorber chamber (duMoulin and Saubermann, 1977).

A review of the literature, then, seems to reveal that there are indeed postoperative infections, that they vary in incidence from 1 to over 20 per cent, and that there is no acceptable evidence of endemic or epidemic infections resulting from contaminated anesthesia circuits.

We have then a controversy consisting of a highly attractive but untested theory, seemingly based on common sense opposed by observations that application of the theory is expensive and the lack of evidence that the supposed problem exists. There can be little objection to instituting change — even if expensive — if the change can be shown to be effective. There is no justification to instituting change — even if reasonably priced — to attack a nonexistent problem. This controversy is solvable. The incidence of postoperative infection can be accurately determined. It should be possible to measure the effectiveness of prophylactic procedures.

To establish the effectiveness of apparatus designed to reduce bacterial respiratory tract infections, an investigation must demonstrate a significant related reduction in *clinical infection* in an actual patient population. This study would of course require that patients be randomly selected, that other aspects of clinical care be the same in both groups, that bacterial cause and effect relationships do in fact exist, and that the diagnosis of respiratory infection is confirmed according to preset standards. This sounds complicated and perhaps pretentious but really is not that difficult and follows only simple rules of experimentation. Such a study has not been reported.

Protagonists of sterile disposable equipment often ask, "Wouldn't you personally rather be anesthetized using a sterile, preferably single-use, system?" The answer to such a question proves nothing except personal likes and dislikes. It is more illogical to note that we often pay dearly to share the plates and utensils of restaurants that use only soap and water cleansing — and these often come in direct contact with us.

This discussion must include some remarks about viral infections, although these have not been studied extensively related to anesthesia equipment. Postoperative viral infections of the respiratory tract seem not to be a serious problem. Respiratory viruses are fragile organisms and postoperative viral respiratory tract infections are rare. The situation concerning viral hepatitis, however, might be quite a different matter. The incidence of postoperative hepatitis is difficult to establish because of a long and variable incubation period. None of the "disposable circle" literature data shed light on this matter. We are informed by virologists, however, that this infection seems to relate to transmission from material that comes in *direct contact* with patients, such as needles, endotracheal tubes, and attendants' hands. We know of no information suggesting transmission of the hepatitis virus by inhalation *per se*.

These remarks must not be interpreted as support for or belief in carelessness in cleaning anesthesia equipment. Neither are we campaigning to revoke the theories of bacterial transmission of disease. We actually adhere to the belief that "cleanliness is next to godliness." This, however, does not force us to surrender our right and responsibility to be discretionary in our practice, to pursue solid clinical research, or to recognize and pursue unanswered questions.

Anesthetists must never neglect the problem of nosocomial infections. We must accept an active role in reducing these complications. We must base our practices on solid evidence whereever it can be obtained and not passively yield to unproved, yet attractive, theories that extract a high price from society and delude us into thinking we are accomplishing something. We must stand firm against those who pressure us with incomplete evidence and inaccurate information.

REFERENCES

Adriani, J., and Rovenstine, E.A.: Experimental studies on carbon dioxide absorbers for anesthesia. Anesthesiology, 2:1–19, 1941.

Albrecht, W.H., and Dryden, G.E.: Five-year experience with development of individually clean anesthesia system. Anesth. Analg. 53:24–28, 1974.

Atik, M., and Hanson, B.: Gram-negative pneumonitis: A new postoperative menace. Am. Surg., 36:198–204, 1970.

Dryden, G.: Uncleaned anesthesia equipment. J.A.M.A., 233:1297–1298, 1975.

duMoulin, G.C., and Hedley-Whyte, J.: A plea for moderation in anesthesia standards. A.O.R.N., 26:1025–1026, 1977.

duMoulin, G.C., and Saubermann, A.J.: The anesthesia machine and circle system are not likely to be sources of bacterial contamination. Anesthesiology, 47:353–358, 1977.

Editorial: Infected anaesthetic apparatus. Br. Med. J., 2:873, 1952.

Editorial: Cross infecting during anaesthesia. Br. J. Anaesth., 36:465, 1964.

Hebert, C.L.: Control of microbial contamination of anesthesia equipment. Proceedings of the International Conference on Nosocomial Infections (Atlanta: Center for Disease Control, 1970), 259–264.

Joseph, J.M.: Disease transmission by inefficiently sanitized anesthetizing apparatus. J.A.M.A., 149:1196–1198, 1952.

Olds, J.W., Kisch, A.L., and Eberle, B.J.: Pseudomonas aeruginosa respiratory tract infection acquired from a contaminated anesthesia machine. Ann. Rev. Resp. Dis., 105:628–632, 1972.

Pandit, S.K., Melita, S., and Agarwal, S.C.: Risk of cross infection from inhalation anaesthetic equipment. Br. J. Anaesth., 39:838–844, 1967.

Snow, J.C., Mangiaracine, A.B., and Anderson, M.L.: Sterilization of anesthesia equipment with ethylene oxide. N. Engl. J. Med. 266:443–445, 1962.

Standards for cleaning and processing anesthesia equipment. A.O.R.N., 25:1268–1272, 1977.

Stark, D.C.C., Green, C.A., and Pask, E.A.: Anaesthesia machines and cross-infection. Anaesthesia, 17:12–20, 1962.

Tinne, J.E., Gordon, A.M., Bain, W.H., and Mackey, W.A.: Cross infection by Pseudomonas aeruginosa as a hazard of intensive surgery. Br. Med. J., 4:313–315, 1967.

STERILIZATION OF ANESTHETIC EQUIPMENT

EDITORIAL COMMENT

The editor's first continuous and intimate involvement with anesthesia was in early 1944 when, as a young physician who had to forgo a surgical residency and enter the Army to be ultimately transferred to an evacuation hospital, he bargained successfully with an ophthalmologist assigned to anesthesia and traded ward medicine for anesthesia (directed by a gynecologist with three months training in anesthesia). The anesthesia machines were portable field Heidbrink models with crudely metered oxygen and nitrous oxide and a glass container with a wick to vaporise (if warm enough) ether. Now, looking back at anesthesia machines and their attachments over a 35-year span, I am fascinated by some changes in some parts but equally impressed by a lack of appreciable change in other parts. Flow meters, reducing valves, and fail safe systems are of a different era; multiple sophisticated vaporizers make the ether jar covered with frozen condensate seem like a bad dream; built-in monitors for circulation and respiration are a pleasure; but the basic design and constituents of the breathing system are unchanged. True, canisters have gone from little to big and back to medium-sized; directional valves have fluttered, flapped, and tilted; and the smell is gone because exhaust valves connect to scavenger systems; but the masks, corrugated tubing, and bags are the same, although antistatic, and what is more, are not cleaned or prepared for the next case much differently on the average. That is what this controversy is all about, with a champion for radical change tilting with a "prove it to me" pair.

The very fact that so much change has occurred in most aspects of machines but not in another has great significance. Changes have occurred in those components that demanded attention and for which data existed to prove the need. One can only conclude that anesthetists as a group have not voiced sufficient concern about breathing systems or do not have data to back up a request for a wholesale change of existing practices. Nor have other practitioners of medicine, because if they thought anesthesia equipment was a real source of morbidity and mortality, we would have heard about it. Remember the complaints by internists and surgeons about halothane?

Dryden is persuaded by so-called "common sense" arguments and sporadic reports. If we are so careful in the intensive care unit, why not in the operating room? Hamilton and Feeley don't see it that way, want some definitive data before changing, and don't see why we can't get the data. They are concerned about costs and hidden problems (disposal of plastic systems). I can't help but react at Dryden's statement of "less than the charge of typing and crossmatching one unit of blood." Actual? Billed? or Collectible? Any way you look at it, it's not cheap. There has to be proof to go this way, for if there is proof, then the answer is clear. Dryden already thinks proof is there.

I am interested in an area related to spread of infection that neither side discusses. The aseptic habits of anesthetists. How many anesthetists wash their hands before and after each case? Would you go to a dentist a second time who didn't wash the hands before working in your mouth? How often do you see used laryngoscopes, tubes, airways, stylets, and catheters placed on top of machines or the anesthetist's table without subsequently cleaning top or table, followed by surgical-clean equipment being placed thereon. Now there is a real source of cross-infection! Let's get reliable data so we can settle the controversy, but in the meanwhile, let's take care of the obvious and "clean up" our own act.

Part 5

DELIBERATE HYPOTENSION

THE PROPOSITION:

Deliberate hypotension is a safe and accepted anesthetic technique.

ALTERNATIVE POINTS OF VIEW:

by M. Ramez Salem
by James E. Eckenhoff, Michael Lesch

EDITORIAL COMMENT

by Nicholas G. Georgiade

by M. RAMEZ SALEM

Loyola University Stritch School of Medicine

DELIBERATE HYPOTENSION IS A SAFE AND ACCEPTED ANESTHETIC TECHNIQUE

The control of bleeding and the maintenance of an adequate circulating blood volume are fundamental tenets of sound surgical practice, but such control is not always easy. Frequently, bleeding is so excessive as to endanger the life of the patient. A more complex problem is the persistent ooze that makes certain operations difficult or impossible. Anesthetic drugs may contribute to oozing by increasing skin and muscle blood flow. Through the years, the frustrating problems of surgical bleeding have been subjected to numerous studies. One solution that has been offered and has stood the test of time consists of intentional hypotension to achieve a relatively bloodless operative field (Larson, 1964).

Credit goes to Enderby, who first employed ganglion-blocking drugs in surgery, describing the new technique as "controlled circulation with hypotensive drugs and posture to reduce bleeding in surgery" (Leigh, 1975). With the introduction of these new hypotensive drugs, other methods of inducing hypotension (arteriotomy and high spinal block) became of historic interest.

From the beginning, some condemned the technique as physiologic trespass because, as with many other new techniques, there was an initial morbidity and mortality (Larson, 1964; Leigh, 1975). The improved knowledge and skills of those who practice it regularly and the availability of newer monitoring devices have contributed to the safety of the technique.

Today, deliberate hypotension stands as a safe and an accepted anesthetic technique. It has the unique advantage of simplicity. The morbidity and mortality associated with deliberate hypotension should not exceed that of any other anesthetic technique. In this article, I

95

would like to attempt to answer the following questions: What does deliberate hypotension have to offer? How should deliberate hypotension be induced? What are the factors that govern the safety of the technique? Finally, I would like to comment on complications associated with deliberate hypotension.

WHAT DOES DELIBERATE HYPOTENSION HAVE TO OFFER?

Deliberate hypotension is useful in reducing blood loss and in facilitating difficult vessel surgery. Hypotensive drugs have also been employed in the management of threatening hemorrhage and to enhance myocardial performance by reducing the preload and afterload. Only deliberate hypotension aimed at reduction of surgical blood loss and facilitation of vessel surgery will be discussed here.

Blood Loss

The ability of deliberate hypotension to reduce bleeding is one of the greatest surgical triumphs in recent years. By enhancing visualization, hypotension allows accurate delineation of lesions without trauma to delicate structures. With its aid, intricate operations may be performed more easily, more exactly, and therefore more successfully (Enderby, 1975). Hypotension enhances viability of grafts and diminishes hematoma formation, thereby reducing sepsis and fibrosis (Larson, 1964; Enderby, 1975). A well-conducted hypotension will reduce need of massive transfusion and decrease the ever-threatening problems of blood transfusion. The operative time is shortened when deliberate hypotension is matched by skillful surgical technique. All of these advantages are of genuine benefit to patients.

Facilitation of Vessel Surgery

Deliberate hypotension has the most to offer in facilitating vessel surgery; common applications include clipping of an intracranial aneurysm and resection of coarctation and aortic aneurysm. The advantages of blood pressure control in assisting large vessel surgery are best exemplified in the surgical correction of coarctation of the aorta (Dalal et al., 1974). Mobilization of the aorta is made easier when the aorta is lax, and during the period of aortic clamping, blood pressure control decreases the risk of hypertensive crisis, acute ventricular failure, and cerebrovascular hemorrhage. Postoperatively, the incidence and severity of postanastomotic hypertension and necrotizing arteritis are reduced.

HOW TO INDUCE HYPOTENSION

Hypotension should not be induced unless a steady state of light anesthesia and a perfect airway with an endotracheal tube are secured (Larson, 1964; Salem, Ivankovic, and Shaker, 1971; Adams, 1975). Light anesthesia may be provided with nitrous oxide, oxygen, narcotic-relaxant technique, or halothane in oxygen. Ventilation should be controlled or assisted. Hypotension may then be initiated, with the patient in the horizontal position after the anesthesiologist has made certain that the patient is physiologically stable. Gradual induction of hypotension follows four basic steps: (1) intravenous administration of a ganglionic blocking or directly acting vasodilator drug. A beta-receptor-blocking drug (propranolol) may also be given at this stage. (2) Subsequent tilting (if feasible), (3) gradual increase in halothane or enflurane concentration, and (4) positive-end expiratory pressure (rarely needed) as the fine adjustment of blood pressure control.

"The power to initiate and maintain hypotension resides entirely with the anaesthetist who can, by skillful use of gravity and controlled ventilation, maintain almost any level of arterial pressure according to the need of surgery and the safety of the patient. Hypotensive drugs merely allow access to these basic controls" (Enderby, 1974).

Evidence indicates that improved operative conditions (relatively dry operative field) with deliberate hypotension are most closely related to reduction in cardiac output or blood flow at the operative site (Salem et al., 1978). Advantages claimed for certain hypotensive drugs are erroneously based on the fact that the cardiac output, and hence the oxygen delivery, is either unchanged or increased with hypotension. It is a misconception that a dry operative field is automatically accomplished with hypotension (Larson, 1964; Salem et al., 1978); in fact, bleeding may be excessive despite adequate fall in blood pressure. We should be reminded that, in describing the technique, Enderby used the phrase "controlled circulation" rather than hypotension (Leigh, 1975). If a dry operative field is the goal, then the anesthesiologist should use a technique that will reduce cardiac output (if the patient is supine) or blood flow at the operative site (if the patient is in a head-up tilt). For this purpose, a longer acting drug, such as pentolinium tartrate, is ideal. Tachycardia can be prevented by the judicious administration of propranolol or increased halothane concentration, and head-up tilt should be utilized to facilitate peripheral pooling whenever possible (Salem and Ivankovic, 1970; Salem, Ivankovic, and Shaker, 1971). I believe sodium nitroprusside to be a poor choice for long operations in which reduction of bleeding is required.

For facilitating delicate operations on large vessels, the objective is different, since it is the decreased vessel tension and not necessarily decreased blood flow that is desirable (Salem et al., 1978). Under these circumstances, drugs and techniques that result in hypotension without concomitant decrease in cardiac output are to be selected. Drugs that provide minute to minute control of pressure, such as tri-

methaphan and nitroprusside, would be most useful. Unless it coun-
teracts hypotension, tachycardia may be left untreated.

Almost all hypotensive drugs are capable of producing tachycardia (Salem and Ivankovic, 1970). This may counteract the fall in pressure caused by an increase in cardiac output and may necessitate further doses of the drug. Failure to maintain the desired hypotension
upon repeated administration of the drug may then result. Failed hypotension is related to tachycardia initiated through the baroreceptor
mechanism (Larson, 1964; Salem and Ivankovic, 1970; Salem, Ivankovic, and Shaker, 1971) and is commonly seen in children and young
healthy adults, rarely in the elderly.

Tachycardia may necessitate increased halothane concentration or
mean airway pressure to maintain hypotension. Even with what appears to be adequate hypotension, tachycardia may increase oozing.
Tachycardia may increase myocardial oxygen demand and enhance
ischemic electrocardiographic changes (Larson, 1964). With nitroprusside, increasing the rate of infusion in resistant cases has resulted in
cyanide toxicity (Tinker and Michenfelder, 1976). Obviously, tachycardia with or without resistant hypotension demands the immediate control of heart rate, best accomplished by the administration of propranolol in small increments up to a dose of 0.06 mg. per kg. (Salem et al.,
1974). When resistance is predicted (as in cases involving children), it is
best to initiate beta blockade before the hypotensive drug is administered.
I have seen cases in which failure to maintain hypotension was related
to excessive fluids given early in the course of the anesthetic. Fluids
are best restricted at induction of hypotension and should be given
when there is a need to raise the pressure or reverse hypotension.

THE SAFETY OF DELIBERATE HYPOTENSION

Anesthesiologists should be aware of the important factors that
govern the safety of the technique.

Onset of Hypotension

The induction of hypotension must proceed slowly (Larson, 1964;
Salem, Ivankovic, and Shaker, 1971) (10 to 15 minutes at least) (Fig.
1). The vessels of vital organs need time to dilate maximally in order
to maintain adequate perfusion. If blood pressure falls too acutely, a
sharp decrease in cerebral venous oxygen tension to critical levels may
occur. Ischemic ECG changes do not occur if the rate of fall in pressure is gradual (Rollason and Hough, 1969).

Degree of Hypotension

The required level of hypotension depends on the surgical requirements and the condition of the patient. In adults, systolic pres-

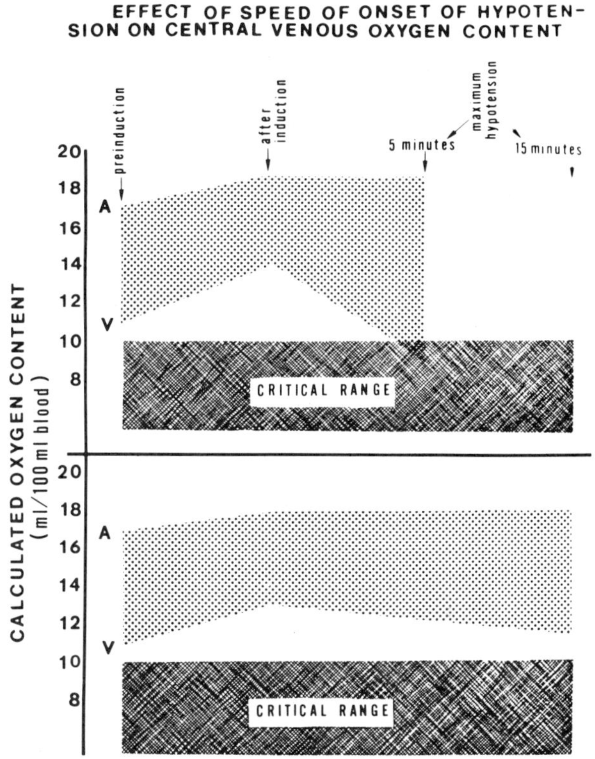

EFFECT OF SPEED OF ONSET OF HYPOTEN-
SION ON CENTRAL VENOUS OXYGEN CONTENT

Figure 1. Upper diagram: Changes in arterial and venous oxygen content when maximum hypotension was achieved in 5 minutes in 6 patients. Note that venous oxygen content fell within the critical range indicating a state of circulatory inadequacy. Lower diagram: In 6 other patients, hypotension was induced slowly (15 minutes). There was no remarkable increase in A-V oxygen content difference and venous oxygen content was above the critical range.

sure should not be allowed to go below 60 torr and not below 75 torr in elderly or hypertensive patients (Larson, 1964). Tilting produces a gradient of about 2 torr for each inch of vertical height above which the arterial pressure is measured. This must be taken into consideration when head-up tilt is used. It is the anesthesiologist's duty to look for warning signs, including too dry an operative field, dark venous blood, decrease in muscle relaxant requirements, and the appearance of apneustic gasps (Salem, Ivankovic, and Shaker, 1971). Any of these signs constitutes an indication to raise the arterial pressure.

Monitoring the Arterial Pressure

Frequent and accurate monitoring of blood pressure is essential during hypotension. Ordinary means of blood pressure measurements are unreliable at low pressures. One of three methods is suggested: oscillotonometry, Dobbler ultrasonic, or direct measurement via arterial cannulation. Oscillometers are sufficiently accurate and are unaffected by electromagnetic interference in the operating room. The apparatus is reasonably cheap, and various cuff sizes are available for children. Provided certain precautions are observed, it is very easy to obtain accurate and reliable readings of systolic and diastolic pressures (Corall and Strunin, 1975). Arterial cannulation serves the double function of continuous monitoring as well as permitting arterial blood analysis. This method is desirable in long operations, when excessive blood loss is anticipated, in critically ill patients, or when profound hypotension is necessary.

Ventilation, Acid-Base Balance, and Arterial Oxygenation

Maintenance of a near normal $PaCO_2$ is essential during deliberate hypotension. It has been noticed that a $PaCO_2$ around 40 torr helps maintain a normal acid-base status; hypocapnia may result in a base deficit. Eckenhoff and his associates found that the alveolar dead space increases in the hypotensive adult patient in a head-up tilt and with increased airway pressure (Eckenhoff et al., 1963). As a result, they recommended controlling ventilation above levels usually considered adequate during hypotension. Further investigations demonstrated that the increase in alveolar dead space during deliberate hypotension is less than previously thought (Askrog, Pender, and Eckenhoff, 1964). Data from infants and children suggest that alveolar dead space does not increase during controlled hypotension even with head-up tilt (Salem et al., 1974). I believe that an increase in physiologic dead space with hypotension has been overemphasized and may be of significance only when excessive airway pressure and head-up tilt are used in adults. Otherwise, if vigorous ventilation is applied, hypocarbia will result.

Unless indicated, hypocarbia should be avoided in the anesthetized patient, whether normotensive or hypotensive. Provided that adequate oxygenation and near normal PCO_2 are maintained, acidemia is not a feature of the hypotensive state (Salem, Ivankovic, and Shaker, 1971). The acidosis reported when sodium nitroprusside is used is due to decreased oxygen uptake caused by cyanide formation (venous oxygen tension rises), preventable if the initial dose is limited to 1.5 μg. per kg. per minute and the total dose for 4 hours does not exceed 1 mg. per kg. (Tinker and Michenfelder, 1976).

Proper placement of the endotracheal tube and control of the airway are mandatory in the anesthetized patient, and the hypotensive patient is no exception. Some observations indicate that the use of high FiO_2 in excess of 0.9 (accomplished by avoiding nitrous oxide) is preferred during deliberate hypotension: (1) High FiO_2 tends to compensate for intrapulmonary shunting, which might be magnified when cardiac output is decreased. (2) During profound hypotension, the lactate to pyruvate ratio did not increase if PaO_2 was kept above 300 torr. (3) Jugular bulb oxygen tension rises significantly when inspired oxygen concentration is altered from 40 per cent to 100 per cent (Salem, Kim, and Shaker, 1970); in fact, some low values rise to above critical levels when 100 per cent oxygen is given. High oxygen concentration does not have deleterious effects if limited to a few hours of hypotension. I believe that the use of high FiO_2 is an important, but frequently neglected, safety factor in induced hypotension.

Contraindications to Induced Hypotension

At one time, almost all systemic diseases were considered absolute contraindications to induced hypotension. With this stringent rule, many patients have been denied the advantages of the technique. Acute or severe heart, brain, or renal disease constitutes a reasonable contraindication to hypotension, however. Significant reduction in oxygen delivery to the tissues is another contraindication. (Oxygen delivery is dependent on cardiac output, hemoglobin concentration, and arterial oxygen saturation.) Low fixed cardiac output, anemia, or a combination of the two will reduce oxygen delivery to tissue. In patients with sickle cell disease, a decrease in mixed venous oxygen tension below 30 torr due to a reduction in cardiac output may trigger a crisis (Salem, 1978). Uncorrected polycythemia is an additional contraindication since it may enhance thrombosis (Larson, 1964).

Diabetes is not a contraindication provided it is reasonably controlled preoperatively. Fahmy and Battit found that there is striking modification of surgery-induced hyperglycemia during pentolinium-induced hypotension (Fahmy and Battit, 1975). A fall in blood sugar to hypoglycemic levels was not demonstrable in either adults or children, however. The pupillary dilation associated with ganglionic blockade may be undesirable in patients with narrow-angle glaucoma. Persistent cycloplegia in the postoperative period should not be misinterpreted as cerebral hypoxia following ganglionic blockade.

The most important single contraindication to the use of induced hypotension is inexperience. Anesthesiologists and surgeons should be familiar with the pharmacology of drugs used, physiology, and implications of hypotension. Teamwork and cooperation are of great importance in the care of patients undergoing this technique.

Age.   Except in neonates and infants, in whom blood pressure may be difficult to measure accurately, the technique need not be withheld. The following points must be kept in mind when induced hypotension is utilized for pediatric patients (Salem et al., 1974; Salem, 1978): (1) They usually respond to hypotension by tachycardia; therefore, the incidence of failed cases may be high. Prophylactic beta blockade prior to the administration of the hypotensive drug is advisable. (2) Lower arterial pressure may be necessary to achieve a bloodless field. (3) Tilting does not produce as great a pressure gradient or peripheral pooling. (4) There is no need to augment ventilation since alveolar dead space does not increase. (5) Because of their increased oxygen demand, high FiO_2 should be administered.

Elderly patients subjected to induced hypotension do well. The following points, however, need to be remembered: (1) They may exhibit substantial fall in pressure with small doses of hypotensive agents; (2) they tend to respond to hypotension and tilting by bradycardia; and (3) low pressures are rarely needed (they have higher critical pressure).

Prone Position.   Recent experience indicates that hypotension can be safely used in the prone position, as for operative correction of scoliosis (Bennett et al., 1974), provided that the following precautions are taken: (1) The airway should be guarded all the time; (2) inferior vena caval compression must be prevented; (3) blood loss may be excessive (but less than with normotension) and requires replacement. Postoperative oozing from bone may continue. (4) Minute to minute blood pressure monitoring, preferably by arterial cannulation, may be necessary. (Resuscitation frequently fails because of body position.)

Postoperative Hemorrhage

There is no evidence to indicate that this complication, feared by surgeons, occurs more often after hypotension. The following procedures should be adopted when hypotension is used, however: (1) allowing gradual return of pressure without vasopressors, (2) reasonable hemostasis before closure, and (3) application of pressure dressings whenever the operation involves a wide superficial surface area. Prevention of coughing and straining in the early postanesthetic period may also be useful in these cases.

Postoperative Care

Before patients are transferred from the operating room, their airway must be assured, blood pressure near normal, and lost blood replaced. Sudden movement should be avoided, since it may precipitate hypotension or cardiac overloading. Skilled supervision and adequate care are imperative. Narcotic drugs are rarely needed, but if given, the dose should be reduced.

A LOOK AT COMPLICATIONS ASSOCIATED WITH INDUCED HYPOTENSION

The reason that hypotension is not universally practiced is probably related to the bad reputation it gained when first introduced (Enderby, 1975). I have no doubt that the technique would be used more frequently today, when we can guarantee greater safety, than in 1950.

The validity of conclusions on morbidity and mortality drawn from large series must be seriously questioned (Lindop, 1975). Series from single institutions where the technique is commonly practiced offer better comparison and realistic assessment. Since 1950, over 18,000 procedures utilizing hypotension have been performed at the Queen Victoria Hospital in East Grinstead, England.* In this single

---

*G.E. Hale Enderby: Personal communication.

large series, deliberate hypotensive techniques carried no more risks than normotensive ones. Series utilizing control normotensive groups have not been able to show significant differences in complications. Furthermore, it is often not possible to distinguish complications attributable to the hypotensive technique and those that occur after normotensive anesthesia.

Recently, a collaborative retrospective study was undertaken to investigate complications attributed to induced hypotension (Salem et al., 1976), the data gathered from five institutions for the period between 1965 and 1975. The complications recorded fit into one of the following categories: (1) cardiac arrest or uncontrollable and severe fall in pressure, (2) temporary or permanent neurologic deficits, (3) reactionary hemorrhage, and (4) failure of the technique. Critical analysis of the cases revealed that almost all the tragedies were attributed to faulty technique, including: rapid induction of hypotension, maintenance of low pressure for long periods, excessive head-up tilt, underestimation of blood loss, failure to detect important warning signs, hypocarbia, hypoxemia, improper use of drugs, and poor selection of patients.

Unfortunately, when hypotension is used, it frequently becomes the target of criticism for unsuccessful outcome. I have seen a case of reactionary hemorrhage after hypotension for an extensive radical head and neck procedure and was of the opinion that deliberate hypotension contributed to the complication. Six months later, the same patient was subjected to a similar, but less extensive, operation. At no time during operation did the blood pressure fall, but the patient developed the same complication. This example demonstrates our inappropriate tendency to blame deliberate hypotension for the occurrence of complications.

SUMMARY

Skilled anesthesia, technical competence, and constant vigilance are essential prerequisites for the safe conduct of hypotensive techniques. Such skills can be easily mastered by practice and by adherence to the principles that govern safety of the technique. These principles include careful selection of patients, use of high oxygen mixture, avoidance of hypocarbia, gradual onset of hypotension, aiming at a blood pressure level consistent with the patient's physical condition and surgical requirements, accurate measurement of blood pressure, detection of warning signs, and adequate postoperative care. The success of hypotension in achieving its goals is dependent on proper selection of drugs and techniques and control of the heart rate. Complications directly related to the technique are rare if one abides by these rules.

REFERENCES

Adams, A. P.: Techniques of vascular control for deliberate hypotension during surgery. Br. J. Anaesth., 47:777, 1975.

Askrog, V. F., Pender, J. W., and Eckenhoff, J. E.: Changes in physiological dead-space during deliberate hypotension. Anesthesiology, 25:774, 1964.

Bennett, E. J., Salem, M. R., Sakul, P., et al.: Induced hypotension for spinal corrective procedures. Mid. East J. Anaesthesiol., 4:177, 1974.

Corall, I. M., and Strunin, L.: Assessment of the Von Recklinghausen oscillotonometer. Anaesthesia, 20:55, 1975.

Dalal, F. Y., Bennett, E. J., Salem, M. R., et al.: Anaesthesia for coarctation: A new classification for rational anaesthetic management. Anaesthesia, 29:704, 1974.

Eckenhoff, J. E., Enderby, G. E. H., Larson, A., et al.: Pulmonary gas exchange during deliberate hypotension. Br. J. Anaesth., 35:750, 1963.

Enderby, G. E. H.: Pharmacological blockade. Postgrad. Med. J., 50:572, 1974.

Enderby, G. E. H.: Some observations on the practice of deliberate hypotension. Br. J. Anaesth., 47:743, 1975.

Fahmy, N. R., and Battit, G. E.: Effect of pentolinium on blood sugar and serum potassium concentrations during anaesthesia and surgery. Br. J. Anaesth., 47:1309, 1975.

Larson, A. G.: Deliberate hypotension. Anaesthesiology, 25:682, 1964.

Leigh, J. M.: The history of controlled hypotension. Br. J. Anaesth., 47:745, 1975.

Lindop, M. J.: Complications and morbidity of controlled hypotension. Br. J. Anaesth., 47:799, 1975.

Robinson, J. S.: Hypotension without hypoxia. Int. Anesthesiol. Clin., 5:467, 1967.

Rollason, W. N., and Hough, J. M.: A re-examination of some electrocardiographic studies during hypotensive anesthesia: The effect of rate of fall of blood pressure. Br. J. Anaesth., 41:985, 1969.

Salem, M. R.: Therapeutic uses of ganglionic blocking drugs. In Ivankovic, A. D. (ed.): Sodium Nitroprusside and Other Short-acting Hypotensive Agents. Int. Anesthesiol. Clin. 16:171, 1978.

Salem, M. R., Bennett, E. J., Rao, T. L. K., et al.: An examination of complications related to hypotensive anesthesia. Abstract of Scientific Papers, American Society of Anesthesiologists Annual Meeting, 1976.

Salem, M. R., and Ivankovic, A. D.: The place of beta adrenergic blocking drugs in the deliberate induction of hypotension. Anesth. Analg. (Cleve.), 49:427, 1970.

Salem, M. R., Ivankovic, A. D., and Shaker, M. H.: Safety factors in deliberately induced hypotension. M.E.J. Anaesth., 3:107, 1971.

Salem, M. R., Kim, Y., and Shaker, M. H.: Effect of alteration of inspired oxygen concentration on jugular bulb oxygen tension during deliberate hypotension. Anesthesiology, 33:358, 1970.

Salem, M. R., Toyama, T., Wong, A. Y., et al.: Haemodynamic responses to induced arterial hypotension in children. Br. J. Anaesth., 50:489, 1978.

Salem, M. R., Wong, A. Y., Bennett, E. J., et al.: Deliberate hypotension in infants and children. Anesth. Analg. (Cleve.), 53:975, 1974.

Tinker, J. H., and Michenfelder, J. D.: Sodium nitroprusside: Pharmacology, toxicology and therapeutics. Anesthesiology, 45:294, 1976.

by JAMES E. ECKENHOFF

MICHAEL LESCH
Northwestern University Medical School

DELIBERATE HYPOTENSION — A DEVIL'S ADVOCATE ANALYSIS

It is now nearly 30 years since the use of deliberate hypotension was introduced as an adjunctive anesthetic technique. By the end of the first decade of use, early enthusiasm had waned, perhaps from indiscriminate application, as highlighted by Hampton and Little (1953), and the technique remained in active use in only a few centers in the world. A resurgence of interest occurred in the mid-1960's. Although commonly employed today, it is by no means a popular technique in this country, and use of the technique is mainly confined to academic medical centers.

Of greater interest is the frequency with which deliberate hypotension is avoided when specifically indicated. If the technique is as valuable as some believe, why do anesthesiologists not want to use it more often, and why do not more surgeons request its use? The answer must be more than a fear that hypotension may cause organ damage. Halothane was introduced into clinical practice 24 years ago and has been under a yellow cloud for at least 16 of those years, yet it remains immensely popular. Interestingly, and from another point of view, when the editor of this volume sought authors for the deliberate hypotension controversy, there was no difficulty in getting a champion of deliberate hypotension but no one wanted to write the contrary side. Nonetheless, any anesthesiologist knows far more associates who avoid hypotension than those who look for the opportunity to use it.

The value of the technique is unchallenged by any who have become thoroughly conversant with it. Benefits purported obtained with the technique include better surgical conditions, a clearer surgical field, better delineation of tissues, less blood loss and consequently less need for ligatures and use of the cautery, less need for blood replacement, alleged better wound healing, smoother convalescence for the

105

patient, and better results with cosmetic surgery. These are appreciable advantages, and one must ask the obvious question, "Why is the technique not used more widely?"

We believe the principal deterrent is the failure of anesthesiologists and surgeons to understand the physiology of normal circulatory control and tissue perfusion. There is a fear of low blood pressure, a tendency to equate postoperative complications with intraoperative hypotension, and a belief that hypotension and shock are synonymous. Other deterrents include failure to appreciate the specific criteria that judge patients fit for the technique, unwillingness of anesthesiologists to become involved with procedures that require prolonged attention to infinite detail, lack of encouragement by surgeons to use the technique, fear of medicolegal insult, and lack of a sufficient volume of statistics to prove the technique safe. Let us consider these deterrents individually.

CIRCULATORY CONTROL

It is important to understand that one does not equate hypotension and shock. The common denominator of shock is inadequate perfusion of tissues with blood; it is not a pressure phenomenon. Hypotension commonly accompanies shock, but with shock, one will observe all of the signs of poor tissue perfusion: vasoconstriction, sweating, pale skin, tachycardia, and perhaps cyanosis. Hypotension can exist without any of these signs and with normal tissue perfusion. Furthermore, blood pressure varies appreciably during the day, from hypotensive levels during deep sleep to modest hypertensive levels during exercise and emotional outbursts.

The human circulation is a dynamic system, regulated by a series of exquisite controls that maintain the circulation of blood to provide adequate tissue perfusion through a wide range of physiologic situations that include wakefulness versus sleep, exercise versus inactivity, cold environmental temperatures versus hot, agitation versus tranquility, upright body position versus supine, high altitude versus sea level atmospheric pressure, overeating versus fasting, and dehydration versus normal fluid balance. In the course of these varying physiologic states, blood pressure is but one of the determinants of blood flow that change; others include cardiac output, heart rate, peripheral vascular resistance, organ metabolic demands, and blood volume. Only in recent years, with the availability of continuous monitoring devices, have we been able to record data on the extent of variations of these parameters during daily life. We have known for a long time that during sleep a heart rate of 40 beats per minute is common, but less well appreciated is the fact that, at the same time, a blood pressure of 80 torr is equally common, especially in the trained subject. With daytime normal activities, blood pressure and pulse rise, cardiac output increases, and organ metabolic requirements go up. During exercise, muscle blood flow increases appreciably as the metabolic demands of muscle rise, and concomitantly, cardiac output and heart rate are elevated as hypertension develops.

Most recent graduates of medical schools have considered the above in the abstract, yet placed in a clinical setting, the average physician does not examine patients over this range of activity and most often sees patients under stylized conditions — in the office or during the day in a hospital bed. The common clinical measurements of the circulation are blood pressure and pulse and occasionally the electrocardiogram. There is no measured evidence of cardiac output or blood volume, no data on cutaneous vasomotor tone, and blood gases are not recorded except in the acute situation when the results are seldom available less than 10 minutes after the fact. All of these measurements can be made, but the routine clinical use of the necessary equipment is prohibitive for a variety of reasons. In the case of the anesthetized patient, the anesthetist or surgeon makes a judgment of circulatory adequacy from direct evidence by measuring blood pressure and pulse and observing the electrocardiogram and from indirect evidence, equating absence of hypovolemia with full veins; normal vasomotor tone with a warm, dry, and pink skin; adequate oxygen supply with bright arterial blood; and so forth. Judgmental decisions worry many; if difficulty arises, objective evidence other than blood pressure or pulse to support a decision is lacking, and peers and the courts cannot see the indirect evidence on which the judgment was made. Hypotension is frequently induced without intra-arterial blood pressure measurement (although becoming more common), usually with an electrocardiogram, and only occasionally with intermittent blood gas measurements. Indirect evidence therefore supplies much of the basis for judgment.

Unfortunately, we lack clinical data on the acceptable limits of either blood flow or oxygen delivery to assure viability of the heart, brain, and kidney, the organs of greatest concern during hypotension. The blood flow and oxygen requirements of these organs are different.

The brain is a passive organ that usually extracts about 20 to 25 per cent of the oxygen delivered to it, and, therefore, additional oxygen is available in cerebral blood immediately on demand. Cerebral blood flow is dependent on the perfusion pressure of arterial blood, the resistance of cerebral arterioles and capillaries, and the pressure on the venous side of the circulation. In the supine position, arterial perfusion pressure will equal pressure at the heart level and venous pressure will be at or above that at right heart level. In the head down position, arterial pressure will be elevated, but so will venous pressure and resistance to flow across the cerebral circulatory bed owing to increased cerebrospinal fluid pressures. In the head up position, mean perfusing pressure will be lowered, venous pressure may be negative within the skull, and resistance to flow across the brain may be low. Often ignored is the fact that in the upright position, mean arterial perfusing pressure is likely to be 20 to 40 torr or more lower than that at heart level, depending on body height, as compared to the supine position, yet, except when compensating mechanisms fail, diminution in cerebral blood flow is not appreciable. Carbon dioxide excess and oxygen deficit increase the rate of cerebral blood flow. General anesthetics and hypothermia diminish cerebral metabolism, decreasing blood flow and oxygen requirements. Unfortunately, we do not know the minimal limits of blood flow or of oxygen supply required to maintain cerebral integrity and do not have a precise definition of how variables play upon these limits at low levels. It has been written that 60 torr is the minimal blood pressure acceptable to maintain normal brain function. We know this to be wrong because one of us has seen blood pressure maintained at heart level at 60 torr for 1½ hours with the patient in a 30 degree head up tilt without subsequent evidence of brain damage. One of us has also measured blood pressure in the internal carotid artery at the base of the brain in the head up position at 17 torr without residual damage manifest. We have seen appreciable periods of marked hypoxia during anesthesia and operation without cerebral damage, although we would be the first to admit that we have seen relatively short bouts of hypoxia followed by stroke. In short, as far as we have come in 34 years since Kety and Schmidt (1945) first reported directly measured cerebral blood flow and oxygen metabolism in man, we cannot do more than speculate about the permissible lower limits of blood pressure, blood flow, and oxygen delivery to the brain and its components.

The heart poses a greater problem so far as clinical definition of pressure, flow, and oxygen requirements are concerned. The heart is a working muscle; it removes 75 to 80 per cent of the oxygen delivered to it. Increased oxygen demand must therefore be met with more flow, better distribution of flow, or better use of the oxygen delivered. The factors that govern oxygen requirements of the myocardium are complex, however, and include (1) intracardiac systolic pressure and myocardial wall tension, (2) work done by myocardial fiber shortening, (3) inotropic state of the myocardial muscle fiber, and (4) frequency of contraction. Oxygen requirements of the myocardium progressively increase as heart rate and systolic blood pressure rise and with positive inotropic influences (e.g., calcium, digitalis, and isoproterenol). These relationships are diagrammatically presented in Figure 1.

Myocardial oxygen requirements are obviously met by the volume of coronary blood flow. Factors that influence coronary flow include (1) autoregulation, (2) mechanical coronary extravascular pressure, (3) metabolic factors, (4) neural factors, and (5) pharmacologic agents (Braunwald, Ross, and Sonnenblick, 1976). If the oxygen requirements of the heart are maintained in a steady state and only coronary perfusion pressure is altered, coronary flow remains remarkably constant over a wide range of perfusion pressure (termed autoregulation). Clinically, it is impossible to alter any one of these factors, or one of those governing myocardial oxygen requirements, without affecting most of the other factors. Thus, if blood pressure increases, then extravascular coronary artery compression likewise rises, me-

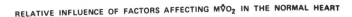

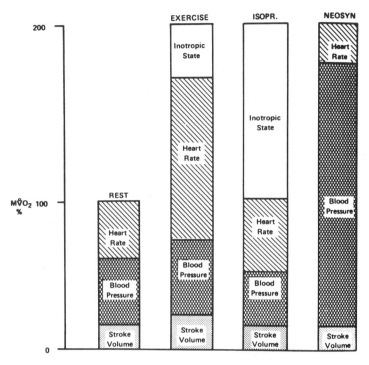

Figure 2. Diagrammatic representation showing myocardial oxygen consumption, first in the resting state (MVo$_2$ = 100%) and then as it is increased under various circulatory conditions. The relative contributions of systolic pressure development by the ventricle (blood pressure), the heart rate, and increases in the inotropic state are shown during mild muscular exercise, isoproterenol infusion (*ISOPR*), and infusion of the pressor agent neosynephrine (*NEOSYN*). (Reproduced from Ross [90], by permission.)

chanically affecting coronary flow, while myocardial oxygen demands are elevated. Similarly, if blood pressure falls, then extravascular compression is reduced and oxygen requirements lessen, although catecholamine liberation and tachycardia, as in shock, elevate the requirements.

It is quickly apparent that the relationship of oxgyen supply and oxygen demand of the myocardium is a dynamic and very complex one. Furthermore, it is not possible to directly monitor the adequacy of oxygen supply to the heart in relation to the oxygen demand of the heart in the clinical situation. The physician is left with indirect evidence and judgmental decisions. It should be obvious, however, that blood pressure *per se* cannot be taken as a guide to adequacy of coronary blood flow.

The kidney has, perhaps, been of the least concern of the three organs and may be better understood so far as flow and oxygen requirements are concerned. That does not imply complete understanding. Under conditions of stress, during hypotension associated with increased vasomotor tone, with hypovolemia and decreased cardiac output, renal blood flow is reduced. There are no data to suggest that a modest degree of hypotension in an anesthetized patient without hypovolemia or unusual stress is likely to damage the normal kidney. There are limits of variability of blood pressure, however, and what are the variables that affect those limits? Again, a 60 torr or lower limit is discussed, but we have seen too many patients with pressures below this level without subsequent damage to believe that pressure alone can be used as a definitive guideline.

From the foregoing, we are relatively ignorant of all of the factors that intrinsically match blood flow and oxygen supply to organ requirements. The three organs of principal concern are not accessible for routine monitoring. We know that blood pressure is one of the variables of blood flow, just as we know that water pressure in a system of rigid pipes will determine how fast a bucket fills with water. We are dealing with systems for which the "pipes" are not rigid and the demands are variable; however, we have the means of determining neither flow versus pressure nor demand versus supply, in the clinical situation. The commonly available measure is blood pressure; therefore, pressure is measured and assumed to be something of primary physiologic significance, which it is not.

THE SELECTION OF PATIENTS FOR DELIBERATE HYPOTENSION

Theoretically, a patient with obvious evidence of vascular insufficiency to brain, kidney, or heart should be excluded from consideration as a candidate for deliberate hypotension. It is unlikely that the technique would be advised for a patient with disease of one of these organs, although we could conceive that such a patient might be a candidate for modified hypotension. We know that there are anesthesiologists with experience in deliberate hypotension who select the technique for a surgical procedure in a patient with known coronary, myocardial, or hypertensive disease on the basis that myocardial oxygen requirements could be reduced and the distribution of coronary flow facilitated, thus protecting the heart. There is no great problem in choosing deliberate hypotension for patients below 40 to 45 years without evidence of coronary, cerebral, or renal disease. This age group is not prone to stroke or myocardial infarction even following short-lived shock.

The real problem comes in middle-aged or elderly patients with neither symptoms of vital organ disease nor laboratory or historical evidence of such disease. Some are reluctant to consider hypotension, fearing undiagnosed vascular disease. Under these circumstances, surgeons, as well as anesthesiologists, are fearful of the technique, believing that as good a surgical operation can be performed without it, and are willing to expose the patient to multiple transfusions. On the other hand, the team experienced with hypotension will use it if it is believed to have advantages to both patient and surgeon. Here, several assumptions must be made: a careful history has not suggested vascular disease; the patient's record has been thoroughly studied and the appropriate work up has been done; and both the surgeon and the anesthesiologist are experienced with the technique, understand its benefits and limitations, and are used to working as a team. Anesthesiologists and surgeons who are not accustomed to working together and who do not have mutual respect should not become involved.

Such decisions lack preciseness. The pathway to a successful outcome is not clearly marked for all to see. The unforeseen may arise. There is no assurance of such statements as "Do not use a spinal anesthetic for a patient in shock" or even "Patients with a history of hepatitis should not be given halothane," as fragile as is the evidence for proving the latter commandment correct and as few such dogmatic beliefs as we have. Lacking rules to judge appropriateness of choice, many surgeons and anesthesiologists avoid hypotension, preferring to go another route. When the surgeon does not want the technique used and the anesthesiologist uses it anyway, the stage is set for conflict should complications arise.

THE WILLINGNESS OF ANESTHESIOLOGISTS TO USE THE TECHNIQUE

The use of the deliberate hypotensive technique requires infinite attention to detail and constant surveillance of patient and operative field by the anesthesiologist. Does not every anesthesiologist always apply attention to detail and constantly survey the operative field? Not always. Some anesthetic techniques have periods requiring great attention, for example, during the first 15 to 20 minutes of a spinal anesthetic or the induction period of a general anesthetic. Once into the maintenance phase, the anesthetic and patient tend to be stable and the anesthesiologist relaxes. Such is never the case with a patient undergoing the hypotensive technique. The anesthesiologist cannot relax attention and should not move his or her eyes from the wound except for the brief moments required to readjust equipment and flows and to check the monitors. It is essential to observe the color of the wound, of arterial bleeding as contrasted with venous. As compared with the usual operation and anesthetic, there can be no question that the margin of safety is reduced with deliberate hypotension; therefore, the anesthesiologist must be more alert. Unsuspected hemorrhage must be seen instantly and measures must be instituted to keep the blood volume normal. Probably no one has had greater success with deliberate hypotension than has G. E. Hale Enderby, of London and East Grinstead, and no one watches patients more continuously or monitors them more closely. This is essential if one is to avoid trouble.

Only one who is willing to study the technique and understand its application, to pay rigid attention to detail, and to monitor the patient continuously throughout and immediately postoperatively and who is able to establish close rapport with surgeons should become involved. We have a surgical acquaintance well versed in deliberate hypotension. We asked if he ever used the technique in his surgical practice. "No." Did he ever ask if the anesthesiologists would use it for his patients? "No." Why not? "They don't understand the technique, have never sought to become trained in it, have never asked to use it even when specifically indicated. I doubt under the circumstances, I would trust them to use the technique."

THE FEAR OF MEDICOLEGAL INSULT SHOULD A COMPLICATION OCCUR

Although threats of malpractice action and settlements on behalf of plaintiffs seem fewer today than they were a few years ago, they nonetheless remain real. There are patients and lawyers willing to file suit for any result other than perfect; there are those who believe surgery and anesthesia to be without risk no matter what the patient's condition; and there are physicians willing to testify against other physicians, regardless of the validity of the claim and only for pecuniary benefit. Most often, the plaintiff claims a deviation from the standard of care normally afforded a patient in a given geographic area. As with the government, too often the law equates all physicians and all hospitals. A physician of consummate skill and experience practicing in an academic institution may find the plaintiff's expert witness to be a generalist with minimal experience in the matter at hand and with a practice confined to a small community hospital. Although the defendant may win, the litigation is harassing and time-consuming and, win or lose, may result in increased malpractice premiums.

Many anesthesiologists and surgeons feel particularly exposed by the use of the hypotensive technique. Since blood pressure is deliberately lowered, when under most circumstances everything is done to sustain it within a "normal" limit, the stage is set for litigation should a complication arise. It is easy to find physicians who will speak learnedly against deliberate hypotension, and there are always "expert witnesses" whose actual experience is confined to a few cases. The number of institutions where the technique is a normal standard of care is not very great in any geographic region. There is an absence of statistics on safety. Add anticipated exposure to litigation to inadequate knowledge of the requirements of vital organs for blood flow and oxygen supply and impreciseness in choice of patients on whom the technique is to be used and we have the conclusion of "Why bother learning about it, let alone use it?"

This situation is likely to prevail until such time as a volume of statistics is available to validate the safety of the technique. As stated in the comment on the acceptance of spinal anesthesia, this acceptance came about only with the accumulation of a large volume of data proving safety and acceptability. We suspect that the continued use of halothane in spite of the rare appearance of posthalothane hepatitis relates to the enormous mass of data proving the overall safety of the agent. We believe that similar data on deliberate hypotension are available and must be reported: Deliberate hypotension is not only feasible but also desirable for some operations.

CONCLUSION

Our conclusion is reproduced from statements pertaining to deliberate hypotension made 14 years ago (Eckenhoff, 1966). We believe they are still appropriate today, perhaps more so.

Deliberate hypotension has a use in surgical procedures whenever the amount of blood lost is of concern or when blood obscures the operative field. The anaesthetist who evades the use of the technique by saying, "It is solely something for the convenience of the surgeon, and that doesn't interest me," reveals himself a fool. For what reason does a patient come for operation — just to have a good sleep? No, he comes to have a specific operation, and everything the anaesthetist or surgeon can do to produce the best possible result is worthy of consideration. Likewise, the surgeon who ignores the possible gain from hypotension suggests he is fully confident in his results and doesn't think they can be improved. It is a pity that there are so few data on the surgical benefits of hypotension and so little published by surgeons who are fully convinced of the value of the technique. . . If, by virtue of deliberate hypotension, a surgeon can accomplish a more complete extirpation of a tumour, a more careful vessel anastomosis or ligation, or a more perfect cosmetic result, then the usefulness of the technique requires careful exploration. The morbidity and mortality associated with its use must be compared in identical groups of patients. However, when deliberate hypotension is used for surgical procedures that can be done as well with normotension, then morbidity and mortality figures must be compared with those from normal and healthy patients.

REFERENCES

Braunwald, L. J., Ross, J., Jr., and Sonnenblick, E. H.: Mechanisms of Contraction of the Normal and Failing Heart. Boston, Little, Brown and Co., Inc., 1976.

Eckenhoff, J. E.: Circulatory control in the surgical patient. Ann. R. Coll. Surg. Engl., 39:67, 1966.

Hampton, L. J., and Little, D. M., Jr.: Complications associated with the use of "controlled hypotension" in anesthesia. Arch. Surg., 67:549, 1953.

Kety, S. S., and Schmidt, C. F.: The determination of cerebral blood flow in man by the use of nitrous oxide in low concentrations. Am. J. Physiol., 143:53, 1945.

Ross, J., Jr.: Factors regulating the oxygen consumption of the heart. In Russek, H. I., and Zohman, B. L. (eds.): Changing Concepts in Cardiovascular Disease. Baltimore, Williams and Wilkins, 1972.

DELIBERATE HYPOTENSION

EDITORIAL COMMENT

by NICHOLAS G. GEORGIADE

Duke University Medical Center

From my own experience with deliberate hypotension over the years, I feel that the surgeon must clearly justify the technique of hypotensive anesthesia and that the benefits derived from its use must be noncontroversial. I had the opportunity to observe these techniques in hypotensive anesthesia at the Plastic Surgical Service in the Queen Victoria Hospital in East Grinstead, England, when Sir Archibald McIndoe was alive. He, of course, was a proponent of this technique. I think that it is an extremely difficult technique to master, particularly with constantly changing anesthesiologists. It is so necessary for the anesthetist to have an intimate knowledge of the physiology of hypotension and the pharmacology of the agents being used to deliberately lower the blood pressure. It is a very challenging and time-consuming type of anesthesia, and the vigilance and monitoring requirements that are necessary are quite formidable. I feel that deliberate hypotension is of value; however, the capability of an anesthetist in any particular institution to carry out this type of anesthesia may be limited. I question whether its usefulness can be expanded until anesthesiologists as a group learn the technique and are able to offer it to the majority of major general hospital operating areas. Trained individuals and back-up teams are required in each of these institutions.

Part 6

ENDOTRACHEAL
ANESTHESIA IN
PARTURIENTS

THE PROPOSITION:

> If a parturient is to be given general anesthesia for vaginal delivery, her
> trachea must be intubated.

ALTERNATIVE POINTS OF VIEW:

> By Jay S. DeVore
> By Otto C. Phillips

EDITORIAL COMMENT

by JAY S. DeVORE

University of California, Irvine

ALL PARTURIENTS RECEIVING GENERAL ANESTHESIA SHOULD HAVE TRACHEAL INTUBATION

The movement toward natural childbirth and concern with maternal-neonatal bonding, which can influence future life, has diminished the request for general anesthesia for routine vaginal delivery. The need for general anesthesia still exists for emergency situations, psychiatric reasons, and cesarean sections, however. Since vaginal delivery is usually brief, does not require muscle relaxants, and is distant from the airway, it has been traditional not to intubate the trachea of these patients. Fortunately, the trend in recent years has been in the opposite direction, and it is my belief that all parturients receiving general anesthesia should have their tracheas intubated. The need for intubation is based on two principles of anesthetic management: airway protection and airway maintenance.

AIRWAY PROTECTION

In order to justify tracheal intubation for airway protection, a discussion of some of the physiologic changes related to pregnancy and labor is necessary.

Maternal Physiology

In the parturient, the standard 4 to 6 hours to empty the stomach after a meal does not apply. During labor, gastric motility is decreased, so that for all practical purposes gastric emptying does not occur (Bonica, 1976). This has been realized for years; anesthetists were taught that if there had been no oral intake for 4 to 6 hours

117

prior to onset of labor, the stomach had time to empty and the patient could be treated accordingly. Gastric secretion at a very low pH continues during labor, however. Even if the parturient does not have solid food in her stomach, she has a variable amount of gastric secretion present (LaSalvia and Steffen, 1950). In 1946, Mendelson, an obstetrician, first described the syndrome of aspiration of gastric content of a low pH. As little as 25 ml. of gastric secretions with pH > 2.5 may lead to chemical pneumonitis, which carries a high morbidity and mortality (Teabeaut, 1952).

It is obvious therefore that the parturient must be considered as having a full stomach, whether of food or of hydrochloric acid. This alone should mandate an endotracheal tube if protective airway reflexes are removed by general anesthesia. Additionally, however, the parturient has increased intra-abdominal pressure due to the mass of the gravid uterus, a pressure further increased if fundal pressure is applied to facilitate vaginal delivery. A full stomach and increased intra-abdominal pressure raise intragastric pressure, a prime factor predisposing to regurgitation and aspiration during general anesthesia. But there is more. The pregnant woman at or near term has an incompetent gastroesophageal sphincter, due to both the mechanical force of the increased intragastric pressure holding the sphincter open and the direct smooth muscle relaxant effect of progesterone. Furthermore, one may administer oxytoxic agents, some of which have a direct emetic effect. Could one ask for a set of circumstances more likely to lead to regurgitation and aspiration? Many practitioners point with pride to personal series of many hundreds of parturients anesthetized by mask without a maternal death. This may be admirable; however, what is the acceptable incidence of maternal death from anesthesia? Even one mother who dies from aspiration during general anesthesia without an endotracheal tube would seem to be too many.

Maternal Mortality

Maternal mortality has been defined by a Council of the American Medical Association as death occurring between the time of conception and 60 days after the expulsion of the products of conception (1957). This figure, according to the National Center for Health Statistics, has steadily decreased in the past 30 years and has plateaued at approximately one to three maternal deaths per 10,000 live births (1969, 1974). Traditionally, hemorrhage, infection, and toxemia have been the major causes of maternal mortality, accounting for approximately 50 per cent of maternal deaths. Ten years ago, anesthesia was fifth among causes of maternal mortality, accounting for approximately 10 per cent (Bonica, 1976). In recent years, the major causes have come under better control, with the result that their relative contribution is less. Anesthesia on the other hand, although not causing more maternal deaths than previously, is not causing fewer deaths either; on a percentage basis, it is now among the leading causes of mortality, actually the most common cause in primiparous and young patients (Hughes, Cochrane, and Czyz, 1976). Over 50 per cent of maternal deaths from anesthesia are due to aspiration of gastric contents (Organe and Crawford, 1974). Based on approximately 3.3 million births per year, a total maternal death rate of 1.5 per 10,000 births, an anesthetic maternal mortality of 15 per cent of maternal deaths, this means that approximately 50 pregnant women die from aspiration each year. Despite the fact that 50 may not seem like a large number, it must be remembered that these are predominantly healthy young women who might not have died had they not received general anesthesia. The sociologic and financial costs of these deaths are immense.

Use of Oral Antacids

Since 1975, emphasis has been placed on the prophylactic use of oral antacids in parturients to reduce the risk of Mendelson's syndrome. Routine use of magnesium or aluminum trisilicates during labor may increase gastric pH above the critical 2.5 level, so that if aspiration occurs, Mendelson's syndrome may not result (Roberts and Shirley, 1974). This has led some to believe that endotracheal tubes are unnecessary; however, although oral antacids may be effective, they are not a guarantee against aspiration.

Patient acceptance is a problem. Oral antacids in general are not palatable, and patients may refuse repeated administration. The acceptability can be improved by keeping antacids cold; at room temperature antacids tend to cause emesis. There is a difference in taste among the available preparations, and experimentation with several types may produce a more acceptable one.

In order to be effective, oral antacids must be given at the proper time. They require at least 30 minutes to effectively alkalize gastric contents, and the alkalization persists for only 3 to 4 hours. Antacids must therefore by repeated every 3 to 4 hours during the course of labor. Despite effectiveness in alkalizing gastric contents, cases of Mendelson's syndrome after antacid administration have been reported (Taylor, 1975). When this is added to the fact that gastric volume does not decrease with use of antacids and that repetitive administration of antacids is often unacceptable, one can see that use of an endotracheal tube is not precluded by antacid therapy.

AIRWAY MAINTENANCE

Airway maintenance is another indication for tracheal intubation in general anesthesia. This is a strong indication in the obstetric patient. The mucosa of the airway is engorged in the parturient, with the result that soft tissue obstruction of the unprotected airway is more likely (Bonica, 1976). Furthermore, light general anesthesia is usually preferred in the parturient in order to minimize anesthetic effects on the fetus. This technique combined with the highly stimulating procedure of delivery or cesarean section is a perfect setting for laryngospasm. Again, this argues for an endotracheal tube.

Muscle relaxants are frequently used in obstetric procedures, particularly in cesarean sections. The use of muscle relaxants, although not mandating an endotracheal tube, certainly is a good indication for one.

In the emergency obstetric situation requiring general anesthesia, there frequently are a minimal number of personnel, particularly anesthesia personnel, available. The use of an endotracheal tube is indicated in order to allow the anesthetist the freedom to use the hands for other than maintaining a mask airway.

A protected airway increases the likelihood of assured oxygenation. Although an endotracheal tube does not guarantee adequate oxygenation, it makes it more likely. Owing to the decrease in functional residual capacity, the parturient is more susceptible to hypoxia, with either short periods of depressed respiration or airway obstruction (Cugell, 1953); therefore, use of an endotracheal tube will maintain the airway and decrease the likelihood of hypoxia. Additionally, the fetus must be considered. Fetal P_{O_2} is responsive to maternal P_{O_2}; it is desirable to maintain maternal oxygenation at a P_{O_2} in the 200 to 300 torr range to assure optimal oxygenation of the fetus (Marx and Mateo, 1971).

TECHNIQUES

Given then that all parturients receiving general anesthesia should have their tracheas intubated, how does one go about this safely? Since we are dealing with an emergency situation in a patient with a full stomach, the rapid sequence induction of anesthesia is the technique of choice. A brief review of the technique is worthwhile. While preparations are being made for delivery, either abdominal or vaginal, the patient should receive 0.4 to 0.6 mg. of atropine intravenously and 100 per cent oxygen by mask. Approximately 1 minute prior to induction, 3 mg. of d-tubocurarine should be administered intravenously. Anesthesia is induced with a sleep dose of thiopental (4 mg./kg.) or ketamine (1 mg./kg.). With loss of consciousness, firm cricoid pressure should be administered by an assistant instructed in this maneuver and maintained until the endotracheal tube is in place with cuff inflated. The hypnotic agent should be followed immediately by a paralyzing dose of succinylcholine, generally 1.5 mg. per kg., a somewhat large dose necessitated by the pretreatment with curare. Artificial ventilation should be omitted during the induction. Once the patient is well relaxed, an endotracheal tube should be placed. A stylet may be helpful to facilitate intubation. Since the parturient has mucosal engorgement of her airway, a smaller than usual endotracheal tube is generally preferred (7.5 mm. inside diameter is usually appropriate). Once the tube has passed the vocal cords, the cuff should be inflated by an assistant, the tube attached to the anesthesia machine, and the patient's lungs inflated with oxygen; only at this point should cricoid pressure be released. The chest should be auscultated to assure the bilateral presence of breath sounds. The surgeon should not begin until the placement of the endotracheal tube is assured. If intubation of the trachea proves difficult, and the surgical procedure has not begun, the patient may be allowed to awaken; if an incision has been made, one is committed to a hazardous course. Although difficult, if absolutely necessary the patient's lungs can be ventilated with oxygen by mask, retaining cricoid pressure. It has been stated that regurgitation will not occur under these circumstances (Sellick, 1961).

As in any patient with a full stomach, the mother should be allowed to awaken completely with the cuffed endotracheal tube in place, since regurgitation and aspiration may occur on emergence as well as during induction. Even though the patient appears to be awake at the end of the procedure, precautions must be taken to prevent aspiration in the recovery period. The patient should be on her side and observed closely. There have been instances in the recovery room of aspiration in patients who were apparently awake but were allowed to remain supine and became obtunded.

CONCLUSION

From the foregoing, it should be patently obvious that all parturients receiving general anesthesia should have their tracheas intubated. The physiologic changes of pregnancy relating to gastric secretion and intra-abdominal pressure as well as the airway alterations and need for increased oxygenation argue for this approach. The fact that general anesthesia without endotracheal tubes accounts for a large percentage of all maternal mortality should preclude argument. Even one maternal death is too many.

REFERENCES

Bonica, J. J.: Principles and Practice of Obstetric Analgesia and Anesthesia. Philadelphia, F. A. Davis Company, 1976.

Cugell, D. W.: Pulmonary function in pregnancy; serial observations in normal women. Am. Rev. Tuberc., 67:568–597, 1953.

A Guide for Maternal Death Studies. Committee on Maternal and Child Care of the Council on Medical Service of the American Medical Association, 1957.

Hughes, E. C., Cochrane, N. E., and

Czyz, P. L.: Maternal mortality study. 1970–1975. N.Y. State J. Med., 76(13):2206–2212, 1976.

La Salvia, L. A., and Steffen, E.: Delayed gastric emptying time in labor. Am. J. Obstet. Gynecol., 59:1075–1081, 1950.

Marx, G. F., and Mateo, C. V.: Effects of different oxygen concentrations during general anesthesia for elective cesarean section. Can. Anaesth. Soc. J., 18:587–593, 1971.

Mendelson, C. L.: Aspiration of stomach contents into the lungs during obstetric anesthesia. Am. J. Obstet. Gynecol., 52:191–205, 1946.

National Center for Health Statistics. Vital Statistics of the United States — 1969. Vol. II, Part A — Mortality. Washington, D.C., U.S. Government Printing Office, 1974, pp. 1–50.

Organe, G., and Crawford, J. S.: The contribution of anaesthesia to maternal mortality. Proc. R. Soc.Med., 67:905–910, 1974.

Roberts, R. B., and Shirley, M. A.: Reducing the risk of acid aspiration during cesarean section. Anesth. Analg., 53:859–868, 1974.

Sellick, B. A.: Cricoid pressure to control regurgitation of stomach contents during induction of anaesthesia. Lancet, 2:404–406, 1961.

Taylor, G.: Acid pulmonary aspiration syndrome after antacids. Br. J. Anaesth., 47:615–616, 1975.

Teabeaut, J. R., II: Aspiration of gastric contents. An experimental study. Am. J. Pathol., 28:51–67, 1952.

by OTTO C. PHILLIPS

University of Pittsburgh School of Medicine

AN ENDOTRACHEAL TUBE IS NOT MANDATORY WHEN GENERAL ANESTHESIA IS GIVEN TO A PARTURIENT

I shall address myself to one specific question: "Should the use of an endotracheal tube be mandatory when general anesthesia is given a parturient?" *Mandatory* is defined as follows: Of the nature of a command; authoritatively ordered; obligatory; permitting no option.* We are therefore discussing the advisability of a mandate making it obligatory that all obstetric patients given a general anesthesia have an endotracheal tube inserted, regardless of the circumstances. It is my firm opinion that, at the present time, such a stance would be ill-advised.

My charge is not to discuss the advantages or disadvantages of the use of endotracheal tubes *per se;* my assignment is to advise on the merits of a manifesto prescribing this technique. The choices are simple: either we do or we do not. The decision for or against should be based on anticipated results — the mortality and morbidity with a mandate and without a mandate. There is not now, there has never been, and there is not likely to be a controlled study comparing the results with and without such an edict. My advice must perforce be based on interpolation of data presented in available studies and surveys. Consideration will therefore be given to the following parameters: population, personnel, results without mandate, and results with mandate.

---

*Stein, Jess (ed.): Random House Dictionary of the English Language. New York, Random House, 1966.

Table 1.   Anesthesia for Vaginal Delivery—Personnel

Personnel	Percentage of Anesthesia
Obstetrician*	26.3
Nurse Anesthetist	30.9
Anesthesiologist*	15.4
Other	27.4
TOTAL	100.0

*Includes residents
(Modified from Phillips, O. C., and Frazier, T. M.: Obstetric anesthetic care in the United States. Obstet. Gynecol., *19*:796–802, 1962.)

THE POPULATION

In 1975, there were 3,153,394 births in the United States. A study by the American College of Obstetricians and Gynecologists in 1970 showed that 95 per cent of deliveries were in hospitals and that 80 per cent of the patients involved received some type of anesthesia. (ACOG, 1970). We may therefore state that annually approximately 2,396,579 obstetric patients are given anesthesia. The ACOG review also showed that in 36 per cent of the hospitals inhalation anesthesia was the most frequently used technique for vaginal delivery. Since this survey indicated that in 12 per cent of the hospitals "other" was the most commonly indicated technique and in 22 per cent it was "no predominant type," we can be certain that the number of patients receiving some type of general anesthesia represents a figure appreciably higher than 36 per cent. In a previous survey, Phillips and Frazier (1962) found that over 62 per cent of obstetric patients received general anesthesia. Even accepting the lower figure of 36 per cent, this means that some 871,396 parturients received general anesthesia each year for vaginal delivery. This is the figure that will be used, and these, therefore, are the patients under consideration.

PERSONNEL

In Table 1, we note from the survey of Phillips and Frazier the percentage of anesthesia given by each category of available personnel. Nurse anesthetists were the most frequent contributors, giving 30.9 per cent of the anesthesia for vaginal delivery. Obstetricians were next with 26.3 per cent; anesthesiologists gave 15.4 per cent. It is noteworthy and alarming, but nonetheless factual, that 27.4 per cent of the anesthesia was given by "other" personnel, including delivery room nurses untrained in anesthesia and assorted categories of people similarly untrained in anesthesia. These figures unfortunately cannot be compared with those in the 1970 survey of the American College of Obstetricians and Gynecologists. In the latter report, classification of personnel is presented as the percentage of hospitals in which each component administered most of the anesthesia. It is interesting to note nonetheless that, according to this survey, untrained persons gave most of the anesthesia for vaginal delivery in approximately 20 per cent of the hospitals. It should be pointed out that data from these two reviews differ notably from those reported in a survey by the American Association of Nurse Anesthetists (Mohler, Biggins, and Kaiser, 1965) that indicated that 13.5 per cent of the anesthesia was given by untrained personnel. In this study, however, only 31.8 per cent of the institutions surveyed submitted usable returns, so that the figures are subject to considerable question. In the Phillips and Frazier report (1962), there was a 90.5 per cent response; in the ACOG survey (1970), 73 per cent of the hospitals contributed data. It is possible that in the AANA review only hospitals with the best coverage submitted returns.

Although the above data are not current, they represent the latest available reports on broad surveys with respectable input. Patterns of anesthesia coverage presented in the ACOG survey in 1970 were not strikingly different from those noted in the Phillips and Frazier review in 1962. There are anecdotal reports of progress in departments of some larger obstetrical units, but there is no sound basis for presuming that there have been significant developments in coverage in the country at large during the past 8 to 10 years.

RESULTS WITHOUT MANDATE

Presently, the decision regarding the use of an endotracheal tube rests with the medical judgment of the professional people in attendance, as it has since the introduction of general anesthesia into obstetric practice. Death from aspiration of vomitus is a well-recognized and continuing cause of obstetric mortality; reports in the literature on this problem are numerous. The real magnitude of the problem, however, is difficult to determine. Most reports simply enumerate the deaths on a service without offering the size of the experience from which they occurred. From a few surveys, however, it is possible to project an approximate number of deaths from this cause occurring each year in this country.

Jacoby reported 33,000 obstetric patients receiving general anesthesia.* Intubation was practically never attempted, and regurgitation and aspiration did occur. A dozen patients developed pneumonitis, three requiring bronchoscopy. There were no deaths. Krantz and Edwards (1973) reported on 37,282 vaginal deliveries; 85 per cent of these were accomplished with general anesthesia without an endotracheal tube. There were five cases of aspiration pneumonitis — 1.34 per 10,000 anesthesia procedures. There were no deaths.

These are exceptional experiences, however, and we know that obstetric deaths from aspiration do occur. Twenty years ago, Phillips

*Jacoby, J.: Personal communication.

and associates (1961) reviewed the records of the Maternal Mortality Committee in the City of Baltimore. From among 298,344 live births during the period 1946 to 1958, the incidence of death from aspiration of vomitus was 0.3 per 10,000 live births. Projecting this figure to the 871,396 or more parturients receiving general anesthesia each year, we might anticipate 26.14 deaths annually in this country from aspiration of vomitus. Phillips and associates (1965) also surveyed the deaths associated with 121,831 live births at a community hospital. There were three deaths from aspiration of vomitus, an incidence of 0.25 death per 10,000 live births. Again, projecting this figure for the 871,396 parturients receiving general anesthesia each year, we might anticipate 21.78 deaths annually due to aspiration of vomitus. We shall round off the larger figure and use an estimated 26 deaths each year in subsequent discussion.

RESULTS WITH MANDATE

The proposal that there be a mandate prescribing tracheal intubation for every parturient given general anesthesia for delivery must be based on the assumption that this would eliminate or at least alleviate aspiration of vomitus. The concept may be sound; the practical aspects of implementation are not, and the net results might increase mortality and morbidity. We must be aware that hundreds of thousands of patients have been anesthetized successfully and uneventfully without the use of an endotracheal tube. In an undefined but real number of these cases, complications could have been precipitated by use of muscle relaxants, laryngoscopy, and intubation.

Coleman and Day (1956) stated that "A cuffed endotracheal tube should be used in all cases where general anesthesia is required for obstetric surgery." They further specified that " . . . there is no place in the labour ward for the inexperienced anaesthetist." They support this position with a report on 100 patients, two of whom had problems (regurgitation, difficult intubation), even though the care was in expert hands.

Smiler and associates (1969) are often cited because of their strong stand on this issue. They state, " . . . we feel its use (endotracheal intubation) is mandatory." The naiveté of such a sweeping, universal conclusion should be obvious when we note that it, too, is based on a series of only 100 patients taken care of by anesthesiologists. Credibility is further lost when the authors state that a cuffed endotracheal tube provides 100 per cent protection against aspiration and that " . . . one day the face mask in the delivery room may seem as outmoded as the ether hook." Even today, 10 years later, I would relish the facial expressions if these authors were to walk into a delivery suite to find that face masks were gone.

Keeping in mind the present state of the art and science of anesthesia and utilizing the personnel presently available practicing this art, let us envision the net result of an attempted tracheal intubation on 871,396 parturients each year. We might hope, and may even pre-sume, that some of the 26 patients now dying annually from aspiration would be saved. We might anticipate, however, an interesting and possibly chaotic scenario with the 871,370 parturients who would survive anyway but for whom intubation must be attempted because of mandate. In a recent report on maternal deaths in England and Wales (Crawford, 1972), there were 50 deaths associated with anesthesia. Five of these patients died from aspiration of gastric contents, and in four, the patient's trachea had been intubated. Difficulties with intubation actually initiated the progress toward death in 10 cases.

Little information is available regarding the magnitude of the problems associated with tracheal intubation or the percentage of cases presenting difficulty. In a prospective review of 1195 intubations, Phillips and Duerksen (1973) reported difficulties due to anatomic aberrations in 19 per cent of the cases, and multiple attempts at intubation were required in 18 per cent. In a retrospective survey of 556 cases, Angiulo and Gibbs accumulated data on difficulty in intubation in 4.9 per cent of the patients; the study encompassed both surgical and obstetric (cesarean section) patients.* The procedures were performed by resident anesthesiologists and nurse anesthetist trainees. The personnel involved in the problem intubations had had an average of 16 months of formal training, and staff anesthesiologists were available for supervision.

If the experience of Angiulo and Gibbs were to be applied to the 871,396 parturients receiving general anesthesia for vaginal delivery, we might anticipate that in about 42,697 parturients each year difficulty would be encountered with tracheal intubation — if these patients were all in the hands of persons with formal training. Recall that 27.4 per cent of obstetric anesthesia is given by "other" or untrained personnel. We can only conjecture as to the results should these people attempt to intubate the tracheas of 238,762 parturients each year owing to a mandatory policy. We could surpass the record in the Crawford report (1972), in which 20 per cent of the obstetric deaths associated with anesthesia were initiated by difficulties at attempted tracheal intubation.

SUMMARY AND CONCLUSIONS

Among the 3,153,394 mothers delivered each year in this country, 2,396,579 (80 per cent) receive anesthesia, 871,396 (35 per cent) of these receiving general anesthesia.

Aspiration of vomitus is a continuing problem in anesthesia, particularly with the obstetric patient. Presuming some consistency between the incidence of death in regional and institutional studies and that on a national level, we might anticipate that there are about 26 deaths annually among obstetric patients from aspiration alone. The proper placement of an endotracheal tube is an important contribution toward minimizing this hazard.

---

*Angiulo, J. P., and Gibbs, C. P.: Unpublished data.

In the hands of trained personnel, some difficulty is encountered with tracheal intubation in about 5 per cent of the cases. Over 25 per cent of the anesthesia for obstetric patients is given by "other" personnel — general duty nurses, medical students, orderlies. If the use of an endotracheal tube were mandatory for all parturients receiving general anesthesia, this would mean that intubation would be attempted on 871,396 parturients each year, on 238,762 by untrained personnel. Since regurgitation and laryngospasm can be triggered by inept efforts at tracheal intubation, we might suspect a higher incidence of morbidity and mortality occurring from inept efforts than the 26 deaths per year currently resulting from aspiration of vomitus.

Although it is recommended that expert anesthesia personnel should be present for every delivery, currently this is simply not the case. Under the prevailing circumstances, the dangers of vomiting are real but probably overestimated, and the hazards of tracheal intubation are either underestimated or possibly not even considered.

An additional consideration to be kept in mind is that a mandate dictating tracheal intubation with all general anesthetics in parturients would render attendants medicolegally vulnerable following general anesthesia without use of a tube even if there were no problems. The anesthesia personnel might be (and have been) accused of not following dictated and "accepted" standards and therefore of being guilty of negligence.

Mandatory use of an endotracheal tube in every general anesthesia administered to parturients would probably increase the risk — to both patients and attendants.

REFERENCES

American College of Obstetricians and Gynecologists: National Study of Maternity Care: Survey of Obstetric Practice and Associated Services in Hospitals in the United States. Chicago, ACOG, 1970.

Coleman, D. J., and Day, B. L.: Anaesthesia for operative obstetrics; value of cuffed endotracheal tube. Lancet, 1:708–709, 1956.

Crawford, J. S.: Maternal mortality associated with anaesthesia. Lancet, 2:918–919, 1972.

Krantz, M. L., and Edwards, W. L.: The incidence of nonfatal aspiration in obstetric patients. Anesthesiology, 39:359, 1973.

Mohler, C. E., Biggins, D. E., and Kaiser, J. A.: Survey of anesthesia service:1965 — a ten-year comparison. J. Am. Assoc. Nurse Anesthetists 33:298–308, 1965.

Phillips, O. C., Frazier, T. M., Davis, G. H., and Nelson, A. T.: The role of anesthesia in obstetric mortality. Anesth. Analg., 40:557–566, 1961.

Phillips, O. C., and Frazier, T. M.: Obstetric anesthetic care in the United States. Obstet. Gynecol., 19:796–802, 1962.

Phillips, O. C., Hulka, J., Vincent, M., and Christy, W. C.: Obstetric mortality: A 26-year survey. Obstet. Gynecol., 25:217–222, 1965.

Phillips, O. C., and Duerksen, R. L.: Endotracheal intubation: A new blade for direct laryngoscopy. Anesth. Analg., 52:691–698, 1973.

Smiler, B. G., Goldberger, R., Sivak, B. J., and Brown, E. M.: Routine endotracheal intubation in obstetrics. Am. J. Obstet Gynecol., 103:947–949, 1969.

ENDOTRACHEAL ANESTHESIA IN PARTURIENTS

EDITORIAL COMMENT

A few years ago, some of us older anesthesiologists were a bit startled by the promulgation of mandatory endotracheal anesthesia if a parturient required or was to be given general anesthesia for vaginal delivery. Many of us recalled thousands of general anesthetics given parturients with minimal difficulty and without mortality. Since the newer generation is adamant, the question is worth pursuing.

Few argue the desirability of regional anesthetic techniques for the parturient, if trained personnel are available. Nor would one question that the practice of obstetrics has changed: mothers are better prepared for both delivery and anesthesia for delivery, operative intervention is more common than was true several decades ago, and high-risk pregnancies are more likely to be referred to academic medicine centers. Nonetheless, as Phillips points out, the last available data would suggest that one third of parturients receive general anesthesia and that an appreciable proportion will be attended by individuals with no or limited training in anesthetics. Although the data are outdated and the need for an accurate updated assessment is obvious, the point is clear: for a variety of reasons, thousands of parturients will continue to receive general anesthesia for vaginal delivery, and some will be attended by individuals not proficient in tracheal intubation. Phillips is concerned about the comparative morbidity of parturients with and without attempted tracheal intubation; he doesn't sound convinced that mortality would be less with an endotracheal tube.

Given the best of all obstetric worlds, the technique DeVore espouses, and the immediate availability of anesthesiologists or nurse anesthetists, both presumably skilled in tracheal intubation, would the mortality following general endotracheal anesthesia for vaginal delivery be less than if general anesthesia were given without a tracheal tube? I am not convinced it would be but look forward to data to prove the point either way. Tracheal intubation is not innocuous and is associated with its own morbidity and mortality. Muscle relaxants are also associated with complications; 1 in 2000 patients is likely to develop apnea after succinylcholine, and the treatment of apnea has its hazards.

The insertion of an endotracheal tube during general anesthesia for vaginal delivery is a judgmental decision; the gain must be equated against the risks involved. Mandated tracheal intubation may not be in either the patient's or the physician's best interests.

129

Part 7

CHOICE OF ANESTHESIA FOR CORONARY BYPASS OPERATIONS

THE PROPOSITION:

Halothane anesthesia is preferable to morphine for coronary bypass operations.

ALTERNATIVE POINTS OF VIEW:

By Carolyn J. Wilkinson
By C. R. Stephen, G. R. Weygandt, E. A. Kopman

EDITORIAL COMMENT

by CAROLYN J. WILKINSON

Northwestern University Medical School

HALOTHANE ANESTHESIA IS PREFERABLE TO MORPHINE

Arteriosclerotic heart disease is still the major cause of death in the United States. It is incurable and is responsible for more than 1,000,000 myocardial infarctions and 600,000 deaths each year. Coronary arteriosclerosis leads to myocardial ischemia and oxygen deprivation secondary to the reduced perfusion. The disease rarely involves only one coronary artery and impairment of flow extends into small vessels. The extent of myocardial infarction after coronary occlusion depends on the balance between the oxygen supply to and the demand of the myocardium. With the advent of surgical measures for treating coronary artery disease, approximately 80,000 patients are being anesthetized annually for aortocoronary bypass operations, now the most prevalent cardiac surgical procedure in the United States.

The indications for an aortocoronary bypass operation vary among surgeons and cardiologists, although most would accept a severe, disabling, chronic, stable angina pectoris that is unresponsive to medical treatment as an indication for coronary arteriography. If arteriography shows two- or three-vessel coronary artery disease and good ventricular function, a 75 per cent chance of symptomatic improvement and an operative risk of less than 5 per cent may be expected with aortocoronary bypass surgery (ACBS). Such surgery is now advocated for patients with unstable angina pectoris or healed myocardial infarctions with left ventricular aneurysms and for some patients with arteriographic evidence of severe coronary artery disease without history of infarction and little or no angina.

The statistics for the risks of operation and improvement of ventricular function and life expectancy vary, a cause for controversy between cardiologists and surgeons. The Veterans Administration Cooperative Study of patients with severe obstruction of the left main coronary artery (Takaro et al., 1976) showed that ACBS *did* improve the survival rate of these patients. The preliminary results of the VA

133

Cooperative Study of patients with chronic stable angina (excluding those with obstructive disease of the left main coronary artery) (Murphy et al., 1977), however, showed no statistically significant difference in survival rate between medically and surgically treated patients, although operation reduced the incidence of severe angina. All studies reported so far comparing the effectiveness of ACBS and medical therapy for angina pectoris have concluded that surgery is effective in reducing symptoms but that it does not significantly improve survival except in patients with obstruction of the left main coronary artery.

In the VA Cooperative Study, the anesthetic technique was not mentioned. Most knowledge of cardiovascular physiology and pharmacology is based on findings obtained from *anesthetized* animals. Too many researchers have assumed that general anesthesia does not alter the response of the circulation to physiologic stresses or pharmacologic interventions and therefore did not modify the conclusions derived from experiments. Anesthetics and adjuvants do have direct or indirect effects upon the heart and circulation; therefore, the anesthesiologist should use an anesthetic technique that minimally impairs cardiac function, alleviates angina or heart failure, and provides the smoothest recovery postoperatively.

Controversy also exists among anesthesiologists as to the choice of anesthetic technique for ACBS. Several principal anesthetic agents are in vogue for patients, the two most popular being the inhalation agent halothane and the intravenous agent morphine, with or without nitrous oxide.

Unfortunately, few data are available concerning current anesthetic practices for cardiac surgery. In 1972, Dalton published data from 63 cardiac surgical centers in Canada and the United States. Of the 14,505 patients for open heart operations reported (the types of surgical procedure were not differentiated), 43 per cent were anesthetized with halothane, 24 per cent with morphine, and 33 per cent with a variety of agents, such as fluroxene, methoxyflurane, nitrous oxide–relaxants, and neuroleptanalgesia (Dalton, 1972). Despite the fact that this study contains the only known survey of various anesthetics used for cardiac surgery, it is not applicable to the situation today. I would guess that halothane is the most commonly used anesthetic agent for cardiac surgery and may be preferred for coronary bypass grafts. There are no data to support this statement.

Except for a prospective random comparison of halothane and morphine for open heart surgery in 1973 (Conahan, 3rd, et al., 1973), there are no published studies comparing the effects of morphine and halothane under cardiac surgical conditions. This study, confined to 128 patients with valvular disease, reported hemodynamic differences between the agents, but comparisons of mortality rates, duration of hospital stay, postoperative stay in the intensive care unit, and need for supplementary inotropic drugs did not demonstrate superiority of one agent to the other.

What, then, influences a cardiac anesthesiologist to choose one agent over another, and why has halothane continued to be popular for ACBS? Does it really matter what agents are used or are skilled monitoring and vigilance the only important factors? Before comparing the two anesthetic agents, I would like to discuss factors that control the balance between myocardial oxygen supply and demand and are basic to understanding the reasons for choice of an agent.

FACTORS AFFECTING MYOCARDIAL OXYGEN SUPPLY AND DEMAND

The heart is an aerobic organ. Its oxygen supply and demand are delicately balanced by autoregulation within the myocardium (Fig. 1). The major determinants of myocardial oxygen supply are: (1) coronary blood flow, (2) ventricular intramural pressure, and (3) oxygen content of arterial blood.

In simplest terms, coronary blood flow is determined by the relationship between coronary vascular resistance and coronary pressure gradient.

$$Q = \frac{P_1 - P_2}{R}$$

Q = coronary blood flow
$P_1 - P_2$ = coronary vascular pressure gradient (the difference between aortic root diastolic pressure and ventricular diastolic pressure, or intramyocardial pressure)
R = resistance to flow

Coronary vascular resistance is a function of blood viscosity and the anatomy of the coronary circulation. High viscosity or diseased small coronary arteries increase the resistance and diminish blood

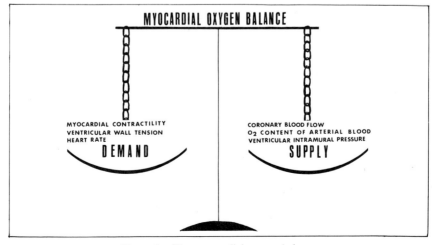

Figure 1. The myocardial oxygen balance.

flow, especially to the subendocardium, a sensitive layer highly vulnerable to ischemia and greatly affected by decreased perfusion pressure and coronary blood flow. This is the area where myocardial ischemia and necrosis appear in patients who had inadequate intraoperative coronary perfusion or myocardial protection.

Coronary vascular resistance is autoregulated; when demand for oxygen increases, vasodilation occurs and blood flow increases. Diseased coronary arteries are incapable of responding to the vasodilatory effects of hypoxia. In myocardial ischemia, the heart releases factors, such as potassium and adenosine, that maintain near maximal coronary vasodilation; coronary blood flow then becomes pressure-dependent.

During cardiopulmonary bypass, intramyocardial (or intramural) pressure may be abnormally high because of ventricular hypertrophy or edema secondary to myocardial injury. Intramyocardial pressure also influences coronary blood flow, especially to the endocardium.

Adequate arterial oxygen content is essential for myocardial oxygenation, but the hemodilution of cardiopulmonary bypass is well tolerated and does not seem to increase the severity of ischemia. The reduced viscosity of the blood may increase collateral flow to the myocardium.

The major determinants of myocardial oxygen demand are as follows (Fig. 1): (1) Ventricular wall tension, (2) heart rate, and (3) myocardial contractility. Ventricular wall tension (T) is *directly* related to the ventricular intracavitary systolic pressure (P) and to the radius of the ventricle (R). An increase in ventricular intracavitary pressure or radius raises the wall tension and myocardial oxygen consumption, and any reduction decreases myocardial oxygen consumption ($T = P \times R$ — Laplace's law). Pressure work by the myocardium requires a greater expenditure of oxygen than flow work does (Braunwald, 1969).

Myocardial oxygen consumption is directly proportional to changes in heart rate, given otherwise stable conditions. Perfusion of the left ventricle diminishes during systole through mechanical compression of the coronary vessels by the contracting myocardium. Coronary perfusion is phasic, in contrast to most other tissues in which perfusion is continuous. During diastole, blood flow increases rapidly. Acceleration of heart rate occurs at the expense of the diastolic interval. Since coronary blood flows mainly in diastole, a fast heart rate may increase myocardial oxygen consumption beyond the capacity of a diseased arterial system. A readily measured hemodynamic product of heart rate and systolic blood pressure, the rate pressure product ($HR \times SBP = RPP$), correlates well with coronary blood flow and myocardial oxygen consumption (Nelson et al., 1974). Ischemic electrocardiographic changes are more common when the RPP exceeds 15,000 to 20,000.

Myocardial contractility is a nebulous term, but the inotropic state of the myocardium is best expressed as the *maximal velocity* at which the left ventricle contracts during systole (Parmley and Sonnenblick, 1970). Increasing myocardial contractility increases oxygen demand;

conversely, decreased contractility decreases demand. This should be kept in mind when anesthetics or adjuvants are used in patients with myocardial ischemia. Beta-adrenergic stimulants increase contractility and oxygen demand. Diuretics, however, decrease the left ventricular radius by lessening the preload (ventricular volume) through blood volume depletion. Beta-adrenergic blockers decrease contractility, blood pressure, heart rate, and left ventricular intracavitary pressure. Nitroglycerin decreases preload, reducing intramyocardial tension. Diuretics, β-adrenergic blockers, and nitroglycerin decrease the oxygen demand of the myocardium.

The regulation of cardiac output is complex but is principally determined by heart rate and stroke volume. The contractile state is only one of the determinants of the heart's ability to eject blood, and one cannot assume that output will be normal if the contractile state is normal and vice versa. Stroke volume, a function of the extent of myocardial fiber shortening, is dependent on

1. *Preload* — filling volume that determines the heart muscle fiber end diastolic length
2. *Afterload* — intramyocardial systolic tension
3. *Contractility* — inotropic state of myocardium

At any given level of contractility, the extent of myocardial fiber shortening varies directly with the preload and inversely with the afterload. Only when the afterload and preload remain constant will the stroke volume depend directly on the contractile state of the heart.

When contractility is impaired, cardiac output can be maintained by increasing either heart rate or stroke volume through the Frank-Starling mechanism. Increases in filling volume (preload) augment stroke volume. The relationship between filling volume (or pressure) and stroke work is best expressed by the ventricular function curve (Fig. 2). Additional stroke work occurs in the normal heart when filling pressures are increased up to 20 mm. Hg.

Cardiac output in a patient with normal ventricular contraction is far more dependent on the influence of peripheral factors on ventric-

Figure 2. Ventricular function curve of the left ventricle (LV). (From Braunwald, R. E., Jr.: Current concepts in cardiology, practical cardiac hemodynamics. N. Engl. J. Med., *296*:203–206, 1977.)

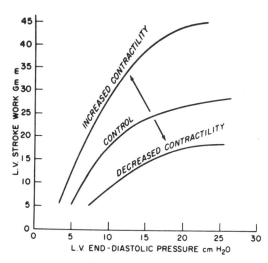

ular preload and afterload than on such central factors as contractile state of the myocardium (Braunwald, 1971). Only in the last few years have the effects of afterload been considered significant in left ventricular heart failure.

Anesthesiologists should have these physiologic principles clearly in mind when attempting to evaluate the effects of anesthetics and techniques during cardiac surgical procedures.

COMPARISON OF ANESTHETIC TECHNIQUES

The ideal anesthetic for ACBS does not exist. An agent that fits the following criteria would be most desirable:
1. Ease of regulating depth of anesthesia
2. Depression of the sympathoadrenal system by the anesthetic
3. Minimal cardiac arrhythmias
4. Ease of control of cardiovascular reflexes
5. Minimal increase in heart rate
6. Minimal changes in myocardial contractility
7. Minimal change in preload
8. Minimal increase in afterload

Let us now consider whether morphine and halothane fulfill these criteria.

Morphine

Narcotics were first recommended as general anesthetics for cardiac surgery by Bailey in 1958. Lowenstein popularized the use of large doses (0.5–3 mg./kg.) of morphine for cardiac surgery in 1969, the idea arising from observations made during the postoperative management of cardiac surgical patients. Morphine was used in large doses to depress respiratory drive and increase tolerance of endotracheal tubes for elective mechanical ventilation (Lowenstein, 1971). Drew, Dripps, and Comroe in 1946 had shown that morphine, 10 to 30 mg., had little effect on the circulation in *normal supine subjects;* however, when supine patients were tilted toward an erect position, blood pressure dropped substantially. The study clearly acknowledged the deleterious circulatory effects of morphine: "It is obvious that morphine produces circulatory changes in man, but as a rule, these changes are revealed only when a strain is placed upon the cardiovascular system. These strains are analogous to tilting, hypertension, certain types of heart disease and any impairment in the vascular regulatory mechanism" (Drew, Dripps, and Comroe, 1946). Lowenstein's data revealed that a 2 mg. per kg. dose of morphine did not affect the cardiac output, systemic vascular resistance, blood pressure, central venous pressure, or heart rate in normal supine subjects. Patients with aortic valvular disease, however, responded with an initial decrease in systemic vascular resistance and a 25 per cent to 50 per cent increase in cardiac index.

After the publication of Lowenstein's article, anesthesiologists were eager to jump on the "morphine band wagon" and use a technique with so few deleterious effects on the heart. Intravenous infusions of epinephrine were often advocated during induction to prevent severe hypotension from morphine. Hypertension appearing during cardiopulmonary bypass often required treatment with vasodilators. The popularity of the morphine technique is amazing because morphine is not an anesthetic and in the 2 mg. per kg. dose range does not produce amnesia or unconsciousness in healthy individuals unless nitrous oxide is added (Wong et al., 1973).

Despite extensive clinical and laboratory studies, morphine's mechanism of action on the cardiovascular system is still poorly understood and therefore subject to controversy. The published data reveal little direct depression of contractility in the blood-perfused mammalian heart (Flacke, 1965) or intact animal (Schmidt and Livingstone, 1933); however, there are data to suggest that morphine may depress contractility in saline-perfused hearts (Schmidt and Livingstone, 1933) and myocardial tissue (Goldburg and Padget, 1969).

The best studies of the effects of morphine on ventricular function and peripheral circulation were done respectively by Vasco and associates (1966a and b) and by Henney and associates (1966). The results of both studies are summarized diagramatically in Figure 3. After the injection of morphine (1 mg./kg.) during the preparation for a right heart bypass in a dog, Vasco (1966b) demonstrated a gradual improvement of myocardial contractile force, a decrease in peripheral vascular resistance, and an increase in the capacity of the peripheral vascular bed, resulting in reduced systemic venous return. The overall response is considered a pharmacologic "phlebotomy" and probably accounts for the effectiveness of morphine in the treatment of pulmonary edema.

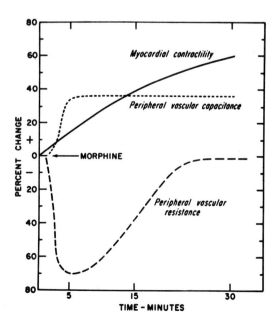

Figure 3. Diagrammatic representation of the independent effects of morphine on the contractile state of the heart and on the peripheral vascular bed. (From Vasco, J. S., Henney, R. P., Oldham, H. N., et al.: Mechanisms of action of morphine in the treatment of experimental pulmonary edema. Am. J. Cardiol., *18*:876–883, 1966.)

The positive inotropic effect on the heart may be an indirect result of release of catecholamines secondary to its action on the spinal cord and supraspinal centers. Vasco (1966a) reports that the action of morphine on contractile force is abolished by beta blockade and by adrenalectomy.

The decrease in total peripheral vascular resistance after intravenous morphine disappears, and values return to, or exceed, control levels after 20 to 30 minutes. The mechanism most likely is a reflexly decreased α-adrenergic tone, since morphine does not act as a peripheral α-adrenergic blocker but seems to attenuate sympathetic discharge at the central nervous system level (Zelis, 1974). No acceptable explanation exists for the prolonged effect on capacitance. Existing data exclude histamine as a major factor in the vasodilation. These studies, however, were carried out in dogs. Although their physiologic responses to morphine resemble those of man, in dogs at least 0.5 mg. per kg. of intravenous morphine is needed to produce a significant effect on the circulation.

Further evidence of catecholamine release during morphine anesthesia and cardiac surgery has been produced by Hasbrouck and associates (1970), who found a 1.3 μg. per liter increase in catecholamines with a morphine dose of 2 mg. per kg. (Hasbrouck, 1970).

Plasma angiotensin II levels rise substantially during morphine-nitrous oxide anesthesia in cardiopulmonary bypass (Taylor et al., 1977). The renin-angiotensin system is thought to play an important role in causing the peripheral vasoconstriction and hypertension seen during cardiopulmonary bypass when morphine is the principal agent. Increases in either catecholamines or angiotensin II may raise myocardial oxygen consumption and increase peripheral vasoconstriction. These may also be important in the production of the low output syndrome and subendocardial ischemia.

Controversy also surrounds the effect of morphine on coronary blood flow. Vatner and associates observed a decrease in coronary blood flow and vasoconstriction after 2 mg. per kg. doses of morphine in awake dogs, even when contractility was elevated and heart rate constant. When the same animals were anesthetized with pentobarbital and given morphine, only coronary vasodilation occurred (Vatner, 1975). Grover and associates found little change in dogs on cardiac bypass with up to 2 mg. per kg. morphine and significant increases in coronary blood flow with 3 to 5 mg. per kg. (Grover et al., 1976).

In Figure 4, some of the cardiovascular parameters recorded during cardiac surgery and morphine anesthesia are summarized. The addition of nitrous oxide reverses the direction of these parameters (Wong et al., 1973; Stoelting and Gibbs, 1973; Lappas et al., 1975). All investigators observed a decrease in cardiac index, but the effect on stroke volume was variable. These data suggest that nitrous oxide depresses left ventricular performance when administered to patients who have received large doses of morphine for heart surgery.

Morphine in the 3 mg. per kg. dose may be an adequate amnesic for heart surgery in critically ill patients, but such is not the case in healthier patients. The effects of very large doses of morphine (8–11

SUBJECTS	Drug&Dose	CI	SV	SVR	CVP	BP	HR
LOWENSTEIN, 1969 AORTIC VALVES	MS 1 mg/kg	↑50%	↑	↓	↑	—	—
NORMAL	MS 1 mg/kg	—		—	—	—	—
WONG, 1973 10 NORMAL	MS 2 mg/kg & N₂O 70%	↑25%	↑	↓	↑	—	←
AFTER 1 HR....	MS 1 mg/kg	↓30%	↓	↑30%	←	—	→
STOELTING, 1973 7 VALVES AFTER 30 MIN....	MS 1 mg/kg & N₂O 60%	←	←←	↓←	↑	→→	|→→
7 CAB AFTER 30 MIN....	MS 1 mg/kg & N₂O 60%	→←	←	→←	←	→→	→→
LAPAS, 1975 12 CAB	MS 2 mg/kg & N₂O 50%	→	→			→	
MC DERMOTT, 1974 16 VALVES or CAB	MS 2 mg/kg & N₂O 10-50%	→	↓	←	—	↓	—

Figure 4. Cardiovascular parameters during morphine anesthesia.

KEY:

CI   — cardiac index
SV   — stroke volume
SVR — systemic vascular resistance
CVP — central venous pressure
BP   — arterial blood pressure
HR   — heart rate

mg./kg.) have therefore been studied (Stanley et al., 1973). Patients treated in this manner required over 2 1/2 times more blood, produced significantly less urine during bypass, and needed significantly more sodium bicarbonate to avoid base deficits. Postoperatively, they needed more crystalloids to maintain urinary output.

In another study comparing blood requirements during morphine-nitrous oxide and halothane-nitrous oxide anesthesia for open-heart surgery (Stanley et al., 1974), patients receiving morphine (1–4 mg./kg.) needed more than twice the amount of blood during bypass, intraoperatively, and the first 24 hours postoperatively than did those given halothane. No significant difference appeared during and after operation between the amounts of crystalloid administered or the amounts of urine produced in the two groups of patients having similar operations. A possible explanation for the increased blood requirement in the patients receiving morphine is likely the increase in vascular capacitance.

Morphine does have some advantages. It lacks arrhythmogenic properties, does not depress myocardial contractility, and does not affect heart rate appreciably. Nevertheless, morphine cannot be used alone, and many other drugs are needed to support and counteract its effects.

Halothane

Halothane was introduced into clinical practice at about the same time as the pump oxygenator. Surgical anesthesia was easily regulated by the administration of 0.5 per cent to 2 per cent halothane in oxygen, and halothane gained wide acceptance as a safe nonexplosive anesthetic for cardiac surgery. The cardiovascular parameters during halothane anesthesia are summarized in Figure 5. The depressive effects on cardiac output are caused by a direct dose-dependent depression of cardiac contractility (Eger, 2d, et al., 1970). Halothane lacks the sympathoadrenal stimulation caused by morphine during cardiopulmonary bypass (Anton, Gravenstein, and Wheat, 1964). Since the contractile state of the myocardium is a major determinant of myocardial oxygen consumption, the decrease in both contractility and adrenergic activity may be advantageous in the ischemic myocardium. In fact, in the nonfailing canine heart, halothane decreases the severity of experimentally induced myocardial ischemia, suggesting that halothane favorably influences the relationship between myocardial oxygen supply and demand when coronary blood flow is limited (Bland and Lowenstein, 1976).

Metabolic acidosis during anesthesia suggests inadequate blood flow and oxygen delivery to the tissues. Blood gas measurements are often used as indirect measurement of adequate blood flow during cardiopulmonary bypass. In a comparison of neuroleptic, narcotic, and halothane anesthetic techniques, metabolic acidosis during and after cardiopulmonary bypass was least with halothane (Maunuksela, 1977).

	SUBJECTS	HALOTHANE	CI	SV	SVR	CVP	BP	HR
McHAFFEY, 1961	18 DOGS	3%	↓	↓	→		↓59%	
	10 PATIENTS	0.6-3%	↓	↓	→			
SEVERINGHAUS, 1958	9 VOLUNTEERS	1.5%	↓31%	↓35%	↑18%	↑	↓25%	—
EGER, 1971	11 VOLUNTEERS	.84% (1st HR.)	↓	↓	—	↓	→	—
		.84% (after 4-5 HRS.)	↑20-40%	↑		↓		↑

Figure 5. Cardiovascular parameters during halothane anesthesia.

Studies by Grover and associates (1976) and Vatner and Smith (1974) have shown little change in coronary blood flow in dogs anesthetized with 0.5 to 1.5 per cent halothane.

SUMMARY

Morphine in large doses became popular for cardiac surgery because myocardial contractility in the intact heart is not depressed. Serious hypotension can occur during induction with morphine, however, because of decreased peripheral vascular resistance and increased vascular capacitance. During cardiopulmonary bypass, hypertension develops in over one third of patients, requiring vasodilator therapy. The hypertension is associated with increased plasma angiotensin II and catecholamine levels, known to augment myocardial oxygen consumption.

Morphine does not consistently cause loss of consciousness without nitrous oxide supplementation. More blood is required during and after bypass when morphine is used than when halothane is used. The rare postoperative complication of "halothane" hepatitis does not compare with the more frequent occurrence of hepatitis after blood transfusions. Mechanical ventilation is necessary postoperatively with large doses of morphine and seldom required with halothane. Morphine must be entirely metabolized whereas halothane is mostly eliminated from the body.

Studies comparing the effects of halothane and morphine on myocardial oxygen consumption during ACBS anesthesia have not been published. These are essential before a final conclusion can be made concerning the superiority of one agent to the other. In the meanwhile, depression of contractility should not be considered a disadvantage if the depression is accompanied by a decrease in oxygen demand.

Anesthesia is still an art, and the basis for the choice of anesthetic technique for coronary bypass surgery remains the skill of the anesthesiologist in using specific agents. According to existing data, halothane has more advantages. I would predict that the use of morphine as the principal anesthetic for cardiac surgery will not continue for many more years.

REFERENCES

Anton, A. H., Gravenstein, J. S., and Wheat, M. W.: Extracorporeal circulation and endogenous epinephrine in plasma, atrium and urine in man — a comparison of halothane and ether. Anesthesiology, 25:262–269, 1964.

Bailey, P., Gerbode, F., and Garlington, L.: An anesthetic technique for cardiac surgery which utilized 100% oxygen as the only inhalant. Arch. Surg., 76:437–440, 1958.

Bland, H. L., and Lowenstein, E.: Halothane induced decrease in experimental myocardial ischemia in the non-failing canine heart. Anesthesiology, 45:287–293, 1976.

Braunwald, E., Ross, J. R., and Sonnenblick, E. H.: Mechanisms of Contraction of the Normal and Failing Heart. Boston, Little, Brown & Co., 1968, p. 57.

Braunwald, E.: The determinants of myocardial oxygen consumption. Physiologist, *12*:65–93, 1969.

Braunwald, E.: On the difference between the heart's output and its contractile state. Circulation, *43*: 171–174, 1971.

Conahan, T. J., 3d, Ominsky, A. G., Wollman, H., and Stroth, R. A.: A prospective random comparison of halothane and morphine for open heart anesthesia: one year's experience. Anesthesiology, *38*:528–535, 1973.

Dalton, B.: Anesthesia for cardiac surgery. Anesthesiology, *36*:521–522, 1972.

Drew, J. H., Dripps, R. D., and Comroe, J. H., Jr.: Clinical studies on morphine; effect of morphine upon circulation of man and upon circulatory and respiratory responses to tilting. Anesthesiology, 7:44–61, 1946.

Eger, E. I., 2d, Smith, N. T., Stoelting, R. K., Cullen, D. J., et al.: Cardiovascular effects of halothane in man. Anesthesiology, *2*:396–409, 1970.

Eger, E. I., Smith, N. T., Cullen, D. H., Cullen, B. F., and Gregory, G. A.: A comparison of the cardiovascular effects of halothane, fluroxene, ether and cyclopropane in man. Anesthesiology, *19*:165–177, 1958.

Flacke, W.: Some actions of morphine on the circulation. Fed. Proc., *24*:613, 1965.

Goldburg, A. H., and Padget, C. H.: Comparative effects of morphine and fentanyl on isolated heart muscle. Anesth. Analg., *48*:978–982, 1969.

Grover, F. L., Webb, G. E., Bevis, V., and Fewel, J. G.: Effects of morphine and halothane anesthesia on coronary blood flow. Ann. Thorac. Surg., *22*:429–435, 1976.

Hasbrouck, J. D.: Morphine anesthesia for open heart surgery. Ann. Thorac. Surg., *10*:364–369, 1970.

Henney, R. P., Vasko, J. S., Brawley, R. K., Oldham, H. N., and Morrow, A. G.: The effects of mor-

phine on the resistance and capacitance vessels of the peripheral circulation. Am. Heart J., *72*:242–250, 1966.

Lappas, D. G., Geha, D., Fischer, J. E., Laver, M. B., and Lowenstein, E.: Filling pressures of the heart and pulmonary circulation of the patient with coronary-artery disease after large intravenous doses of morphine. Anesthesiology, *42*:153–159, 1975.

Lowenstein, E., Hallowell, P., Levin, F. H., Daggett, W. M., Austin, G., and Laver, M. D.: Cardiovascular responses to large doses of intravenous morphine in man. N. Engl. J. Med., *281*:1389–1393, 1969.

Lowenstein, E.: Morphine "anesthesia" — a perspective. Anesthesiology, *35*:563–565, 1971.

Mahaffey, J. C., Aldinger, E. E., Sprouse, J. H., Darby, T. D., and Thrower, W. B.: The cardiovascular effects of halothane. Anesthesiology, *22*:982–986, 1961.

Maunuksela, Eeva-Liisa: Hemodynamic responses to different anesthetics during open-heart surgery. Acta Anaesthesiol. Scand., *65*(Supplement):1–71, 1977.

McDermott, R. W., and Stanley, T. H.: The cardiovascular effects of low concentrations of nitrous oxide during morphine anesthesia. Anesthesiology, *41*:89–91, 1974.

Murphy, M. L., Hultgren, H. N., Detre, K., Thomsen, P. H., Takaro, T., et al.: Treatment of chronic stable angina. A preliminary report of survival data of the randomized Veterans Administration cooperative study. N. Engl. J. Med., *297*:621–627, 1977.

Nelson, R. R., Gobel, F. L., Jorgensen, C. R., Wang, K., Wang, Y., and Taylor, H. L.: Hemodynamic predictors of myocardial oxygen consumption during static and dynamic exercise. Circulation, *50*:1179–1189, 1974.

Parmley, W. W., and Sonnenblick, E. H.: Reevaluation of V max as an index of contractile state: An analysis of different muscle models. Circulation, *42*(Supplement III):3–115, 1970.

Schmidt, C. L., and Livingston, A. E.: The action of morphine on the mammalian circulation. J. Pharmacol. Exp. Ther., *47*:411–441, 1933.

Severinghaus, J. W., and Cullen, S. C.: Depression of myocardium and body oxygen consumption with fluothane. Anesthesiology, *19*:165–177, 1958.

Stanley, T. H., Gray, N. H,, Stanford, W., et al.: The effects of high-dose morphine on fluid and blood requirements in open-heart operations. Anesthesiology, *38*:536–541, 1973.

Stanley, T. H., Gray, N. H., Isern-Amaral, J. H., and Patton, C.: Comparison of blood requirements during morphine and halothane anesthesia for open-heart surgery. Anesthesiology, *41*:34–38, 1974.

Stoelting, R. K., and Gibbs, P. S.: Hemodynamic effects of morphine and morphine-nitrous oxide in valvular heart disease and coronary-artery disease. Anesthesiology, *38*:45–52, 1973.

Takaro, T., Hultgren, N. H., Lipton, M. J., et al.: The VA cooperative randomized study of surgery for coronary arterial occlusive disease. II. Subgroup with significant left main lesions. Circulation, *54*(Supplement 3):III 107–117, 1976.

Taylor, K. M., Morton, I. J., Brown, J. J., Bain, W. H., and Caves, P. K.: Hypertension and the renin-angiotension system following open-heart surgery. J. Thorac.

Cardiovasc. Surg., *74*:849–845, 1977.

Vasco, J. S., Henney, R. P., Brawley, R. K., Oldham, H. N., and Morrow, A. G.: The effects of morphine on ventricular function and myocardial contractile force. Am. J. Physiol., *210*:329–334, 1966a.

Vasco, J. S., Henney, R. P., Oldham, H. N., Brawley, R. K., and Marrow, A. G.: Mechanism of action of morphine in the treatment of experimental pulmonary edema. Am. J. Cardiol., *18*:876–883, 1966b.

Vatner, S., F., and Smith, N. T.: Effects of halothane on left ventricular function and distribution of regional blood flow in dogs and primates. Circ. Res., *34*:155–167, 1974.

Vatner, S. F., Marsh, J. D., and Swain, J. A.: Effects of morphine on coronary and left ventricular dynamics in conscious dogs. J. Clin. Invest., *55*:207–217, 1975.

Wong, K. C., Martin, W. E., Horbein, T. F., Freund, F. G., and Everett, J.: Cardiovascular effects of morphine sulphate with oxygen and nitrous oxide in man. Anesthesiology, *30*:542–549, 1973.

Zelis, R., Mansour, E. J., Capone, R. J., and Mason, D. T.: The cardiovascular effects of morphine. Peripheral capacitance and resistance vessels in human subjects. J. Clin. Invest., *54*:1247–1255, 1974.

by C. R. STEPHEN

G. R. WEYGANDT

E. A. KOPMAN
Washington University School of Medicine

BALANCED ANESTHESIA USING MORPHINE, NEUROMUSCULAR BLOCKERS, AND NITROUS OXIDE IS THE TECHNIQUE OF CHOICE

In choosing an anesthetic technique for heart surgery, the primary concern is to avoid drugs that might impose additional stress and strain on an already compromised cardiopulmonary system. A variety of anesthetic drugs, alone and in combinations, have been employed for this surgical procedure, but today advocates appear to be divided into those recommending a potent inhalation anesthetic and those preferring a "balanced" technique.

The purpose of any general anesthetic is to produce in the patient the degrees of hypnosis (unconsciousness or lack of awareness), analgesia, muscle relaxation, and obtundation of undesirable reflexes required for the particular operation. In heart surgery, significant analgesia is required while the target organ is being exposed, but from that point until closure, the need for analgesia becomes much less because the heart and great vessels are supplied with few sensory nerves, eliminating the need for profound levels of anesthesia for a large part of the operation. Indeed, drugs producing light anesthesia, reducing awareness, and providing amnesia may be the prime requisites. By using a "balanced" pharmacologic approach, the anesthesiologist can choose drugs in doses, learned by experience, that render the patient oblivious and the surgeon content.

Fulfilling the subjective requirements of the patient and the sur-

147

geon are to little avail if the hemodynamic variables of the patient are altered in such a way that organ damage can develop, however. So, in choosing the premedication and the tranquilizing, amnesic, analgesic, and relaxant drugs, one must keep in mind the reactions that the several drugs may exert on the tenuous balance often existing between adequate and inadequate myocardial function.

In the preservation of the sometimes delicate equilibrium between myocardial oxygen supply and oxygen demand, one must consider the following:

1. Hypotension.   If not rapidly corrected, this can lead to a critical decrease of coronary blood flow and oxygen supply to the myocardium.

2. Hypoxemia.   This complication of anesthesia should not develop in a patient who is in the hands of a competent anesthesiologist properly ventilating the patient's lungs with sufficient oxygen. Hypoxia of the heart or brain may develop secondary to inadequate perfusion or oxygenation while the patient is on the pump, however — hence the need for frequent arterial blood gas determinations.

3. Myocardial Depression.   Drugs such as halothane and enflurane produce dose-dependent degrees of direct myocardial depression. Although this probably reduces myocardial oxygen demand, in a heart already functionally impaired the resultant hypotension and diminished blood flow can cancel out the decreased oxygen requirements.

4. Tachycardia.   Heart rate is a chief determinant of myocardial oxygen demand. In patients with coronary artery disease, tachycardia can be injurious because an increase in myocardial oxygen consumption may not be met by a corresponding increase in nutrient flow.

Myocardial wall tension is another important determinant of myocardial oxygen demand. In patients with aortic stenosis, even in the presence of a normal systemic pressure, left ventricular intracavity pressure and thus wall tension and myocardial oxygen demand are high. Tachycardia, by increasing oxygen demand, can cause myocardial hypoxia and arrhythmias even in the absence of coronary artery disease.

In mitral stenosis, the time interval required for effective emptying of the left auricle is critical. Rapid heart rates can so shorten this interval that auricular emptying is incomplete. The resultant decrease in left ventricular stroke volume leads to hypotension, and the increase in left atrial pressure may precipitate pulmonary edema.

5. Hypertension.   This change always increases wall tension, and hence myocardial oxygen demand; therefore, it is hazardous in patients with coronary artery disease and severe aortic stenosis. In mitral insufficiency, hypertension increases regurgitant flow into the left auricle, which can increase pulmonary venous pressure, leading to an increase in lung water.

6. Arrhythmias.   In the damaged heart, arrhythmias, particularly those ventricular in origin, may lead to ventricular fibrillation. Avoidance of drugs that sensitize the myocardium and conduction system of the heart will reduce the incidence of such complications.

Taking the above factors into consideration, it is our premise that anesthesia for cardiac surgery can best be provided by a balanced technique that includes the use of morphine, scopolamine, diazepam, thiopental, nitrous oxide, oxygen, and d-tubocurarine. The rationale for using each drug will be discussed, along with the use of certain other drugs that may be necessary to provide an optimum physiologic state.

MORPHINE

In this balanced technique, morphine plays the leading role. Since the middle of the 19th century, morphine has been used predominantly in anesthetic practice as a premedicant prior to induction of anesthesia. Approximately 10 years ago (Lowenstein, 1971), the cardiac anesthesia group at the Massachusetts General Hospital recommended relatively large doses of morphine (0.5 to 3.0 mg. per kg.) intravenously as the principal analgesic drug for cardiac surgery. The report stated that when the drug was given in small incremental doses (5 mg. per minute), the large total dose had little deleterious effect on cardiac output in normal subjects or in patients with valvular heart or coronary artery disease (Lowenstein et al., 1969; Stoelting and Gibbs, 1973).

In some patients, however, hypotension is associated with these doses of morphine, particularly if the circulating blood volume is low or if incremental doses are given rapidly. The reasons for this fall in blood pressure are poorly understood; transient decreases in peripheral vascular resistance have been noted in man (Wong, 1973) and suggestive evidence of venodilation has been seen in animals (Henney et al., 1966). Nonetheless, the Boston group believed that the incidence of hypotension in cardiac patients was less with morphine than with potent inhalation anesthetics. Our clinical impressions coincide, particularly for patients with advanced valvular or coronary disease.

The principal contribution of morphine to the anesthetic state is the intense analgesia that it provides. It also induces tranquility, relieving the subject of anxiety and permitting the environment to be viewed with a "roseate hue." Even with large total doses, however, some degree of consciousness and awareness may remain, so that other drugs must be given to assure the "anesthetic" state.

The long duration of action of morphine is of benefit in cardiac surgery, not because the operation is usually lengthy but because patients subjected to this operation usually benefit from ventilatory support for 24 hours or more postoperatively. The residual effects of morphine provide continuing tranquility, depressing the respiratory center and suppressing the cough reflex so that an endotracheal tube and positive pressure ventilation are more easily tolerated. During this period, patients are usually responsive when stimulated but otherwise quiet and pain free.

Premedication is usually with morphine 0.2 mg. per kg. and scopolamine 0.4 to 0.6 mg. intramuscularly an hour before the patient is brought to the operating room. Scopolamine is an important supplement to morphine in apprehensive patients because of the cerebral sedation and significant amnesia it provides. When the patient arrives in the anesthesia induction room, a peripheral intravenous cannula is inserted, a radial artery cannula is placed, and a Swan-Ganz catheter is inserted through the internal jugular vein. The premedication provides comfort for the patient during these procedures.

Anesthesia is induced with diazepam 10 to 20 mg. and thiopental 2 to 3 mg. per kg. intravenously. In this dose, diazepam provides significant sedation but does not consistently induce unconsciousness, with the result that a "sleep" dose of thiopental is required. Diazepam does not affect the cardiovascular system in this dose, and its amnesic action is a real contribution to the technique. Thiopental is a myocardial depressant, but in the small doses used this is not readily apparent.

Tracheal intubation using "light" anesthesia is accompanied in the majority of patients with coronary artery disease by an increase in blood pressure. To combat this hypertension, isosorbide dinitrate, 10 mg. dissolved in 1 ml. of normal saline, is placed sublingually immediately after the patient becomes unconscious. This drug, like nitroglycerin, acts primarily on the venous bed, causing vasodilation (Alfonso et al., 1963) with resulting decrease in venous return and stroke volume. The patient's lungs are then ventilated with 50:50 nitrous oxide-oxygen, and succinylcholine 100 mg. is given intravenously to facilitate tracheal intubation. When a fall in arterial blood pressure is noted on the oscilloscope, the endotracheal tube is passed. In a study of 36 patients with coronary artery disease in whom this technique was used, we observed only eight develop a systolic pressure above 150 torr, and only once was it above this level five minutes after intubation. We believe that this prophylactic measure is beneficial in patients having coronary artery surgery.

In patients for cardiac valve surgery, isosorbide is not administered routinely because hypertension does not consistently occur with tracheal intubation.

Following tracheal intubation, nitrous oxide-oxygen is continued and *d*-tubocurarine is administered intermittently to a total dose of 0.8 mg. per kg. This drug also can cause vasodepressor responses because of its ganglion-blocking action; therefore, it is given intermittently while observing the blood pressure response. *D*-tubocurarine is preferred to pancuronium because the latter precipitates tachycardia in some patients.

At this time, the patient is moved to the operating room and an infusion of morphine is begun. The dose of 1 to 1.5 mg. per kg. is mixed with 100 ml. of 5 per cent dextrose in water and administered via a microdrip set while observing the blood pressure on the oscilloscope. If the systolic pressure rises to 150 torr, the drip is run rapidly; otherwise, it is run continuously. If hypertension cannot be controlled with morphine, sodium nitroprusside (50 mg. in 500 ml. of 5 per cent dextrose in water) is administered by microdrip. This drug reduces peripheral resistance (Tinker and Michenfelder, 1976) and is effective in small doses.

During the operation, controlled ventilation with nitrous oxide and oxygen is maintained using an Emerson anesthesia ventilator. A carbon dioxide absorber is not used, and normal carbon dioxide elimination is achieved by high gas flows. Usually, with a tidal volume of 10 ml. per kg. and a respiratory rate of 20 per minute, the total flow required to maintain normocapnia is 4 to 6 liters per minute (60 ml. per kg.). Blood gases are determined frequently to ensure maintenance of a stable state.

Cardiac output tends to fall when nitrous oxide is administered to patients with valvular or coronary artery disease who have received morphine 1 to 2 mg. per kg. (Wong, 1973; Stoelting and Gibbs, 1973). The reason for this change is not clear, and a comparison with potent inhalation drugs was not studied. From the practical viewpoint, we find the analgesia and hypnosis provided by nitrous oxide to be an important part of this technique. During the prebypass part of the operation, if a concern develops for the patient with coronary artery disease, it usually relates to hypertension rather than hypotension. The most crucial time in the procedure so far as cardiac output is concerned is the immediate postbypass period. We have usually found it unnecessary to use nitrous oxide at this time and especially avoid it if concerned about cardiac output. In patients with poor ventricular function, we have administered oxygen alone during the entire postbypass period without later indication of awareness by the patient.

Stanley and associates (1974) compared the amount of blood transfused during and after bypass in patients who had received morphine 1 to 4 mg. per kg. with that of those receiving halothane anesthesia. The morphine group required considerably more blood. These authors believe that venodilation produced by morphine, but not by halothane, accounted for the difference. Their criteria for transfusion were as follows: During bypass, enough blood was added to the heart-lung machine to maintain flows of 40 to 70 ml. per kg.; after bypass, blood was given to maintain venous pressure at preoperative levels. To our knowledge, there is no refutation of this report. There are three pertinent considerations, however. (1) The dose of morphine was large (mean of 2.75 mg. per kg.) and the relationship may be dose-dependent (Stanley et al., 1973). We believe that doses above 1.5 mg. per kg. are rarely necessary. (2) A significant amount of blood was given during bypass, a practice that has been largely abandoned. (3) The choice of preoperative venous pressure as a guideline to transfusion after bypass may have been unfortunate because a heart depressed by halothane may produce higher venous pressures (Stoelting, Reis, and Longnecker, 1972). Thus, the guidelines for transfusion might account for the differences noted.

SUMMARY

Anesthesia for patients requiring cardiac surgery is not easy to administer. The drugs chosen should interfere minimally with the delicate balance that the patient has established, in spite of cardiac pathology, as his or her "best" myocardial efficiency. We believe that the balance achieved with morphine as the anchor and nitrous oxide, diazepam, thiopental, scopolamine, and *d*-tubocurarine as the satellites best fulfills the objectives. The use of drugs that are not direct myocardial depressants, the avoidance of wide fluctuations in arterial pressure, the adequate provision of analgesia and amnesia, and the maintenance of a tranquil state postoperatively are desirable requisites for the cardiac patient.

REFERENCES

Afonso, S., Rowe, G. G., Lowe, W. C., et al.: Systemic and coronary hemodynamic effects of isosorbide dinitrate. Am. J. Med. Sci., *246*:584, 1963.

Henney, R. P., Vasko, J. S., Brawley, R. K., et al.: The effects of morphine on the resistance and capacitance vessels of the peripheral circulation. Am. Heart J., *72*:242, 1966.

Lowenstein, E.: Morphine "anesthesia" — a perspective. Anesthesiology, *35*:563, 1971.

Lowenstein, E., Hallowel, P., Levine, F. H., et al.: Cardiovascular response to large doses of intravenous morphine in man. N. Engl. J. Med., *281*:1389, 1969.

Stanley, T. H., Gray, N. H., Isern-Amarol, J. H., and Patton, C.: Comparison of blood requirements during morphine and halothane anesthesia for open heart surgery. Anesthesiology, *41*:34, 1974.

Stanley, T. H., Gray, N. H., Stanford, W., et al.: The effects of high-dose morphine on fluid and blood requirements of open-heart operations. Anesthesiology, *38*:536, 1973.

Stoelting, R. K., and Gibbs, P. S.: Hemodynamic effects of morphine and morphine-nitrous oxide in valvular heart disease and coronary artery disease. Anesthesiology, *38*:45, 1973.

Stoelting, R. K., Reis, R. R., and Longnecker, D. E.: Hemodynamic responses to nitrous oxide-halothane and halothane in patients with valvular heart disease. Anesthesiology, *37*:430, 1972.

Tinker, J. H., and Michenfelder, J. D.: Sodium nitroprusside: pharmacology, toxicology and therapeutics. Anesthesiology, *45*:340, 1976.

Wong, K. C., Martin, W. E., Hornbein, T. F., et al.: The cardiovascular effects of morphine sulfate with oxygen and with nitrous oxide in man. Anesthesiology, *38*:542, 1973.

CHOICE OF ANESTHESIA FOR CORONARY BYPASS OPERATIONS

EDITORIAL COMMENT

Twenty years ago, Phillip Woodbridge* dissected the components of anesthesia and pointed out that the old ideas of loss of various functions in the descending planes and stages of anesthesia first enunciated by Arthur Guedel were only appropriate for a complete anesthetic, such as diethyl ether, not for the then modern anesthetics or anesthesia. He proposed that there were four essential components of anesthesia: loss of pain perception, unconsciousness, loss of motor power, and elimination of reflex activity. Specific drugs were considered available to manage each of these components; thus, deep anesthesia with volatile anesthetics was no longer needed. We have moved far since then — so far, in fact, that few of the products of our anesthesia training programs in the last 20 years have ever used a single anesthetic agent to manage all four components.

Stephen and his associates have presented a technique that follows Woodbridge's concepts: narcotics to control pain perception, nitrous oxide and thiopental to produce unconsciousness, muscle relaxants to paralyze motor responses, and a variety of drugs to eliminate reflex activity. Wilkinson, on the other hand, advocates the principal use of the volatile anesthetic halothane to control the various components, thereby placing less reliance on many substances to control each specific component. She believes that it is easier to obtain the balance required and that at the termination of anesthesia and operation, the patient can more quickly regain control of his or her own body systems.

Definitive data to conclusively prove one technique superior to the other in the clinical situation are lacking. Wilkinson's method is less complicated and the patients do appear to regain a near normal state more rapidly. The observation that patients given morphine require more blood during and following operation is significant but requires better documentation. Considering the volume of cardiac operations performed in academic centers, where the resources and talents exist to gather the needed data, the controversy is solvable.

---

*Woodbridge, P. D.: Changing concepts concerning depth of anesthesia. Anesthesiology, 18:536, 1958.

Part 8

TRACHEAL INTUBATION IN INFANTS

THE PROPOSITION:

> Endotracheal anesthesia is obligatory if an infant less than one year of age is to have general anesthesia.

ALTERNATIVE POINTS OF VIEW:

> By Joseph H. Marcy
> By Anne E. P. Jones

EDITORIAL COMMENT

by JOSEPH H. MARCY

University of Pittsburgh School of Medicine

ENDOTRACHEAL ANESTHESIA SHOULD BE USED IN ALL ANESTHETIZED INFANTS LESS THAN ONE YEAR OF AGE

The anatomic and physiologic limitations of the young infant during general anesthesia are of such significance that age itself is an indication for tracheal intubation. Moreover, intubation can be accomplished in infants with sufficiently low morbidity that the advantages of safety and smooth conduct of anesthesia outweigh the disadvantages.

Attempting to defend the premise that endotracheal anesthesia should be used in all anesthetized infants less than one year of age is hazardous for several reasons, however. Absolutes are seldom appropriate in medicine; there are bound to be exceptions. A greater difficulty arises in attempting to group pediatric patients by precise age limits. The child, and particularly the infant, is in a continuum of rapid growth and development, the stages of which defy precise classification. What may be advisable (or inadvisable) during the first year of life does not cease to be true on the morning of his first birthday! Thus, a "strict constructionist" approach to this controversy may well be indefensible.

CRITERIA FOR INTUBATION

Tracheal intubation is not required for every general anesthetic. Thus, criteria for intubation are necessary. The usual mandatory indications for intubation involve procedures in the chest and in the head and neck, those in which the body position is other than supine, and

157

the like. Many of the procedures unique to the newborn period and early months of life fall into this group. Techniques of anesthesia may also make intubation mandatory. The popularity of nitrous oxide-muscle relaxant techniques has increased the number of pediatric surgical procedures that fall into this category. A secure airway, excellent muscular relaxation, controlled ventilation, avoidance of the potent volatile anesthetics, and rapid emergence are significant benefits for these patients and justify the required use of tracheal intubation.

There are, however, other indications for intubation. Smith (1968) has suggested three other categories: *definitely preferable, optional,* and *unjustified.* Such a classification is useful but arbitrary. Anesthetists depending on training and experience have their own ideas of what patients and which procedures belong in each group. It is apparent, however, that today the use of tracheal intubation in all ages of patients has increased and that procedures that once fell into the unjustified or optional categories are now considered to be highly preferable or even mandatory. In pediatric anesthesia, a similar, if slower, change in attitude has occurred. This delayed wider acceptance of intubation for infants and children is no doubt related to the relatively smaller number of infants and children being operated on in a general hospital setting, the disappearance of "open ether" techniques involving spontaneous breathing, and the fear of complications, such as laryngeal edema. Tonsillectomy in children and pyloromyotomy in infants are but two examples of procedures for which intubation is now, but has not always been, considered mandatory by most anesthetists. Yet, many anesthetists remain reluctant to employ tracheal intubation in infants unless absolutely indicated by the type of procedure or anesthetic technique. This view is neither *wise,* since it deprives many infants of the advantages and safety of an assured airway, nor *necessary,* since the risk of intubation is low. The infant under one year of age presents special problems in airway management not shared by the adult that make the first few months of life themselves a criterion for intubation.

INFANCY AS A CRITERION FOR INTUBATION

Many anatomic characteristics complicate the anesthetist's task of assuring adequate ventilation through an unobstructed airway in the unconscious infant.

The lack of prominent features on the infant's face makes it difficult to achieve and maintain a reasonably gas-tight fit with a mask. Inordinate pressure of the mask upon the face is at times required to prevent gross leaks, especially with positive pressure ventilation. The difficulties in achieving a good fit are most troublesome if partial or complete airway obstruction develops during induction or maintenance. Anatomically contoured masks, such as the Rendell Baker-Soucek, offer some advantages over conventional types but are of little use if an oral airway or gastric tube is in place.

The infant's head is large in proportion to the body and is poorly supported by weak neck muscles; the neck is short. Extension of the head to an optimal position for airway maintenance frequently lifts the shoulders from the table — an unstable position and difficult to maintain. A head ring and a pad under the scapulae are often required to achieve a degree of immobilization.

With loss of muscle tone, the tongue, which is relatively larger in the infant in relation to the oral cavity and pharynx, tends to fall against the posterior pharyngeal wall. This posterior displacement of the tongue is exaggerated by upward pressure on the mandible — a maneuver that usually improves the adult airway but more often obstructs the airway in the infant. This paradoxical effect is seen not only in the infant but also often in children up to the age of four or five years. The airway obstruction thus inadvertently created by the anesthetist is often misinterpreted as laryngeal spasm. Keeping the fingers free of the mandible tends to improve the airway but then makes maintenance of proper extension of the head and fit of the mask more difficult. The triple airway maneuver may be helpful but is difficult to maintain. If both hands are required, the anesthetist can do little else.

The larynx of the infant is more susceptible to reflex spasm than that of the adult. In the lightly anesthetized infant, sudden increase in concentration of anesthetic gases, secretions from the pharynx or stomach, or reflex stimulus from pain or traction may evoke severe glottic spasm. Premature insertion of a pharyngeal airway in an attempt to cope with soft tissue obstruction is a common source of such stimulation. Thus, a deeper plane of anesthesia may be required to prevent laryngeal spasm than is necessary for the surgical procedure.

It is not known whether the tone of the cricopharyngeal sphincter is as great in the infant as in the adult. Isolated measurements by Sieber* have shown a wide range of values and are inconclusive. Nevertheless, dilation of the stomach with inspired gases under positive pressure is more common and more serious during infant anesthesia and resuscitation than in the adult. The volume of gas entering the infant's stomach readily elevates the diaphragm and interferes with ventilation. Because of the frequency with which dilation of the stomach occurs, even during routine induction in infants and children, it is our standard practice following tracheal intubation or induction to pass a 12 or 14 French catheter (an oxygen catheter is quite suitable) into the stomach to aspirate any gastric air as well as secretions or residual ingested material. When anesthesia is maintained by mask, gastric distention frequently recurs.

Immaturity causes several respiratory deficiencies in the infant. Examples are the relatively ineffective role of the ribs and intercostal muscles in respiration and the residual atelectasis and persistent right-to-left shunting in the first few weeks of life. High closing volumes in the newborn period (Nelson, 1976) and perhaps in the older infant

*Sieber, W. K.: Personal communication, 1978.

and child as well (Mansell et al., 1972) are also suggestive of the ventilatory disadvantage of the infant. It is difficult to evaluate the role of these factors in the anesthetic management of the healthy term infant, however.

What is of more certain anesthetic significance is that the infant's oxygen consumption is twice that of the adult on a body weight basis. Respiratory frequency twice as great and "turnover" ventilation two to three times as rapid as the adult's are required for the infant to meet the greater metabolic requirements (Nelson, 1976). Not only does hypoxia develop more quickly with airway obstruction or hypoventilation but bradycardia and the metabolic effects of hypoxia also develop.

Usually, none of these characteristics of the anesthetized infant are insurmountable problems in and of themselves, nor do they constitute an indication for the use of an endotracheal tube. Taken together, however, they present a constant threat to the patient, and since they are all interrelated, one seemingly small problem frequently has a domino effect on the others. The results in such cases run the gamut from simply a poorly conducted anesthetic to a serious accident with tragic consequences. The irony is that such misadventures may occur in healthy patients undergoing elective surgery when there was no "indication" for intubation.

Intubation of course does not guarantee freedom from airway problems; it does, however, effectively eliminate most of the potential hazards described. The anesthetist is relieved of constant concern with the airway and is able to devote more attention to other aspects of the anesthesia and operation. With the airway assured, there is greater flexibility in choice of anesthetic techniques through use of muscle relaxants and controlled ventilation. When emergency ventilatory problems arise, intubation provides the best possible means of coping with them.

THE MORBIDITY AND RISK OF INTUBATION

Intubation of the trachea in the pediatric age group carries a low but tangible morbidity. A small percentage of the complications are unpredictable and presumably are not preventable, but for the most part, they can be prevented and readily treated when they do occur.

Traditionally, the specter of subglottic edema has been a deterrent to the unrestricted use of intubation. Edema is indeed by far the most common problem. The overall reported incidence of postintubation croup varies from 1 per cent to 6 per cent (Pender, 1954; Bachman, 1962; Goddard et al., 1967; Jordan et al., 1970; Koka et al., 1977) (Table 1). It is difficult, as Koka and coworkers state, to compare these studies or to draw firm conclusions from them, since they do not utilize uniform definitions of postintubation croup.

In a review of 2372 consecutive intubations at the Children's Hospital of Pittsburgh, Cook* found the overall incidence of croup was 6.5 per cent and 3.1 per cent in patients under one year of age.

---

*Cook, D. R.: Personal Communication, 1978.

Table 1.   Incidence of Postintubation Croup

	Percentage All Infants and Children	Percentage Infants Less Than One Year
Bachman	<9.7*	2.6
Cook‡	6.5	3.1
Goddard	6.0**	<1.0**
Jordan	3.7	3.3
Koka	1.0	0.025†
Pender	1.6	4.6

*No figure is given for all infants and children. This percentage is for highest incidence in any age group.
**All patients received prophylactic betamethasone.
†Incidence of airway obstruction only.
‡Cook, D. R.: Personal communication, 1978.

Croup was defined as evidence of brassy cough with or without evidence of stridor or retraction. Cough without other signs, although suggestive of edema as a result of intubation, poses no threat of airway obstruction. When stridor and retraction alone were used as criteria of croup, the incidence in this series was reduced to 3.0 per cent overall and 2.2 per cent for those under one year of age (Table 2).

In all but one of the reports (Pender, 1954), the incidence of croup was lower in the first year of life than in the overall group. In their series, Koka and associates reported only two instances, and Goddard and coworkers but one. The difference is even more striking if the first 12 months are contrasted with the succeeding years. For example, Bachman found an incidence of 2.6 per cent in infants under one year, as opposed to one of 9.7 per cent in the third year of life.

The relative importance of the causative factors of postintubation croup is difficult to determine. Cook's series showed the highest incidence in operations involving the head and neck. Similarly, Koka

Table 2.   Incidence of Postintubation Croup in 2372 Patients at the Children's Hospital of Pittsburgh

Age	Percentage of Cough, Stridor, and/or Retractions	Percentage of Stridor and/or Retractions
Neonates	0.0	0.0
2–6 months	1.8	1.2
7–12 months	9.2	6.7
0–1 year	3.0	2.2
1–2 years	19.7	11.9
2–3 years	12.0	5.7
4–6 years	8.6	3.5
7–10 years	7.1	2.2
11–15 years	1.7	0.2
0–15	6.5	3.1

and colleagues found a higher morbidity in patients who required an intraoperative change in position, in those whose procedures were about the neck, and in those who were in positions other than supine. Most of these procedures in both series would meet criteria for mandatory intubation. On the other hand, it is significant that none of the 145 patients intubated for herniorrhaphy in the Children's Hospital of Pittsburgh series* developed signs of croup.

Trauma to the larynx is generally conceded to be one of the causes of croup. Both Bachman (1962) and Koka and associates (1977) report higher incidence with prolonged intubation and with positions other than supine. Again, most patients in these categories were likely to be intubated in any case by traditional criteria. Trauma as a result of ineptness in laryngoscopy and intubation no doubt plays a role but is a factor controllable with skill and experience. Lack of these virtues, however, poses equal hazards to the patient whether or not intubation is used.

Chemical irritation and infection introduced by the endotracheal tube have been suggested as causes of croup. This problem has been satisfactorily eliminated with the sterile, implantation-tested endotracheal tubes readily available today. Existing or recent respiratory infection has also been incriminated. We have therefore considered elective intubation in such patients to be relatively contraindicated. Koka and coworkers (1977), however, found no correlation between the incidence of croup and upper respiratory infection.

The treatment of postintubation croup, when it occurs, has been dramatically facilitated with the use of nebulized racemic epinephrine. Jordan and associates (1970) were able to relieve airway obstruction in this manner in all cases of postintubation croup without recourse to reintubation or tracheotomy. In our hands, this form of treatment has been very effective and is being used increasingly, even in minor degrees of tracheitis after intubation. The role of steroids in the management of postintubation croup (Deming and Oech, 1961) is less certain but is included in Jordan's protocol (1970) and recommended by Goddard and associates (1967).

It is evident that the infant under one year of age is less likely to develop postintubation croup and that this complication occurs most frequently in those procedures for which intubation would be required in any case. The causative factors of postintubation edema have largely been identified and some, at least, eliminated by use of sterile, tissue-safe tubes and, of course, by skill and experience. Treatment of croup, when it occurs, is effective and readily available. The risk of tracheal intubation in these young patients is not a cause for concern.

CONTROVERSY, COMPROMISE AND CONCERN

We believe that tracheal intubation is a means of providing safer anesthesia at minimal "cost" to a group of patients who are at greater

---

*Cook, D. R.: Unpublished data, 1978.

risk than their older counterparts, from the point of view of airway management, and that the advantages of intubation outweigh the disadvantages. Presumably, those who would dispute our approach do not argue so much against "intubation" as against "all." There are indeed some procedures of such minor nature and of such short duration that intubation is perhaps unnecessary. Other patients in this age range will be intubated by virtue of mandatory criteria; these patients are not under consideration here. Our concern is directed to the larger number of infants, many healthy and undergoing elective procedures that ordinarily are not among the criteria for intubation. There is a tendency among surgeons and anesthetists to underestimate the anesthetic problems of these patients, placing more emphasis on the minor nature of the procedure than on the care of the patient. It is in this group that there is the greatest potential for anesthetic complications and disaster. Such misadventures, when they occur, are seldom reported (in contrast to the incidence of complications of intubation) but are familiar to any supervisor in a teaching department or other active service. A safer and more conservative approach is an understanding among all concerned that all infants, whether less than one year of age or some other arbitrary limit, be considered candidates for intubation. When such a philosophy of care becomes policy, it is an acknowledgment of the risk, and there is a safe method at hand to meet that risk. Such a policy should in no way exclude sound medical judgment in each case — there will be exceptions. The fact that some of these patients will not be intubated may mean the loss of a debate but does not invalidate the concept of utilizing an accepted and proved technique when it can provide better anesthesia, and more importantly, greater safety.

REFERENCES

Bachman, L., cited in Hallowell, P.: Endotracheal intubation of infants and children. Int. Anesthesiol. Clin., 1:135, 1962.

Deming, M. V., and Oech, S. R.: Steroid and antihistaminic therapy for postintubation subglottic edema in infants and children. Anesthesiology, 22:933, 1961.

Goddard, J. E., Phillips, O. C., and Marcy, J. H.: Betamethasone for prophylaxis of postintubation inflammation. A double-blind study. Anesth. Analg. (Cleve.), 46:348, 1967.

Jordan, W. S., Graves, C. L., and Elwyn, R. A.: New therapy for postintubation laryngeal edema and tracheitis in children. J.A.M.A., 212:585, 1970.

Koka, B. V., Jeon, I. S., Andre, J. M., et al.: Postintubation croup in children. Anesth. Analg. (Cleve.), 56:501, 1977.

Mansell, A., Bryan, C., and Levison, H.: Airway closure in children. J. Appl. Physiol., 33:711, 1972.

Nelson, N. M.: Respiration and circulation after birth. In Smith, C. A., and Nelson, N. M. (eds.): The Physiology of the Newborn Infant. 4th ed. Springfield, Illinois, Charles C Thomas, 1976.

Pender, J. W.: Endotracheal anesthesia in children: advantages and disadvantages. Anesthesiology, 15:495, 1954.

Smith, R. M.: Anesthesia for Infants and Children. 3rd ed. St. Louis, The C. V. Mosby Company, 1968.

by ANNE E. P. JONES
University of California, Irvine

TRACHEAL INTUBATION IS NOT MANDATORY IN INFANTS LESS THAN ONE YEAR OF AGE

The decision whether or not to intubate the trachea of a child under one year of age undergoing general anesthesia is in many cases simple and obvious — do so specifically when the site or nature of the surgical procedure demands that it be done. There remain some patients, however, for whom the decision is less obvious unless one takes the point of view that all patients in this age group must have endotracheal anesthesia regardless of the procedure planned.

In the last few years, the pendulum has swung from the necessity to justify tracheal intubation to the need to justify its avoidance. The reasons for this change in attitude are several:

1. Improved materials, disposability, and ensured sterility of endotracheal tubes.

2. Increased familiarity with the technique of tracheal intubation in children by practitioners of anesthesia.

3. The feeling that intubation requires less skill than good airway management with mask techniques.

4. Possibly, the inclination toward the practice of defensive medicine encouraged by the present medicolegal climate.

The soundest basis for this change in philosophy is the technical improvement in endotracheal tubes. The red rubber, thick-walled tubes requiring use of metal stylets for insertion have been replaced by the thin-walled but fairly firm tubes constructed of tissue implantation–tested plastic materials that are used once and then thrown away.

Regardless of the improved technology and increased familiarity with technique, to state that intubation should be mandatory in all patients in this age group is to assume that the benefit to the patient always outweighs the hazards of intubation. It also discounts the use of anesthetic methods, such as the use of ketamine for short procedures, in which the main benefit may be the avoidance of intubation.

In examining this problem, the anatomic differences between the infant and the adult larynges will be considered, and the complications of and indications for tracheal intubation will be reviewed. In children, as in adults, the incidence of all complications can be lessened by good judgment and careful management. Consequently, the decision to perform any given procedure should be determined by rational choice based on relative indication rather than dictated by habit, custom, or regulation.

THE ANATOMY OF THE INFANT LARYNX

In 1951, Eckenhoff published a classic paper that described the salient differences in the structure of the infant larynx as compared with that of the adult larynx and included a discussion of their significance in the performance of tracheal intubation (Eckenhoff, 1951).

In brief, he stated that visualization of the larynx in the infant may be difficult because its position in the neck is more cephalad, leading to greater angulation of the trachea with the upper airway, the relatively larger tongue offering further hindrance. The epiglottis is long, stiff, and U-shaped, and instead of being flat and tucked up behind the base of the tongue, it protrudes at an angle to partially cover the glottic opening during normal breathing. This is possibly an evolutionary adaptation to protect the larynx from aspiration in the early months of life. In infants, it is usually necessary to pass the laryngoscope blade posterior to the epiglottis in order to visualize the laryngeal opening. In the older child and adult, the tip of the blade is frequently placed anterior to the epiglottis, lifting it forward indirectly, and avoiding trauma to the mucosa overlying the cartilage of the structure.

The glottic opening, the first narrow area through which the endotracheal tube is passed, is bounded by the ligamentous vocal cords and the arytenoid cartilages. The cartilaginous portion of this boundary is greater in the infant, relative to the more compliant ligamentous part, than in the adult, with the accompanying possibility of increased pressure and mucosal damage by passage of a semirigid endotracheal tube.

The most important anatomic feature in the infant is that the narrowest diameter of the airway is at the cricoid ring. It is essential to choose a tube around which a gas leak is apparent when the tube is in position, because the narrowest area cannot be seen.

The implications of these anatomic features will be further reviewed when the complications of intubation are discussed.

COMPLICATIONS OF INTUBATION

Several papers have been published recently referring to the trauma caused by the process of intubation and by short-term contact between tube and tissue. Although many refer to the sequelae of long-term intubation, they are, in general, not germane to the discussion of intubation for surgical procedures. In surveying the literature on the complications of tracheal intubation, articles published before 1970 were excluded because they pertained to endotracheal tubes made of nonstandardized materials that were commonly resterilized and reused. Papers were included, however, that described trauma produced experimentally in animals or clinically in adults, when the mechanism described was common to techniques used in children. Many of the reported complications in infants would appear to be avoidable by the use of skill and good technique, but this does not invalidate their consideration when evaluating the overall benefits and hazards of the procedure. The complications of intubation discussed are presented in chronologic order with experimental data included when appropriate.

The Process of Tracheal Intubation

Complications occurring during this initial period include trauma, both minor and major, and harmful reflex responses. The minor hazards of bruised gingiva and abraded mucous membranes are well recognized. More serious accidents include perforation of the pharynx or trachea, several incidences of which have been reported in neonates since 1975 (Serlin and Daily, 1975; Schild et al., 1975; Touloukian et al., 1977; Talbert et al., 1977).

The pyriform sinus is the most frequently reported site of pharyngeal perforation; the initial submucosal injury extends into the posterior mediastinum in a majority of cases, giving the appearance of "pseudodiverticulum." Perforation of the trachea occurs anteriorly, the tip of the endotracheal tube entering the anterior mediastinum. Both accidents are common during emergency intubation, which may be performed hurriedly or with excessive vigor. The use of a stylet adds to the risk, although the bevel of a fairly rigid polyvinyl tube alone can cause a submucosal tear. Another contributing factor is hyperextension of the head and neck, which stretches the pharyngeal tissues and tends to angulate the trachea forward so that the tip of the tube impinges on the anterior wall, which may then be perforated with the use of excessive force.

In patients in whom no gross injury of this type occurs, it is likely that the trachea is traumatized to a lesser degree (Klainer et al., 1975). Hilding (1971) described lesions produced in experimental animals by short-term intubation (less than six hours) and compared them with those seen in postmortem specimens from patients intubated just prior to death. Macroscopically, all these specimens showed desquamation over the posterior plate of the cricoid and arytenoids in the larynx, with lesions over the cartilaginous rings along the anterior wall of the trachea for the distance reached by the tube. This tracheal trauma, varying from loss of cilia to total absence of epithelium and basement membrane, was seen in all the specimens. Because of the site and length of the area involved, the trauma must have occurred during intubation or extubation. The injury to the posterior larynx may have been due to abrasion during intubation or to continued pressure as the tube lay *in situ,* the lesions being most severe in those patients intubated for the longest time.

Laryngotracheal stimulation during laryngoscopy and intubation may give rise to vagal reflexes that cause coughing, vomiting, laryngospasm, apnea, bradycardia and cardiac arrhythmias and sympathetic reflexes, including tachycardia, arrhythmias, and hypertension.

Coughing, vomiting, and laryngospasm are generally precipitated by an attempt to intubate during too light a plane of general anesthesia without the aid of muscle relaxants. Vagal cardiac reflexes may be prevented by the use of atropine. Deeper general anesthesia will also help protect the patient against the sympathetic reflexes.

Tube in Place

Complications arising while the patient's trachea is intubated are mainly those of obstruction, endobronchial intubation, and accidental extubation.

Respiratory obstruction may result from kinking of the tube, occlusion of its lumen by secretions or blood clots, and, occasionally, malpositioning the tube so that its bevel lies against the tracheal wall. Adequate monitoring will quickly alert the anesthetist to the respiratory obstruction; the cause must then be determined and treated.

Vascular anomaly is an unusual cause of respiratory obstruction in the intubated child. Congenital abnormalities of the aortic arch and its branches may result in the formation of vascular rings with varying degrees of compression around the trachea and esophagus. Vascular rings may be asymptomatic preoperatively but cause occlusion of the endotracheal tube opening because they compress the trachea in the area in which the bevel of the endotracheal tube lies. If the presence of such an anomaly is unsuspected, diagnosis may be difficult (Vaughan and McKay, 1975).

The accidental insertion of the endotracheal tube into a main stem bronchus, or its dislodgment into that position by repositioning the patient during an operation, is common and unless recognized may lead to serious hypoxemia, cardiac arrhythmias, and postoperative atelectasis (Tisi, Twigg, and Moser, 1968). Tube position should be checked after intubation and repositioning of the head, especially with flexion of the neck, by listening to both sides of the chest. In the newborn infant, the distance between the larynx and the carina is only 4 cm., allowing little room for error in placement. In children under the age of one year, there is a more equal angulation of right and left main bronchi with the trachea, so that it is possible to cannulate either bronchus with an overlong tube.

Accidental extubation during an operation is likely to occur when the patient is in the prone or lateral position. Secure fixation of the tube is vital.

Extubation

The most commonly seen complication during extubation is laryngospasm caused by removal of the tube during a light plane of anesthesia, when laryngeal reflexes are sensitive. Clinically, laryngospasm following extubation seems to be less common in those less than one year of age than in older age groups, possibly because awake extubation is performed in the younger group more frequently. If it does occur, hypoxia and bradycardia ensue, necessitating rapid reintubation with its attendant trauma. If the child is allowed to emerge from anesthesia breathing oxygen without stimulation, such as repeated pharyngeal suctioning, it is generally possible to perform an awake extubation without the patient bucking and coughing on the tube.

Postextubation

The most important complication following intubation in children is the occurrence of edema of the airways, leading to varying degrees of respiratory obstruction, with stridor, rib retraction, and possible hypoxia. It is probable that some degree of mucosal edema of the airway, particularly at the subglottic level, occurs following even the most gentle introduction of an endotracheal tube. Supraglottic edema affecting the epiglottis and arytenoid folds may result from the trauma of initial laryngoscopy and intubation and be manifest as respiratory obstruction after extubation. In these cases the tissues will be visibly swollen. Subglottic edema at the level of the cricoid ring is probably the most serious problem of this type, however.

The diameter of the cricoid ring in this age group, as previously mentioned, is the smallest diameter to be encountered in the upper airways. It is also unyielding and cannot be distended by a tube that is too large. The mucosa in this region is ciliated columnar epithelium loosely attached to the cartilage by areolar connective tissue prone to edema.

The significance of even a small amount of edema in this region becomes apparent when the cross sectional area of the cricoid ring is considered. Resistance to laminar flow through a tube, according to Poiseuille's Law, is inversely proportional to the fourth power of the radius. With turbulent flow, as occurs in the larynx, the influence of size increases to the fifth power of the radius. One millimeter of edema will therefore reduce the flow through an infant larynx proportionally far more than in the older child or adult, readily accounting for the relative frequency of respiratory distress in infants and its rarity in adults (Table 1).

The most significant cause of subglottic edema appears to be the

Table 1.   Effect of 1 mm. of Uniform Edema on Reducing the Cross
Sectional Area of Larynx at Cricoid Ring

Diameter at cricoid ring, mm.	Area, mm²	Area if 1 mm. Uniform Edema, mm²	Decrease in Area, per cent
4	12.6	3.14	75
5	19.6	7.1	64
6	28.3	12.6	55.5
7	38.6	19.6	49.2
8	50.2	28.3	43.6
9	63.3	38.6	39.0
10	78.6	50.2	36.2
12	113.0	78.6	30.4
14	154.0	113.0	26.7
16	202.0	154.0	23.4
20	314.1	259.0	19.0

(From Eckenhoff, J. E.: Some anatomic considerations of the infant larynx influencing endotracheal anesthesia. Anesthesiology, *12*:401–410, 1951.)

use of too large an endotracheal tube. Other factors include the irritant effect of the tube on the mucosa, reduced by the use of materials reaching the Z-79 tissue implantation standard, and movement of the tube within the larynx due to coughing and straining or repositioning the patient.

Biller and associates (1970) have produced laryngeal edema experimentally in young squirrel monkeys by using polyethylene tubes one size too large. The edema caused a rise in subglottic pressure, maximal about one hour postextubation with gradual improvement thereafter (Biller et al., 1970). The initial rise was reduced, and recovery was hastened by the administration of intravenous dexamethasone, 6 to 7 mg. per kg.

Laryngeal edema may necessitate reintubation with a smaller tube until the edema resolves. Other less drastic measures include humidification and increased inspired oxygen and the use of nebulized racemic epinephrine (Jordan, Graves, and Elwyn, 1971; McGovern, Fitz-Hugh, and Edgemon, 1971).

Late Sequelae

Postintubation subglottic tracheal stenosis is becoming more frequently reported as a complication of improved methods of respiratory support in the newborn period. It appears to occur following long-term intubation of 24 hours or more, however. A survey of the literature did not reveal any reports of this serious problem following intubation for surgical procedures (Johnson and Jones, 1976).

The Incidence of Complications

The incidence of postintubation complications is difficult to determine from the literature. Catastrophic complications, such as perfora-

Table 2.   Incidence of Complications

Jordan	3.9%	"objective morbidity"	1970
Goddard	6.0%		1967
Pender	1.6%		1954

tion of the airways, are described in single case reports and are obviously rare. The incidence of the most immediate postoperative complication, laryngeal edema and obstruction, has been studied by several authors. These reports, however, date from the era prior to the use of disposable, tissue implantation–tested tubes. The use of other materials and various methods of resterilization, including ethylene oxide, probably increased tissue irritation and the incidence of complications.

As can be seen in Table 2, the incidence of postoperative laryngeal edema in children varies between 2 and 6 per cent. This cannot be regarded as negligible.

Data from experimental and postmortem studies suggest that some degree of trauma, demonstrated histologically, occurs during every intubation, so that the presence of obvious morbidity represents only one end of the scale. Subjective differences in assessment of seriousness could account for the considerable variation in reported incidence.

THE INDICATIONS FOR INTUBATION

There can be no dispute over the necessity for tracheal intubation for the majority, probably a large majority, of children less than one year of age requiring anesthesia. It may be dictated by the patient's condition; the full stomach or intestinal obstruction, anatomic airway anomalies, or poor physical status, including immaturity, may determine that the safety of intubation far outweighs its disadvantages.

For many surgical procedures, intubation is essential, for example, any major surgical procedure of thorax and abdomen, neurosurgical procedures, and operations on the head and neck that would be technically impossible to perform with anesthesia given by mask. Similarly, surgery involving the airways — the cleft lip and palate repairs, surgery for choanal atresia, adenoidectomy, and tonsillectomy — requires the passage of an endotracheal tube.

There are circumstances for which intubation is indicated in the majority of cases, although it may not be regarded as mandatory. One is the necessity for anesthesia in the infant less than one month of age, or older in the case of babies born prematurely. The majority of procedures performed in this age group will be such that intubation is required by the criteria described previously. The reason for including these children in the group for which intubation is necessary, however, is their small size and immaturity. Their response to the inhalation agents required for the maintenance of mask anesthesia is resistance to the anesthetic effects but sensitivity to the respiratory and cardiovascular depressant effects, with a tendency to periods of apnea and hypotension that become progressively less as the child matures.

Intubation is also generally indicated in children for whom surgery, although of a minor nature and without field avoidance problems, is likely to be prolonged. This requires maintenance of an uncompromised airway and respiratory status for a longer time than can be easily accomplished by mask techniques. Individual anesthesiologists will have their own limits for this parameter.

There remains a group of patients, however, for whom tracheal intubation is unnecessary and should be avoided. Since intubation is commonly performed in the age group using deep anesthesia with inhalation agents rather than with muscle relaxants, it would seem sensible to continue the anesthesia for the performance of short and relatively minor procedures, such as circumcision, herniorraphy, and removal of small accessible tumors and extra digits, rather than subject the child to the risk of intubation. This is especially the case for procedures performed on an out-patient basis. In these patients, the conditions required for an operation often need no greater depth and little greater length of general anesthesia than would be required for the performance of intubation alone. Likewise, the occurrence of even a minor complication of intubation, such as postintubation laryngeal spasm or croup, becomes of relatively greater importance when compared with the minor nature of the surgical procedure.

The patients for whom intubation should be avoided, if possible, are those few for whom repeated general anesthetics are necessary. Two particular instances come to mind: children requiring daily radiotherapy for a malignancy, such as retinoblastoma or Wilm's tumor, and burned children who need daily dressing and debridement too painful to experience without anesthesia. The incidence of complications increases with repeat intubations, and frequently the anesthetic requirements of these short repeated procedures can be well met by the use of ketamine in a dosage low enough to avoid respiratory depression or airway compromise.

CONCLUSION

The indications for tracheal intubation are many. Although serious complications are relatively rare, there remain times when intubation is unnecessary and occasions when it should be avoided if possible. The practice of anesthesia is always an exercise in judgment — a choice between the many different pharmacologic and mechanical methods available to us in our efforts to ensure safe and pleasant conditions for the patient undergoing surgery. I believe that, in children less than one year of age, the decision to intubate the trachea should be based upon specific indications in each instance, the single most important factor in the conduct of these cases being that the person administering the anesthetic is skilled and experienced in dealing with this age group and thus competent to make the choice.

REFERENCES

Biller, H. F., Harvey, J. F., Bone, R. C., et al.: Laryngeal edema — an experimental study. Ann. Otol., 79:1084–1087, 1970.

Blanc, V. F., and Tremblay, N. A.: The complications of tracheal intubation: a new classification with a review of the literature. Anesth. Analg. (Cleve.), 53:203–213, 1974.

Eckenhoff, J. E.: Some anatomic considerations of the infant larynx influencing endotracheal anesthesia. Anesthesiology, 12:401–410, 1951.

Goddard, J. E., Jr., Phillips, O. C., and Marcy, J. H.: Betamethasone for prophylaxis of postintubation inflammation: a double-blind study. Anesth. Analg. (Cleve.), 46:348–353, 1967.

Hilding, A. C.: Laryngotracheal damage during intratracheal anesthesia. Ann. Otol., 80:565–581, 1971.

Johnson, D. G., and Jones, R.: Surgical aspects of airway management in infants and children. Surg. Clin. North Am., 56(2):263–279, 1976.

Jordan, W. S., Graves, C. L., and Elwyn, R. A.: New therapy for postintubation laryngeal edema and tracheitis in children. J.A.M.A., 212:585–588, 1970.

Katz, R. L., and Bigger, J. T.: Cardiac arrhythmias during anesthesia and operation. Anesthesiology, 33(2):193–213, 1970.

Klainer, A. S., Turndorf, H., Wen-hsien, W., Krishi, M., and Allender, P.: Surface alterations due to endotracheal intubation. Am. J. Med., 58(5):674–683, 1975.

McGovern, F. H., Fitz-Hugh, G. S., and Edgemon, L. J.: The hazards of endotracheal intubation. Ann. Otol., 80:556–564, 1971.

Pender, J. W.: Endotracheal anesthesia in children: advantages and disadvantages. Anesthesiology, 15:-495–505, 1954.

Schild, J. P., Wuilloud, A., Kollberg, H., and Bossi, E.: Tracheal perforation as a complication of nasotracheal intubation in a neonate. J. Pediatr., 88:631–632, 1976.

Serlin, S. P., and Daily, W. J. R.: Tracheal perforation in the neonate: a complication of endotracheal intubation. J. Pediatr., 86:596–597, 1975.

Talbert, J. L., Rodgers, B. M., Felman, A. H., and Moazam, F.: Traumatic perforation of hypopharynx in infants. J. Thorac. Cardiovasc. Surg., 74(1):152–156, 1977.

Tisi, G. H., Twigg, H. L., and Moser, K. M.: Collapse of left lung induced by artificial airway. Lancet, 1:791–793, 1968.

Touloukian, R. J., Beardsley, G. P., Ablow, R. C., and Effman, E. L.: Traumatic perforation of the pharynx in the newborn. Pediatrics, 59(Supplement 6):1019–1022, 1977.

Vaughan, V. C., III, and McKay, R. J. (eds.): Nelson Textbook of Pediatrics. 10th ed. Philadelphia, W. B. Saunders Company, 1975, pp. 1067–1069.

TRACHEAL INTUBATION IN INFANTS

EDITORIAL COMMENT

A controversy regarding the need for endotracheal anesthesia when infants are to be anesthetized has existed for years. There are those who would hardly consider anesthetizing an infant without intubation of the trachea and others who avoid the technique for many procedures in normal, healthy patients. Are there reasons for both positions, and is compromise possible?

Jones takes the traditional position — that of concern about potential postintubation tracheal edema. Although she points out that tracheal intubation should not be withheld if indicated, she nonetheless indicates that there are an appreciable number of healthy, normal infants for routine operation who do not require endotracheal anesthesia. She recognizes that there are hazards inherent in the technique itself, in addition to postintubation tracheal edema, especially in the hands of the inept.

Marcy dwells more on the reasons for widespread use of endotracheal anesthesia that are related to the anatomic underdevelopment of the infant lungs and airways, presents data to support a contention that the incidence of tracheal edema is lower in the one-year-old or less infant than in older children, and speaks of effective and readily available therapy for croup should it appear. He does not believe that concern, as expressed by Jones, is valid.

Neither author comes to grips with the distribution of infants requiring surgical care, although Marcy suggests that today more of these patients are being treated in a children's hospital setting, nor are data presented as to the technical facility of the anesthetist related to appearance of tracheal edema, although Jones points out that technically, tracheal intubation in the infant is more difficult than in the average adult. I am comfortable with Marcy's position in a well-equipped children's hospital with an experienced staff of anesthetists and recovery room nurses but am less assured in the community hospital with surgeons and anesthetists treating occasional infant surgical cases, often with a meager choice of equipment and with recovery rooms not attuned to infant care. But then I recall the case of the occasional pediatric anesthetist who neither was sufficiently adept technically to get the tube in the trachea nor understood the limitations of infant dead space without a tube — with resultant cerebral hypoxia. The reader will have to take it from there.

Part 9

ACUPUNCTURE IN ANESTHESIOLOGY

THE PROPOSITION:

Acupuncture is an important anesthetic technique and should be taught in anesthesiology training programs.

ALTERNATIVE POINTS OF VIEW:

By Max S. Sadove
By John J. Bonica

EDITORIAL COMMENT

by MAX S. SADOVE

Rush Medical College

ACUPUNCTURE IS USEFUL IN PAIN MANAGEMENT

In 1959, while working for several months in a developing nation in Indo-China, I saw Oriental medical practice involving some "Western" and some "Oriental" techniques. The pharmacopeia of the East was not understandable to me because it included flowers, pods, roots, organics, powdered rhinoceros horn, mandragora, and the like. The "back-up" pharmacologic explanation was at best very poor; largely it was, "we use this for that," and it frequently worked. The observations of Oriental anesthesia and analgesia were even more confusing. At that time I did not see acupuncture *anesthesia;* there was only *analgesia,* not for pain relief of childbirth, dental extraction, or surgical procedures but for a variety of nonsurgical painful states that seemed to respond. Was this another form of mesmerism? I watched, read, and discussed procedures and techniques through interpreters but finally lost interest because it was all too confusing.

Approximately 10 years later, I learned of Dr. Masayoshi Hyodo of Japan and his use of acupuncture for treatment of patients in a pain clinic. Why should this skilled anesthesiologist be treating nearly one half of the patients in his clinic with acupuncture? He was an excellent clinician, was skilled in regional anesthesia techniques, had excellent physical therapists available, and was knowledgeable about drugs of the West as well as the East. But, he frequently used acupuncture! Why?

Six years ago, Dr. Hyodo was invited to be a Visiting Professor at the Rush University Medical School and the Presbyterian-St. Luke's Hospital. We arranged for 30 to 40 patients to be treated daily for various painful states for just over a month on an experimental basis. No one was charged. One of Dr. Hyodo's associates remained for a year so that we could continue treatment and follow the patients being treated. It was obvious from the results that something was happening that justified continuation of the use of acupuncture. Many of these patients had the usual therapy available at a major teaching institution's pain clinic, but for some, the referring physician and the

177

patient preferred acupuncture. Since then, over five years of experience have been gained at the Rush University Pain Center. Well-trained doctors of Oriental medicine with long years of experience with acupuncture have participated with continuous analysis and review of results and registration of the satisfaction of patients, referring physicians, and staff.

WHAT IS ACUPUNCTURE?

Acupuncture is another method of pain therapy to be considered along with transcutaneous stimulators, biofeedback, hypnosis, regional nerve blocks, and perhaps 20 other means of treating pain. Many of these therapeutic techniques are not really understood, and perhaps theories of their actions are erroneous as well as unproved. This applies to many forms of physical therapy as well, all really not better understood than acupuncture.

Many patients are referred to our Pain Center for acupuncture because of the failure of conventional methods. After recording the usual medical history and doing a physical examination, we may or may not utilize acupuncture. Consultation with appropriate services is requested. Occasionally, acupuncture is used initially because the referring physician or patient requests it, but this method also gives us time to better evaluate the patient. Frequently, the response is pleasantly surprising. Many patients have arthritis or myofascial pain or are in a similar state. We have little else to recommend that is specific and has not already been tried.

There is little doubt that acupuncture has great potentiality for abuse, both intentional and unintentional. There is also no doubt that, as with other forms of therapy, it has a psychotherapeutic effect. Once the confidence of the patient is gained, which hopefully is rapidly, specific therapy must be used if identifiable and available. Many patients with such syndromes as postlaminectomy syndromes, myofascitis, bursitis, and tendonitis respond just as well to acupuncture as to conventional epidural injection of corticoids or the use of local anesthetics with corticoids. Thus, one is faced with the dilemma of when to stop acupuncture and try more specific therapy. The earlier one starts specific therapy, the less vulnerable one is medicolegally, scientifically, and academically. Often, however, this is a gray area. In the absence of clearly defined therapy, acupuncture may have a real place, if used with propriety.

Abuse can be unintentional. In one instance, an anesthesiologist utilized acupuncture for a patient with causalgia. There was good response and the anesthesiologist was convinced that the patient was improving. The local medical society asked for my opinion as to the ethics of this approach. I responded that a therapeutic nerve block would have been my preferred method of therapy, but the anesthesiologist subsequently reported that he had had good response from acupuncture, equally as good as with regional nerve blocks. Was he correct? I doubt it, and he had no controls or recorded data. Another anesthesiologist reported on television that excellent results could be obtained with ear acupuncture in the treatment of obesity. We decided to see if we could reproduce his results. Our carefully controlled study showed that there was essentially no difference between therapeutic and placebo loci, with very insignificant overall results. I suspect that this is true of many of the studies on the use of acupuncture for treatment of narcotic addiction. I can understand the enthusiasm of acupuncturists and why they do not do controlled studies, but without these studies, truth is evasive.

At times one regrets one's inability to pursue these projects. On hearing of the "studies" in China on the treatment of the deaf with acupuncture, we attempted a study in this area. Although the changes in audiometry showed slight and occasional change, overall, the results of audiometry suggested that this method of treatment was ineffective. Many patients claimed improvement of speech discrimination, however. Our investigation of speech discrimination was inconclusive and was abandoned because of the large volume of patients in the pain clinic. Recommendations were made that the study be continued with large numbers of deaf children, but for many reasons this did not occur. I should like to see the study repeated, improved, and greatly enlarged. After much thought, I doubt that the results will be positive but believe that it should be completed in large institutions, but not by the average acupuncturist avialable today — the potential for abuse is too great. Many patients claim that they "heard better," but I wonder. It is interesting that patients with tinnitus repeatedly assure us of the diminution of this complaint. We have never engaged in the acupuncture treatment of drug abuse or impotence at the Pain Center, nor do we permit acupuncture for many other diseases that are claimed in the Oriental texts to be benefited by its use.

ACUPUNCTURE ANESTHESIA

We have utilized this technique on only five patients; it was successful in three, partially successful in one, and failed in the other. I doubt that we will use it again, even though we think that it could be used in some cases. We have reliable and safe techniques that are superior to acupuncture! In almost all of the films we have seen from various parts of the world, acupuncture is spectacular in providing pain relief in some, just as in three of our patients, but is 60 per cent effectiveness adequate? Certainly not! It is of note that when acupuncture fails, conventional anesthesia succeeds. But, what is going on? This is not intentional hypnosis, and I wish that I knew what hypnosis is, after practicing it often over a period of 20 years. One can review the excellent movie that Melzak filmed of an African tribesman having a trephine operation on his skull, the patient sitting holding a bowl to collect blood freely flowing from his scalp, neither uncomfortable nor seemingly having pain (Melzak and Wall, 1965). He has not had drugs or "needles" but probably has had some type of psychic preparation for this extensive and painful operation. How much does an operation really hurt? Why did the patient not have pain? Certainly acupuncture should not be called *anesthesia,* since the patient can feel pressure, heat, touch, and the cut of the knife. Does it produce analgesia? Yes! The analgesia takes time to develop, approximately 20 or more minutes. Electrical stimulation of the needles at sensitive points is more effective than their simple insertion and manipulation.

Are we positive that this is so? Yes, because in rats in our laboratory, we can produce analgesia and measure its gradual increase in intensity, reaching a maximum in about 25 minutes to one hour (Fig. 1). Reversal of this analgesia occurs in two minutes if naloxone is injected (Fig. 2). The pattern of analgesia is very similar to that developed after a usual therapeutic dose of narcotic and is reversed similarly by naloxone.

Now that the scientific world has learned of endorphins and enkephalins, one may assume that these or similar molecules are synthesized or mobilized by electrical acupuncture. In man and rat, development of analgesia after acupuncture and its immediate neutralization

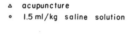

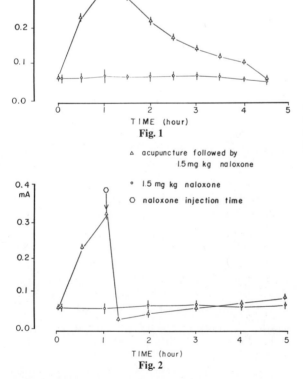

Fig. 1

Fig. 2

Figures 1 and 2. These are recordings of a group of 10 rats using electrical acupuncture. It is essentially equal to 5 mg./kg. of morphine as measured by the Rush Algesimeter in our Pain Laboratory.

by antagonists is striking. Can the release of endorphins be one of the ways that acupuncture causes analgesia? We believe this is probable. On bioassay in the rat and comparing the degree of analgesia with that produced by meperidine or morphine, however, we are still not clear what occurs in the patient being operated on during acupuncture anesthesia because the amount of analgesia seen in the rat appears inadequate for a surgical procedure.

We hope to repeat the laboratory study on human beings, comparing the analgesia developed by acupuncture to that produced by a narcotic. In a few cases we have studied acupuncture analgesia in man and the data derived are very similar to those obtained from the rat. There is little doubt that this technique can develop analgesia sufficient for a surgical procedure in an unknown proportion of the population. But can it be used in the West? Only for purposes of study or curiosity! We do not believe that it has a significant place in our future. The fact that we can produce analgesia in the rat, however, means that we should realize that something is happening that is real and measurable and that it can be antagonized. Can it also be potentiated? If so, how and how much? The analgesia that has been developed in the patients in China and Japan is significant.

WHAT IS THE MECHANISM OF ACTION OF ACUPUNCTURE?

Simply stated, I don't know. After many years of working daily with different highly trained doctors of Oriental medicine from China, Korea, and Taiwan and after extended discussions with world authorities who specialize in ear acupuncture, others who extensively use moxibustion, and with the Japanese group represented by Dr. Hyodo, who has published excellent texts on Japanese acupuncture techniques, we are impressed (Hyodo, 1975). The electrical activity in the meridia has been measured at representative points as has the electrical effects of cupping and scalp needle therapy. I have read the various acupuncture texts repeatedly. Do meridia exist? I have seen no evidence that they do. Are there acupuncture points? If one visualizes the points in the Oriental texts and measures conductivity of the skin by the use of a voltmeter at these points, one can detect changes that could be significant. If one reads Bonica's excellent text on pain (Bonica, 1954), one can see an interesting coincidence in the trigger points of the West and the acupuncture points of the East; even the recommended injection sites are similar.

In several patients we have done classic acupuncture and simultaneously measured thermal changes in distal areas using liquid crystals with photographic recording. These records clearly show that as postthoracotomy chest pain diminishes, the previously painful skin area increased in temperature. What does this change signify? It is unclear but is highly suggestive of an organic change. This study must be expanded to become significant. We have described the technique in a recent publication, for those who wish to explore it (Lee, Sadove, and Kim, 1976).

In a few patients, we have studied the development of analgesia in classic versus neutral points, as measured by a recording algesimeter (Lee and Sadove, 1977) (Figs. 3 and 4). The analgesia seemed appreciably better in the classic points; the curve developed in man was similar to that observed in rats. We have not attempted to neutralize human analgesia with naloxone, but from experience gained with rats, we are confident that analgesia will be antagonized in man. Further studies to prove statistical significance are indicated. This work corroborates that of Pomeranz and Chiu at the University of Toronto (1976).

The classic acupuncturists never heard of endorphins or enkephalins, nor did they do research or measure the changes that occurred. The possibility that reflex arcs are affected by acupuncture were also not disucssed in the classic acupuncture literature. It is obvious that pain causes harmful reflexes both locally and distally. The

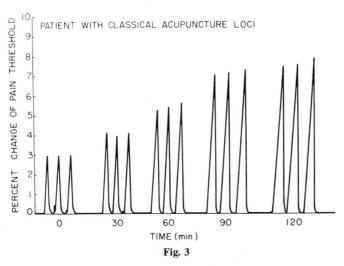

Fig. 3

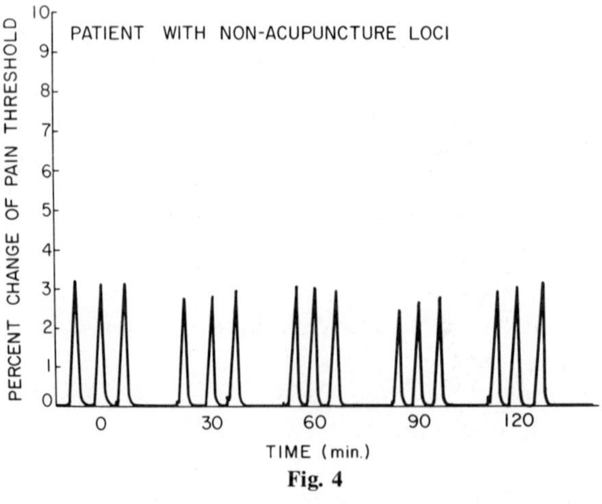

Fig. 4

Figures 3 and 4. Typical recorded charts. (Patient: R.M.)

pain relief within a few minutes after acupuncture in some patients with tennis elbow, tendonitis, and bursitis is probably based on a reflex vascular response and is not a result of endorphin release. In an asthmatic, relief is likely due to a local reflexogenic activity combined with the interruption of distal reflexes and interference with endocrine activity as well as an overall psychologic effect.

What does acupuncture do? I do not know, but I do know that it is clinically useful similar to other commonly used and little understood therapies, such as the application of heat, counterirritation, and the like.

Can there be abuse? Certainly! Should acupuncturists work alone? Definitely not! Should chiropractors, psychologists, and the like use it? I believe that acupuncture is useful and should not be employed by those only interested in financial gain. It is so easy to treat with acupuncture needlessly and thus delay specific and proved therapy. New techniques like acupuncture, biofeedback, and transcutaneous stimulation should be done under the supervision of those with proved skills in medical practice, with knowledge of investigative techniques, and those who have the ability to employ other accepted methods of providing pain relief just as easily as acupuncture.

CONCLUSION

Acupuncture has a useful place in a pain clinic but not to provide analgesia for surgical procedures in Western countries. It has a psychic effect just like any other modality in pain management. It also has multiple effects on reflexes, the endocrine system, immunologic systems, and endorphins and enkephalins, and other bodily systems. Should classic acupuncture be ignored? No! It must be studied and used by those interested in pain therapy. Its greatest potential for harm is its misuse.

REFERENCES

Bonica, J. J.: The Management of Pain. Philadelphia, Lea and Febiger, 1954.

Hyodo, M.: Ryodoraku treatment. Japan Ryodoraku, Autonomic Nerve System society, 1–4, Nakatsu-Handori, Oyodoku, Osaka, 531, Japan, 1975.

Lee, M. H., Sadove, M. S., and Kim, S. I.: Liquid crystal thermography in acupuncture therapy. Am. J. Acupuncture, 4:145–148, 1976.

Lee, M. H., and Sadove, M. S.: Use of the rush algesimeter in acupuncture. Am. J. Acupuncture, 5:249–256, 1977.

Melzack, R., and P. D. Wall: Pain mechanisms: a new theory. Science, 150:971–979, 1965.

Pomeranz, B., and Chiu, D.: Naloxone blockade of acupuncture analgesia: endorphin implicated. Life Sci., 19:1757–1762, 1976.

by JOHN J. BONICA

University of Washington School of Medicine

ACUPUNCTURE ANALGESIA AND ANESTHESIA

The purposes of this article are to review the use of acupuncture in the People's Republic of China (PRC), to summarize its current status in the United States, and to offer conclusions that will help the reader place this procedure in proper perspective. It is important to emphasize that the use of acupuncture for the therapy of chronic pain and other medical disorders, referred to as "therapeutic acupuncture," and its use to produce surgical anesthesia, or "acupuncture anesthesia," are quite different phenomena. The material will be presented in the following order: a review of Chinese traditional medicine to provide a background for the discussion of the use of acupuncture, a review and evaluation of therapeutic acupuncture and of acupuncture anesthesia, and a review of speculations concerning the mechanisms and action of acupuncture. The information is based on personal observation during a three-week visit to PRC, communication with other physicians and scientists who have visited China, activities as chairman of the Ad Hoc Committee on Acupuncture of the National Institutes of Health and the American Society of Anesthesiologists, and the information contained in relevant publications. Detailed accounts can be found in national reports (American Acupuncture Anesthesia Group, 1976; Bonica, 1974; Hogness, 1973; McLoud, Sainsbury, and Joseph, 1974).

TRADITIONAL CHINESE MEDICINE

Medicine in China dates back several millennia. The *Huang Ti Nei Ching Su Wen,* or the *Yellow Emperor's Classic of Internal Medicine,* written between the 8th and 5th centuries B.C., is the earliest extant medical classic in China. It consists of 18 volumes covering a great variety of subjects, including the theory of diseases and their etiology, diagnosis, and treatment (Yellow Emperor's Classic, 1972).

184

In the book, man is seen as a microcosm of the universe, subject to the same tension disruptions as nature itself. The immutable course of nature, the *Tao,* is believed to act through two opposing and unifying forces, the *Yin* (the feminine, negative, and passive force) and the *Yang* (the masculine, positive, and active force). In a normal person, the two opposing forces are in balance and assist the vital energy, called the *chi,* to circulate to all parts of the body via a network of 14 channels *(ching-10),* or meridians, each connected to an important internal organ or function to which it branches. Obstruction (deficiency) and outpouring (excess) in the circulation of the *chi* causes imbalance of the two forces, resulting in disease.

Diagnosis is made by studying the patient's behavior, coloration, respiration, and expressed complaints and, most importantly, by palpating the radial pulse. Six pulses, each representing an organ or system, are located at each wrist. Therapy consists primarily of acupuncture, moxibustion, massage, physical exercises, and dietary regimens. Acupuncture therapy at one or more of the 365 specific points located along the meridians corrects the imbalance and eliminates the disease. Disease is not a local process but affects the entire body and is often influenced by emotional and behavioral factors.

During the ensuing two millennia, the book underwent numerous revisions but remained a standard work in traditional medicine. Moreover, therapeutic acupuncture continued to be refined. Many books exclusively devoted to the subject were published, and the method spread to Japan and other Asiatic countries. In the 17th century, it was introduced to Europe (Kao, 1972).

With the introduction of Western medicine in China, traditional medicine in general and acupuncture in particular began to fall into disrepute as being nonscientific. In 1822, the Great Imperial Medical Board ordered the virtual abandonment of acupuncture on ethical grounds. Chinese intellectuals came to regard Chinese medicine as old-fashioned and a hindrance to the modernization and development of their country. In 1929, the Kuomintung government banned the practice of traditional Chinese medicine, including acupuncture. Despite this, the populace, particularly in rural areas, continued to believe in and use acupuncture and traditional medicine. Moreover, before the Chinese communists' victory in 1949, which they call the "War of Liberation," there were only about 20,000 to 30,000 Western-trained physicians, most of whom practiced in the large coastal cities and cared only for the foreign and rich Chinese population. Since 80 per cent of the 550,000,000 people in China at the time lived in rural areas, they had virtually no benefit from Western-trained doctors but relied on the estimated 400,000 traditional practitioners (Orleans, 1969). Before the "War of Liberation," inadequate health care, poverty, frequent famines, chronic malnutrition, and poor housing were the reasons China had one of the highest mortality rates and lowest life expectancies in the world (Quinn, 1973).

Soon after liberation, intensive programs to improve food production, housing, and medicine were initiated. Mao Tse-tung set forth four concepts of health care: (1) to serve the workers, peasants, and soldiers, (2) to put prevention first, (3) to unite Western and traditional Chinese medicine, and (4) to coordinate medical campaigns with mass movements. With help from Russia, new hospitals were built, old ones were rehabilitated, and medical school enrollment increased manyfold. At the same time, the Chinese increased the number of nurses, midwives, and assistant doctors and developed a new type of paraprofessional called "barefoot doctor," "worker doctor," and "Red Guard doctor" — peasants, factory workers, or soldiers given approximately three months training and subsequent on-the-job training in the provision of basic health care (Sidel, 1972).

The integration of traditional and Western medicine was repeatedly stressed by Chairman Mao, who stated, "Chinese medicine and pharmacology are a great treasure house; efforts should be made to explore them and raise them to higher levels." The old-type doctors were urged to abandon conservative prejudices, accept new knowledge, study science, and cooperate with Western-style doctors in order to increase their competence. By the same token, Western medicine "must study the popular and widespread spirit of Chinese medicine" (Shanghai, 1971). As a result, "Chinese medicine improvement schools" and "Chinese medicine research centers" were instituted, and, in 1954, the Chinese Academy of Traditional Medicine was established. Moreover, a concerted effort was begun to introduce courses on traditional medicine into medical school curricula, practicing physicians were required to take special courses in traditional medicine, and both types of doctors began to work side-by-side in hospitals and clinics.

The Great Proletariat Cultural Revolution during the years 1966 to 1969 affected the radical changes proposed by Chairman Mao. It influenced every aspect of life, including health care. It moved China away from the elitist bureaucracy that had pervaded until 1965, allegedly under the influence of former President Liu Shao-Chi, and replaced it with the egalitarian society espoused by Mao. During the revolution, universities and medical schools were closed, scientific publication was suspended, and students and professors were sent to the countryside for re-education, which included physical labor in the fields as well as medical work. When medical schools reopened, the curriculum, formerly taking six years, was reduced to three, and "theoretical" teaching was abandoned in favor of "practical training" outside the classroom.

One of the most important results of the nationalism and ferment of the Cultural Revolution was the renewed emphasis on traditional medicine. It was given equal status with Western science and medicine, its practitioners were restored to favor, and a vigorous program was mounted to effect a true merger of the two schools. The curricula of Western-type schools contained many courses on various aspects of traditional medicine, including acupuncture, while students in traditional medical schools studied certain basic sciences and the use of "Western therapeutic methods." Moreover, hospital staffs now have both Western-type and traditional practitioners, the ratio varying with the type and specific function of the hospital. The outpatient clinics of these hospitals and the health stations in factories, communes, and villages offer the patient a choice between the two types of doctors.

THERAPEUTIC ACUPUNCTURE

In compliance with the aforementioned health policies and due in part to the influence of Western medicine, therapeutic acupuncture has undergone significant changes during the past several years, but especially since the Cultural Revolution. Much effort has been devoted to improving the selection of patients and to techniques by means of clinical trials. Moreover, there has been a significant change in attitude toward traditional concepts in order to make acupuncture acceptable to Western physicians (Shanghai, 1971; Hogness, 1973).

Techniques

There are now several methods of therapeutic acupuncture, but the method involving insertion of needles in specific acupuncutre points is most commonly used. The needles are of stainless steel, usually 1 to 10 cm. long, and are of four or five standard sizes, with diameters ranging from 0.4 to 0.28 mm.

The selection of acupuncture points varies, depending on the disease being treated and the acupuncture school followed. The old traditional schools used acupuncture points throughout the body, the number varying from source to source (although there is some uniformity with regard to certain points). Practice of the old traditional type could involve the use of as many as 800 of these points distributed around the body surface or as few as one or two discrete points. The traditional practitioners related these points to organ meridians as dermal representations of internal organs, both real (e.g., heart) and unreal (e.g., "triple warmer"). More contemporary acupuncture "science" views these points as aggregations of nerve endings, the stimulation of which produces patterns of activity within the nervous system that is allegedly responsible for its effects.

The practice of acupuncture is difficult to define because of an incomplete transition of what was originally a philosophy into a scientific practice. By and large, however, it appears to involve the insertion of needles into points following one of three patterns. They may be inserted into specific points along the organ meridians, the points bearing little anatomic relation to the organ being treated, or needles may be inserted only in an ear. This technique, developed by Nogier (1972) of Lyon, France, maintains that the whole body image is projected on the ear, and therefore needling can be restricted to this organ. Finally, there are those who insert needles into appropriate areas of the body where pain is felt, e.g., for arm pain the needle would be inserted in the arm, that is, into structures supplied by the same spinal cord segments as the painful area.

In many instances, a combination of acupuncture points is used. The needle is inserted and advanced until the *te ch'i* is experienced by the patient. This is described as a feeling of tingling, distention, heaviness, and numbness. Stimulation is achieved either manually, through a push-pull and rotatory movement, or by electroacupuncture. Manual stimulation is carried out for 10 to 15 minutes, the needle either removed or left in place, and after an interval of time the procedure is repeated. In recent years. electroacupuncture has gained widespread use because it produces continuous stimulation over longer periods of time with less effort on the part of the operator because the strength of stimulation can be adjusted according to the needs of the patient and a stronger stimulation can be achieved than with manual stimulation.

The number of treatments depends on the type of disease and its severity. Acute diseases are treated one to three times daily until the condition improves. In chronic diseases, acupuncture is done daily or two to three times weekly for a total of 10 to 20 treatments.

Other forms of acupuncture include the injection of sterile water, saline, procaine hydrochloride, morphine sulfate, vitamins, or other medication into acupuncture points (Shanghai, 1972). "Thread acupuncture" involves the insertion of a surgical needle threaded with catgut through one acupuncture point and out another. The catgut thread is left in place to produce persistent stimulation for several weeks until it is absorbed. "Pressure acupuncture" or "acupressure" consists of the application of pressure on the skin overlying the appropriate acupuncture points for a period of several minutes. Cutaneous needle acupuncture involves the application of numerous short (0.5 cm.) needles placed either on a roller or on sticks and applied lightly on the skin overlying the acupuncture points. Moxibustion involves the use of a smoldering piece of dried moss (*Artemisia vulgaris*) that may be applied directly on the skin over the acupuncture points, held at a distance from the skin, or placed on the shaft of an acupuncture needle. It is important when discussing acupuncture therapy to define the specific modes and sites of stimulation, since it varies considerably in use by different practitioners.

Clinical Applications

Acupuncture therapy has been advocated and used for treatment of virtually every disorder or disease in man and animals (Shanghai, 1972). In contrast to acupuncture anesthesia, often done by medical personnel, therapeutic acupuncture is generally performed by traditional practitioners, assistant doctors, and barefoot doctors and at times, by teachers or nurses in health stations or schools (Bonica, 1974b; Orleans, 1969). currently, its therapeutic role varies, depending on training of the practitioner and facilities available. In health stations, communes, factories, and villages, it is used empirically as the initial phase of treatment of symptoms, often without a diagnosis. In fact, it is employed in many instances as a primary diagnostic tool. Acupuncture is tried on the assumption that the symptom is due to a particular disease; if the symptom disappears after therapy, this confirms the diagnosis. In the event benefit is not derived, other forms of treatment are given.

Traditional practitioners use acupuncture alone or in combination with moxibustion, herbs, and massage. In major hospitals staffed by "integrated" practitioners, it is usually employed after the diagnosis is established and is often used in conjunction with drugs, chemotherapy, and other well-established "Western" forms of therapy.

Relief of Pain. Pain is the most frequent indication for acupuncture therapy. It is said to be highly effective in relieving pain due to a variety of post-traumatic, musculoskeletal, visceral, and other disorders. Unfortunately, controlled trials have not been done, and all reports claiming efficacy of acupuncture in relieving pain are anecdotal (Bonica, 1974b).

Acute Pain. Two injured patients I saw after admission to hospital were not given acupuncture for pain relief but were managed with narcotics or regional analgesia. I was told that acupuncture is not so effective in emergency conditions when the patient is apprehensive (Bonica, 1974b). Since acupuncture analgesia used for surgery is said to persist for several hours after the operations and thus obviates the use of narcotics, I was disappointed to learn that because of insufficient manpower, acupuncture is not used to relieve postoperative pain in patients who have been managed with regional or general anesthesia.

Musculoskeletal Pain. Pain due to various musculoskeletal disorders is probably the most frequent indication for therapeutic acupuncture. It is the primary form of therapy in chronic back pain, muscular pain, periarthritis of the shoulder, and cervical spondylosis. Although excellent results were claimed, no data on long-term effects were available (Bonica, 1974b; McLoud, 1974).

Arthritis Pain. Arthritis pain is a common indication for acupuncture therapy in China. In general, the needles are inserted in points near the affected joint and stimulation is applied either manually or with electroacupuncture. The series of treatments vary from 10 to 30 or more. Excellent relief was claimed by all, and some indicated that acupuncture caused regression of the disease process, but, again, data were not available to substantiate the claims (Bonica, 1974b; McLoud, 1974).

Neuralgia. Control of trigeminal neuralgia is another important indication for acupuncture therapy. The needles are inserted into local points in the face, depending on which nerve branch is affected, or into ear points. Although in most traditional hospitals acupuncture therapy is considered highly effective and the primary form of treatment, in one hospital I visited it was considered inferior to the use of drugs and neurosurgery (Bonica, 1974b).

Sciatic neuralgia has been widely treated with acupuncture with varying success. The needles are usually placed in the lower lumbar paravertebral region, gluteal region, and lower limbs. In addition to needle stimulation either manually or by electroacupuncture, moxibustion is used by some. Some practitioners inject procaine, 10 per cent glucose, or 25 per cent magnesium sulfate; others use ear acupuncture, inserting the needles into one or two hypersensitive spots; and still others use cutaneous acupuncture or heavy tapping and cupping in the paravertebral region. In discussing results, the Shanghai group (1971) emphasized the importance of differential diagnosis and reported that acupuncture is most effective in "primary sciatica"; others reported better results in acute and chronic cases or in those patients who had undergone previous disc surgery.

Headache.   Acupuncture is widely used and considered very effective in the treatment of migraine and headache due to emotional tension, spasm of neck muscles, physiologic dysfunctions, hypertension, and disorders of the ear, nose, and throat (Shanghai, 1971; Bonica, 1974b). Needles are inserted in different positions in the scalp, face, and upper limbs. The points selected and type of stimulation used vary according to the site and nature of the headache and apparently vary considerably from hospital to hospital.

Visceral Pain.   In rural areas and traditional hospitals, acupuncture is considered the primary treatment of acute cholecystitis, cholelithiasis, appendicitis, and gastritis and for peptic ulcer and renal colic (Shanghai, 1971; Bonica, 1974b; McLoud, 1974). It is claimed that acupuncture is effective not only in relieving the pain but also in causing the regression of the disease process of "simple, acute appendicitis" or cholecystitis. The treatment is repeated two to three times a day and continued until the symptoms disappear. Due emphasis is placed on the need to carefully observe the patient, on the concomitant use of drugs, and on emergency surgery if the symptoms do not improve. One group in Canton claimed that of 250 patients with peptic ulcer treated with acupuncture, symptomatic and radiologic improvement had occurred in 95 per cent (McLoud, 1974). It is of interest that all patients had been admitted to hospital for six weeks and treatment had included dietary restriction and medical therapy.

Cancer Pain.   Among the many traditional practitioners and Western-type internists, surgeons, and anesthesiologists, there was unanimity that acupuncture has no value in the treatment of chronic pain of malignant disorders. These patients are usually managed with narcotics and chemotherapy; a few undergo neurosurgical operations for the relief of pain.

Therapeutic Acupuncture in the U.S.A.

Acupuncture as a therapeutic modality was mentioned by Weir Mitchell during the Civil War and advocated by Sir William Osler as the most effective therapy for acute lumbago (Osler, 1916). Moreover, there was widespread, albeit unofficial, use in the Chinese sections of New York, San Francisco, Seattle, and other large cities that have Oriental communities. Until 1971, however, the American medical profession showed little interest in the procedure. Initial reports by Snow and Reston in the lay press (N.Y. Times, August 1, 1971) and Dimond in the Journal of the American Medical Association (1971) aroused the interest of the American public and medical profession. This was greatly engendered by subsequent visits to China by other physicians (Signer and Galston, 1972) and President Nixon. In the course of the ensuing year, there developed an enormous, almost incredible interest in acupuncture therapy that was accompanied by many misconceptions among the American public and by confusion among physicians as to its role. This was, in part, due to the early reports made by Americans, including some highly respected scientists, who although well-meaning, did not have the expertise to critically evaluate their observations (Bonica, 1974b). Moreover, many reports appeared in the lay press about the success of acupuncture therapy. These reports misled some Americans to believe that therapeutic acupuncture was a well-tested, thoroughly proved, therapeutic modality that was a panacea for all illnesses. This, in turn, generated immense public pressure on the medical profession and state legislatures to permit the widespread indiscriminate use of therapeutic acupuncture.

As a result, acupuncture was practiced extensively by physicians and other health professionals and acupuncturists. Although some used the method in an ethical, albeit empirical, fashion and a few did clinical studies and made observations, many unscrupulous persons exploited the public's interest by operating their acupuncture "clinics" or "centers" like "mills," where several hundred patients were treated daily at exorbitant fees. The interest and curiosity of many physicians were exploited by groups who sponsored "mini-courses" and by the acupuncture equipment companies, who sold charts, needles, and "do-it-yourself" kits.

Public interest was partly responsible for the National Institutes of Health appointing an Ad Hoc Advisory Committee on Acupuncture and sponsoring two conferences devoted to reports of laboratory and clinical studies. As a result of the conferences, the committee concluded that although acupuncture held some promise as a therapeutic modality, it was clearly no panacea and well-designed and controlled scientific studies would be needed before it could be considered for widespread clinical use in the United States (Jenerick, 1973). In a comprehensive report, I re-emphasized that the widespread use of acupuncture was unwarranted until scientific evidence derived from well-controlled clinical trials became available (Bonica, 1974b), particularly in relation to its use for the therapy of chronic pain, which is influenced by many factors, including culture, tradition, education, and background. Moreover, because acupuncture was a new therapeutic modality in American medicine, it was essential that it be tested on American patients, using well-established scientific principles. I further suggested that each state allow such studies to be carried out until sufficient data are available to ascertain whether acupuncture is better than, as good as, or inferior to well-tested drugs and procedures. Unfortunately, these suggestions were generally ignored and acupuncture therapy continued to be used widely. Subsequently, many reports were published, most extolling the efficacy and virtues of acupuncture therapy in the management of chronic pain syndromes. In time, however, data from well-controlled clinical trials were published, suggesting that therapeutic acupuncture has limited usefulness in the management of pain. Lee and associates (1975) demonstrated that it did not matter if the needles were inserted in traditional meridian points or in "control" points and that relief was usually temporary; 18 of their 261 patients obtained good relief (15 per cent) beyond four weeks after a series of four acupuncture treatments. At the University of Washington Pain Clinic, a self-selected series of 100 patients suffering from chronic pain refractory to other forms of conventional therapy undertook a trial of acupuncture analgesia at weekly intervals (Murphy, 1976). Although initial results were often spectacularly successful, after the third treatment, long-term benefit from acupuncture analgesia was as disappointing as that from other forms of therapy. None of the 100 patients showed any continued objective evidence of pain relief; i.e., medication intake and functional impairment continued despite claimed subjective relief in a small percentage of patients. Only three of the 100 patients claimed long-term (upwards of three months) pain relief from a course of acupuncture therapy. Fifteen per cent maintained subjective relief, provided they underwent acupuncture at approximately weekly intervals, but they did not, as a result of this claimed relief, decrease analgesic medicines or improve activity levels. Similar patterns of response to acupuncture therapy for chronic pain have been noted by others (Kepes, Chen, and Schapira, 1976; Levine, Gormley, and Fields, 1976).

The results of these and other well-controlled trials suggest that acupuncture can be effective in relieving pain temporarily in self-limited musculoskeletal problems, such as post-traumatic pain after sport injuries. Whether this is an improvement on conventional therapy remains to be proved. The limited usefulness of therapeutic acupuncture is further attested to by the fact that the enthusiasm among the public and medical profession has waned. Many (the majority or most?) of the acupuncture clinics have closed.

ACUPUNCTURE ANESTHESIA

Acupuncture anesthesia is not really anesthesia but more correctly analgesia, since sensations other than pain are maintained. In contrast to its use for therapy, which goes back several millennia, acupuncture anesthesia is relatively new, first used in 1958 (Bonica, 1974b; Shanghai, 1971). Every report on the subject published in China credits "Chairman Mao's proletarian Medical and Public Health Line" as the impetus for its development. Apparently prompted by the question, "If acupuncture relieves pain of medical disorders, why not use it to prevent pain of surgery," it was first employed to relieve post-tonsillectomy pain and, subsequently, during the changing of wound and burn dressings and for teeth extractions, tonsillectomy, and other simple operations (Shanghai, 1971; Bonica, 1974a).

The initial reports created excitement and interest among health care professionals and the Chinese public for two reasons. First, acupuncture anesthesia held the promise of helping to solve a serious health care problem — the lack of trained anesthetic personnel. At this time, anesthesiology, which started as a discipline a few years earlier, was at an early stage of development, and virtually all of the anesthesiologists and nurse anesthetists practiced in large hospitals in urban areas (Bonica, 1974a). Consequently, the anesthetics given in rural areas (where 80 per cent of the population lived) were usually administered by untrained personnel, resulting in a high incidence of complications. A second and equally important reason for the interest generated was the fact that acupuncture anesthesia was an exclusively Chinese invention unrelated to Western medicine, which still bore the taint of "Western imperialism."

Despite the initial favorable impact, acupuncture anesthesia did not become widely used. In fact, during the early 1960's, it was virtually abandoned in many hospitals. One authoritative textbook states that less than 10,000 cases were done in the entire country during the first eight years (Shanghai, 1971). During the Cultural Revolution, however, there was great impetus to reintroduce acupuncture anesthesia and expand its clinical use as part of Chairman Mao's movement to integrate Western and traditional medicine.

Current Status

Reports by most early visitors to China gave the lay public and the medical profession of the United States and other Western countries the impression that acupuncture anesthesia was being used widely for many, if not most, operations and that it was highly effective in most cases. During my visit to PRC, however, I found this not to be the case as did others who visited that country subsequently (Capperauld, 1972; Dimond, 1971; Gingras and Geekie, 1973; Jain, 1972; Kao, 1972). On the basis of data provided by anesthesiologists and surgeons in hospitals visited by our delegation and statistics published by the Chinese, I estimated that acupuncture was being used in less than 10 per cent of surgical operations in China (Bonica, 1974b). In fact, based on a Chinese report that about 600,000 operations with acupuncture anesthesia were done in China up to 1973 (Shanghai, 1971) and using other data on the incidence of surgical operations in other countries, I speculated that this figure represented about 1 to 2 per cent of the operations done in China during the seven-year period prior to 1973.

The claim that acupuncture anesthesia is effective in about 90 per cent of patients, a figure accepted by many other visitors to China, is also incorrect. This is based on personal observations and those of others (Bonica, 1974a and 1974b; McLoud, 1974) and is also suggested by data published by the Shanghai group (1971), which involved 80,000 patients given acupuncture anesthesia for more than 100 different types of operations. Table 1 lists the criteria used by the Shanghai group, and Table 2 contains data on their results (Bonica, 1974b). The Chinese considered grades 1, 2, and 3 as effective, and when added, they give the

Table 1. Criteria for Evaluation of Results of Acupuncture Anesthesia

Grade	Pain	Changes in Blood pressure, Heart rate, and Respiration	Supplementation Meperidine (mg./kg./2 hrs.)	Local Anesthetics	Operating Conditions
I Excellent	Brief periods of mild pain; patient calm	Little or no	1.0–1.5	None	Good
II Good	Periods of moderate pain; groaning	Mild	1.0–1.5	Small dose	Satisfactory
III Moderate	Obvious pain during operation but could still be accomplished	Moderate	1.5–2.0	Moderate dose	Fair
IV Pain (failure)	Severe pain	Marked	Necessary to change to drug anesthesia		

Table 2. Results of Acupuncture Anesthesia

Operation	Number of Cases	Grade (in percentage of cases) I	II	III	IV	Effective Rate I + II + III (Percentage)
Craniotomy	606	34	35	26	4	96
Thyroid operations	670	54	31	10	5	95
Pulmonary resection	656	17	26	52	4	97
Heart operations	172	24	51	16	8	92
Subtotal gastrectomy	763	16	45	34	4	96
Hysterectomy	590	34	40	11	14	87
Total Cases	3,457					
Mean percentage of total		31	37	27	6	94

overall success rate of 94 per cent. The data, particularly of those operations on the head, neck, and thorax, which are considered the most suitable for acupuncture, show that the pain and reflex responses to noxious stimulation occurred in most of the patients, and therefore acupuncture must be considered as unsatisfactory when compared with successful regional or general anesthesia. Chapman and Fink (in press) analyzed the results obtained with acupuncture anesthesia in about 11,000 patients and found that approximately 41 per cent had grade 1, 35 per cent grade 2, 16 per cent grade 3, and 8 per cent grade 4. According to the Chinese criteria, the overall success rate was 92 per cent. The American Acupuncture Anesthesia Study Group, which visited China for three weeks in May 1974, evaluated the results in 48 operations, which they observed using their own criteria. They noted 52 per cent of the patients who were rated grade 1, 21 per cent grade 2, 2 per cent grade 3, and 25 per cent grade 4. All of these computations suggest that only 30 to 50 per cent of the Chinese patients had pain relief that would be considered acceptable to American patients.

EXPERIENCES IN THE U.S. AND OTHER COUNTRIES

In Japan, Taiwan, Hong Kong, and other Asiatic countries where therapeutic acupuncture has been used for centuries and is still widely employed even by Western-type physicians, attempts to induce acupuncture anesthesia have mostly failed (Bonica, 1974b). Yet, most of the people who have attempted the procedure are highly qualified anesthesiologists and experienced with therapeutic acupuncture. In Taiwan and Hong Kong, where the population is ethnically, genetically, and culturally similar to that of PRC, attempts to produce acupuncture anesthesia have generally failed, according to data obtained through personal communication with anesthesiologists and scientists in Asia, Europe, Great Britain, and the United States as part of a survey for the NIH Ad Hoc Committee on Acupuncture.

In Britain, Mann, the leading exponent of therapeutic acupuncture, and others have been unsuccessful in producing consistently effective analgesia, even for minor operations. Nguyen Van Nghi (1973), one of the best known acupuncturists in France, reported that 32 of the first 50 patients operated on with acupuncture in that country had satisfactory analgesia. Roccia (1973) of Italy reported that of 33 patients operated on with acupuncture analgesia, only four required supplementation with drug anesthesia. Sporadic reports from other European medical centers have appeared, but the total number of successful procedures published thus far represents a miniscule proportion of the operations done.

The exact number of patients operated on with acupuncture anesthesia in the United States is unknown, but one can speculate that the procedure has been attempted in several hundred surgical and obstetric patients and a larger number of dental patients. Few, if any, of the anesthesiologists who have used acupuncture anesthesia on an experimental basis have seen fit to continue its application. This is undoubtedly due to the high failure rate and unpredictable results, especially compared with the certainty of regional and general anesthesia. Most American physicians who have attempted the procedure have not had training in acupuncture anesthesia for surgery but have relied on experience with therapeutic acupuncture.

CONCLUSIONS

The foregoing information and data permit certain conclusions, speculations, and suggestions. First, in China, operations are being performed with acupuncture alone as analgesia. As one who has seen American patients complain of pain and become unmanageable when an incision is made with inadequate drug anesthesia, I was impressed to see Chinese patients wide awake, lying quietly while surgery was performed. In selected and prepared patients, acupuncture apparently decreases or eliminates the pain of surgical operations. Acupuncture analgesia is not used as frequently or as effectively as claimed by the Chinese and most American visitors, however.

These comments are intended to place the procedure in perspective and *not* to detract in any way from this important Chinese achievement. The fact that acupuncture analgesia permits completion of surgical operations in some patients is an important gain in a country with a severe shortage of anesthetic personnel. The Chinese are more successful with the procedure than are others for many reasons, including intense preoperative counseling and preparation, their admirable ability to tolerate moderate to severe pain, the intense motivation provoked in the patient and surgical team by shortage of anesthetic personnel and by political and ideologic factors, and the skill, gentleness, and dexterity of Chinese surgeons, who are willing to accept less than optimal operating conditions.

MECHANISMS OF ACUPUNCTURE ANALGESIA

The traditional explanation of restoration of energy balance is not an acceptable explanation for contemporary understanding of acupuncture. This is somewhat akin to the caloric and phlogiston theories as explanations of inflammatory processes and would invoke the existence of an alternative biologic system other than those of conventional physiology and anatomy.

It is, perhaps, with neuronal interaction that any mechanisms of acupuncture might be best explained physiologically, and the efficacy of acupuncture anesthesia certainly appears to be dependent on the integrity of the nervous system (Chiang et al., 1973). Data suggest that the afferent input generated by acupuncture stimulation somehow interferes with and suppresses the appreciation of pain. The mechanism of acupuncture analgesia may well work within the framework of some of the recent explanations for the phenomenon of pain extending from the initial concept of the "gate theory" (Melzack and Wall, 1965). The basic principle of this theory involves the concept that one stimulus can be modified, perhaps suppressed, by the input of an alternative stimulation.

This gate theory and its subsequent modification have led to a therapeutic approach to relieving pain by administering an alternative sensory input to the pain via the use of dorsal column stimulators and, more recently, transcutaneous nerve stimulators that apply an electrical current, usually to the site of the pain. Transcutaneous somatic stimulation can relieve pain and yield therapeutic benefits that outlast their brief duration (Melzack, 1975). It is conceivable that acupuncture analgesia might work via similar mechanisms, especially when the needles are stimulated electrically (Fox and Melzack, 1976). It would also appear that the maximal effect of electroacupuncture is obtained with stimulation in the same dermatome as the pain. This has been shown experimentally with dental pain, for which there was a substantial analgesic effect after electroacupuncture when the needles were placed in the same dermatome as the teeth, but there was trivial analgesic effect if they were used at a remote dermatome (Andersson, et al., 1973; Chapman, Chen, and Bonica, 1977).

Most theories of the appreciation of pain attest that the pain experience depends on more than activity in the afferent ascending pathways and that such factors as the psychologic make-up and the cultural background of the individual play a role (Chapman, 1975). It is almost certain that the analgesia that follows acupuncture is dependent on such factors. Certainly, our interpretation as to whether an afferent impulse is painful or not depends not only on direct sensory pathways but also on "response bias" or interpretation of this afferent input.

Clarke and Yang (1974) have shown, by using a signal detection theory experimentally with a radiant heat source on the arm, that acupuncture did not decrease sensory discrimination but produced a substantial shift in response bias. The subjects interpreted the heat stimuli as less painful following an acupuncture trial, so that acupuncture may not produce true analgesia but an attitudinal change towards sensory input resulting in a diminution of the pain experience.

More recently Chapman (1977) confirmed that intrasegmental stimulation is more effective than extrasegmental meridian point stimulation in dental pain. In contrast to the study of Clarke and Yang, the resulting analgesia was a relatively pure sensory change not due to modifications of response bias.

A further possible mechanism of acupuncture anesthesia is that acupuncture stimulation liberates a neurohumoral analgesic substance. This was first suggested in China on the basis of analgesia obtained by (a) the transfer of plasmal or cerebrospinal fluid from a donor (acupunctured) to a "receptor" (nonacupunctured) rabbit and (b) closed circulation experiments in which only one animal was acupunctured but both showed analgesia (Research Group of Acupuncture Anesthesia, 1973). The recent discovery of endorphins, substances that bind to opiate receptors, and the fact that analgesic effects of acupuncture are blocked by naloxone and hypophysectomy support this thesis. The sequence characteristics of acupuncture anesthesia, i.e., a gradual rise in pain threshold with the onset of needling and a gradual decrease of analgesia after needling is stopped, is compatible with the time course of production and decay of endogenous pain-relieving substances probably produced in the pituitary and midbrain in response to acupuncture stimulation. Since this newly discovered antinociception system receives input from the cortex, it is likely influenced by psychologic factors.

In view of these considerations and the evidence seen in China, I believe that decrease or elimination of acute pain inherent in surgical operations is due to several factors. The peripheral nerve stimulation probably increases the activity of the antinociception system to neurophysiologic mechanisms. This is reinforced by psychophysiologic mechanisms that may further increase the activity of the antinociception system and other, as yet undiscovered, supraspinal descending modulating systems. Providing the type of information that the Chinese patient receives decreases or eliminates anxiety that in turn lowers nociceptive transmission, probably through psychophysiologic mechanisms that may involve stimulation of descending inhibitory systems. This is reinforced by other psychophysiologic mechanisms initiated by the intense motivation provoked by political ideology, the "esprit de corps" engendered by the intense interaction of patient and members of the surgical team, by discussions with other patients who have had acupuncture, and by the strong suggestions inherent in the full preparation of the patient. In a relatively small percentage of patients, all of these factors appear to decrease or eliminate the perception of pain and even the segmental and suprasegmental reflex responses to the noxious stimulus of the operation. In others, these processes are less effective, the patient feels some pain, but the reflex responses shown by rise in blood pressure, increase in heart rate and dilation of the pupils are not affected. In a final group, the process has little or no effect on nociceptive transmission; consequently, the patient feels moderate to severe pain and manifests most of the reflex responses produced by noxious stimulation.

REFERENCES

American Acupuncture Anesthesia Group: Acupuncture in the People's Republic of China. Washington, D.C., National Academy of Sciences, 1976.

Andersson, S. A., Ericson, R., Holmgren, E., et al.: Electro-acupuncture: effect on pain threshold measured with electrical stimulation of teeth. Brain Res., *63*:393–396, 1973.

Bonica, J. J.: Anesthesiology in the People's Republic of China. Anesthesiology, *40*:175–186, 1974a.

Bonica, J. J.: Therapeutic acupuncture in the People's Republic of China. J.A.M.A,, *228*:1544–1551; *229*: 1317–1325, 1974b.

Capperauld, I.: Acupuncture anesthesia and medicine in China today. Surg. Gynecol. Obstet., *135*:440–445, 1972.

Chapman, C. R.: Psychophysical evaluation of acupunctural analgesia. Anesthesiology, *43*:501–506, 1975.

Chapman, C. R., Chen, A. C., and Bonica, J. J.: Effects of intra-segmental electrical acupuncture on dental pain: evaluation by threshold estimation and sensory decision theory. Pain, *3*:213–227, 1977.

Chapman, C. R., and Fink, B. R.: Acupuncture anesthesia in China. *In* Wollman, H., and Larson, C. P. (eds.): Anesthesiology. Philadelphia, J. B. Lippincott Co., in press.

Chiang, C. Y. Chang, C. T., Chiu, H. L., et al.: Analysis of peripheral afferent pathway for effect of acupuncture analgesia. Sci. Sin., *16*:210, 1973.

Clarke, W. C., and Yang, Y. C.: Acupunctural analgesia? Evaluation by signal detection theory. Science, *184*:1096–1098, 1974.

Dimond, E. G.: Acupuncture anesthesia: western medicine and Chinese traditional medicine. J.A.M.A., *218*:1558–1563, 1971.

Fox, E. J., and Melzack, R.: Transcutaneous stimulation and acupuncture: comparison of treatment for low back pain. Pain, *2*:141–148, 1976.

Gingras, G., and Geekie, D. A.: China report: health care in the world's most populous country. Can. Med. Assoc. J., *109*:150A–150P, 1973.

Hogness, J. R. (ed.): Report of the Medical Delegation to the People's Republic of China. National Academy of Sciences Institute of Medicine, 1973.

Jain, K. K.: Glimpses of neurosurgery in the People's Republic of China. Lancet, *1*:1328–1330, 1972.

Jenerick, H. P.: Proceedings of the NIH Acupuncture Research Conference, Publication No. 74–165. (Washington, D.C., Department of Health, Education, and Welfare)

Kao, F. F.: China, Chinese medicine, and the Chinese medical system. Am. J. Chin. Med., *1*:1–59, 1972.

Kepes, E. R., Chen, M., and Schapira, M.: A critical evaluation of acupuncture in the treatment of chronic pain. *In* Bonica, J. J., and Albe-Fessard, D. (eds.): Advances in Pain Research and Therapy. Vol. 1. New York, Raven Press, 1976, pp. 817–822.

Lee, P. K., Anderson, T. W., Modell, J. H., et al.: Treatment of chronic pain with acupuncture. J.A.M.A., *232*:1133–1135, 1975.

Levine, J. D., Gormley, J., and Fields,

M. L.: Observations on analgesic effects of needle puncture (acupuncture). Pain, *2*:149–159, 1976.

McLoud, J. G., Sainsbury, M. J., and Joseph, D.: Acupuncture: A Report to the National Health and Research Council of Australia. Canberra, Australian Government Publishing Services, 1974.

Melzack, R., and Wall, P. D.: Pain mechanisms: a new theory. Science, *150*:971–979, 1965.

Melzack, R.: Prolonged relief of pain by brief intense transcutaneous somatic stimulation. Pain, *1*:357–373, 1975.

Murphy, T. M.: Subjective and objective follow-up assessment of acupuncture therapy without suggestion in 100 chronic pain patients. *In* Bonica, J. J., and Albe-Fessard, D. (eds.): Advances in Pain Research and Therapy. Vol. 1. New York, Raven Press, 1976, pp. 811–815.

Nogier, P. F. M.: Treatise of Auruolo Therapy. Moulin-les-Metz, Moulinneuve, 1972.

Orleans, L. A.: Medical education and manpower in communist China. *In* Hugh, C. T. (ed.): Aspects of China's Education. New York, Teachers College Press, Columbia University, 1969.

Osler, W.: Principles and Practice of Medicine. New York, D. Appleton & Co., 1916, p. 1131.

Quinn, J. R. (ed.): Medicine and Public Health in the People's Republic of China. Publication No. 73–67. Fogarty International Center, National Institutes of Health. Department of Health, Education, and Welfare, 1973.

Research Group of Acupuncture Anesthesia, Peking Medical College: Effect of acupuncture on pain threshold of human skin. Chin. Med. J., *3*:151–157, 1973.

Roccia, L.: A'azione analgesica dell'agopuntura in chirurgia generale. G. Accad. Med. Torino 135:1–6, 1973.

Shanghai Acupuncture and Moxibustion Research Laboratory: Handbook of Acupuncture and Moxibustion Therapy. Translated and edited by H. Agren. Hong Kong, Commercial Press, 1971.

Sidel, V. W.: The barefoot doctors of

the People's Republic of China. N. Engl. J. Med., *286*:1292–1300, 1972.

Signer, E., and Galston, A. W.: Education and science in China. Science, *175*:15–23, 1972.

Van Nghi, N.: Acupuncture anesthesia concerning the first 40 cases conducted in France. Am. J. Chin. Med., *1*:135–142, 1973.

The Yellow Emperor's Classic of Internal Medicine. Translated and edited by I. Veith. Berkeley, University of California, 1972.

ACUPUNCTURE IN ANESTHESIOLOGY

EDITORIAL COMMENT

The use of acupuncture as a method of pain relief is well outlined in the contributions of Bonica and Sadove. The result of the insinuation of political objectives and pressure by the lay press on medical judgment is apparent.

Both authors clearly indicate that the effectiveness of acupuncture for the relief of pain associated with surgical procedures is inferior to more reliable and proven anesthetic techniques. Neither deny that in *some* patients, appropriately selected and prepared, the techniques may succeed. Can one afford a technique that *may* succeed?

Similarly, both authors agree that in the treatment of acute and chronic painful syndromes, acupuncture will provide pain relief in *some* patients. Both strive to define which syndromes are susceptible. The answers are not clear and data are needed. Both agree that acupuncture does effect physiologic and pharmacologic change. However, men and women are prone to many subjective influences, ill defined. The more chronic the pain, the less definitive the explanation for relief.

The technique is worthy of study by those who seek valid data. The demonstration of release of endorphins after acupuncture and the reversal of acupuncture analgesia by naloxone are striking observations begging further study. Interestingly, even some patients respond to placebos with the release of endorphins. Unfortunately, as Sadove repeatedly stresses, acupuncture can be exploited by the unscrupulous, by those who seek personal gain, and by those indifferent to the results of controlled studies.

Part 10

THE TRAINING
AND SUPERVISION
OF NURSE
ANESTHETISTS

THE PROPOSITION:

Anesthesiologists should be responsible for teaching and
supervising nurse anesthetists.

ALTERNATIVE POINTS OF VIEW

By John W. Ditzler
By Ira P. Gunn

EDITORIAL COMMENT

by JOHN W. DITZLER

The Veterans Administration

NURSE ANESTHETISTS SHOULD BE TRAINED AND SUPERVISED BY ANESTHESIOLOGISTS

Delivery of anesthetic care in the United States in 1900 largely resided with the paramedical anesthetist. Early in the century principal training emphasis was on programs for nurses and even today they show continued growth. Nurse anesthesia training programs seem now to be outdistanced by physician (anesthesiologist) training programs and even appear to be challenged by other paramedical anesthetists (nonphysician) programs. The *raison d'etre* for all of these programs, although subject to debate over merits for each, seems clearly to be one of manpower (person power). A serious student of the needs of the patient (sic) American public will soon discover that complexity of tasks, rapid advance of basic science knowledge, and changing moods in health care delivery contribute to what used to be a "them or us" controversy. It is unfortunate that rational postures of various groups seem to have made intransigence the theme, rather than enlightened discussion leading toward rational solutions. To that end, the following may help. Despite the fact that I believe the board-certified anesthesiologist is nonpareil on today's medical horizon, the realities suggest that appropriate training and medical direction of the nonphysician anesthetist with a team approach are now the emerging national pattern.

THEME

I believe it naturally follows that nurse anesthetists should not only be trained by anesthesiologists and work under the medical direction of anesthesiologists but that they should also be trained by anesthesiologists in an academic environment. That this approach has been undertaken successfully in a few institutions in this country over the past quarter of a century seems to have escaped an earlier practi-

205

cal implementation by their academic colleagues. What some of us believed 15 years ago now seems to have been acknowledged from several directions.

Hear now the American Board of Anesthesiology (1977):

> . . . the Board believes that the increasing complexity of anesthetic care, the management of more profoundly sick patients, and the development of commensurate abilities of the specialty to provide the necessary care should provide the impetus to an increasing use of a team approach for the delivery of anesthesia care. To ensure that the public receives the full measure of knowledge and skills which the specialty can bring to bear for the benefits of patients, all anesthetic administration should be by or under the direction of an anesthesiologist. Both the physician and the nonphysician members of the anesthesia care team must possess the requisite skills, reliability and commitment to patient care.

The Board further recognized "anesthesia subspecialty training, training for direction of intensive care, *and training for the leadership of the anesthesia care team** represent additional elements of education which cannot stand alone." The positions that I have previously taken with respect to the training and development of the anesthesia care team seem best highlighted in the conclusion of this article, ". . . the board believes that the anesthesiologist as the leader of the anesthesia care team must be trained to assume responsibility for the performance and the educational standards to be met by the nonphysician anesthetist."

Nicholas M. Greene (1975) indicates that ". . . the public has decided that a great deal of medical care in the future years will be provided by paramedical and allied health science personnel. It is incumbent upon academic anesthesiologists to assure high quality of this care." That this can be safely and effectively accomplished in a medical school environment has been attested to by Peter J. Cohen and others from the Department of Anesthesiology at the University of Michigan, where a program for training nurse anesthetists exists. They stated:

> About two years ago when a new program of anesthesiology was established at the University of Michigan, we inherited a delicate and potentially incompatible situation where a resident training program and a school of nurse anesthetists both existed under the same roof. In spite of our absolute commitment to establish a superior resident training program, we decided to retain the nurse anesthesia school and experiment on a new approach to deal with it in an effort to give a new direction to the perplexing situation of the anesthesia care system in this country. . . . The experience of the system during the last one and one-half years has been gratifying. Analysis of cases done by each group shows proportionality in quantity and quality. The interpersonal relationship between the two groups has been good. The morale of the Department as a whole has been improved (Pandit, Brown, and Cohen, 1977).

Although this brief synopsis of a controversial and continuing program may not do either party justice, it is my position that this is a valid approach and should be duplicated in greater numbers.

---

*Emphasis is mine.

A TEAM EVEN IN 1932

It is perhaps well to go back in time and review the statements of one of the pioneers of our profession. In 1916, Paluel J. Flagg, a physician specialist in anesthesia in a period when principally nurse anesthetist training and practice abounded, wrote the following in the introduction to his textbook: "... a layman who administers an anaesthetic is like a blind guide who is led by the patient instead of leading him. Those who relegate anaesthesia to the layman place the responsibility of the outcome on their own shoulders. . . . " Sixteen years later, in the preface to his fifth edition, Flagg indicated that

In well organized medical groups with a large volume of material susceptible to routine treatment the technician is useful and safe. Intelligent direction and responsibility for the anaesthetic or the practical integration of the facts of a given case is here adequately met and safely is preserved by the operating surgeon . . . . The employment of a nurse to give an anaesthetic implies a knowledge of anaesthesia on the part of the surgeon. The man who makes use of technical assistance outside of a large well organized group must be trained to meet his responsibility. . . . (Flagg, 1932)

In the 1900's, when anesthesiologists were few, training for the practice of surgery consisted of either practical experimentation or some training by preceptorial means concerning the complexities and the practical problems of anesthesia. Many surgeons of the day were most knowledgeable concerning the body of information then present, to wit, Babcock, Mataas, Lemon, and Jones in spinal anesthesia and Crile, with his concern of the influence of pain on metabolism (anoci-association). Although young surgical house officers of today are well trained in modern medicine and surgery, their knowledge of the complex field of anesthesia is often lacking, due most often to the presence of anesthesia physicians, trained or in training in the same environment in which they are receiving surgical training. Therefore, when these surgical colleagues enter practice in areas in which physician anesthetists are scarce, they are likely to be in the position envisioned by Flagg in 1916—without the requisite skills to integrate "... medical judgment, direction, and legal responsibility. . . ."

The definitions of anesthesiology vary according to those addressing the subject. As described by the American Board of Anesthesiology, it can be defined as a practice of medicine dealing with but not limited to management of procedures for rendering patients insensible to pain during surgical, obstetric, and other procedures; support of life functions under the stress of anesthetic and surgical manipulations; the management of patients unconscious from whatever cause; management of problems in pain relief and in cardiac and respiratory resuscitation; the development of research supporting new and improved methodologies; applications of research methods as well as clinical methods in respiratory therapy; and various fluid and electrolyte and metabolic disturbances.

Ira Gunn, in an article on training for nurse anesthetists, stated that

... the contemporary role of the nurse anesthetist has evolved into that of an anesthesiologist nurse practitioner, one who provides selective medical services of an anesthesiological nature as the agent of the physician while providing nursing services for which he or she bears an independent professional responsibility. (Gunn, 1974)

In 1977, Newsweek magazine (in the December 5 issue) discussed "the supernurse." Subsequently, a letter to the editor of Newsweek (in the December 26, 1977 issue) contained the following interesting letter: "I was glad to see your coverage of the 'supernurses'. This 'new kind of professional' is demonstrating that nursing is indeed an independent discipline in which the nurse functions as the doctor's professional colleague rather than as his loyal and helpful subordinate." I suspect that some of the same attitudes prevail and are reflected in Ms. Gunn's article on the preparation of the nonphysician anesthetist. The word "colleague" from the Latin is defined as "one chosen to serve with another." It also has the meaning, from the French, of "associate" and in common usage is synonymous with partner, ally, confederate, and even the derogatory term of accomplice.

When Ms. Gunn states that health care is not synonymous with medical care, one need be reminded that anesthesiology by definition at law, as well as conceptual agreement throughout the medical profession, is the practice of medicine. As such, there *must* be an insistence on "mere dependency" (Gunn, 1974) for appropriate medical and legal responsibilities when often the individuals have not been adequately trained and are not even prepared to follow medical direction.

In December 1974, the number of approved nurse anesthesia schools was 206, with only 206 physician faculty members, 154 of whom were Diplomates of the American Board of Anesthesiology. This suggests inadequate physician input into the educational mileau for the nurse anesthetist, and failure of modern surgical programs to provide in depth anesthesia training and experience and an environment to seek the best possible team approach recommends further consideration of the best way to provide the educational training to the nonphysician anesthetist.

Thoughtful educators in the field of nurse anesthesia today agree that the two- or three-year school of nurses followed by a 12- or 18-month course in an anesthesia educational environment *is inadequate* for preparing today's nurse anesthetist to meet contemporary need. I am sure that nurse educators would agree that baccalaureate training is preferred and that a masters degree in the science and practice of anesthesia should be a minimum sought for future education. This begs the question of *medical direction,* however; moreover, it begs the question of how the *attitudinal* minimums may be best achieved. It especially ignores history and the continuing fact that only physicians, particularly those from great academic departments, ensure the developments that have provided the agents and tools for the nonphysician anesthestist.

Sidestepping for the moment the method whereby such training may be guaranteed and accreditation of appropriate nonphysician schools achieved, there is the traditional argument by nurse anesthetists that they need to be independent of physician specialists in anesthesia in geographic areas when direction by these specialists is not feasible. Through the concerns of hospital staffs, principally urged by the Joint Commission on Accreditation of Hospitals, there must be at least a responsible figurehead in small hospitals, often an internist or general surgeon without training in anesthesia. Although it is true that the surgeon whose patients are anesthetized by the nonphysician anesthetist has a legal and moral responsibility, there is a distinction between administrative (and legal) *supervision* and the urgent need for *medical direction*. Unfortunately, the combination of a desire to have "any anesthetist" and a surgeon inadequately trained in anesthesia judgments serves but to emphasize the need for a better way in the future.

ACADEME RESPONDS

I recently asked 15 chairmen of anesthesiology departments in prominent medical schools to define their attitudes with respect to obligations for the training of nurse anesthetists in the same institution in which residents are trained in anesthesiology. My selection of individuals to be queried was prejudiced by the knowledge that they believed in such programs. In general, they were unanimous in their belief that schools of nurse anesthesia could be satisfactorily conducted simultaneously at the same institution, in a medical school environment, where physician residents were training. Most indicated that there was no adverse effect on recruitment into residency training programs. Several responses suggested a greater concern; one indicated that "the sorriest of programs for nurse anesthesia have at times been run by anesthesiologists." In my view, this is a challenge to anesthesiology, academic anesthesiology in particular, to provide the impetus for improved education of the nonphysician anesthetist. According to one person, the "stronger the residency program and the better quality physician and specialist one is dealing with, then the less problem there will be with this type of combined program. The converse is also true, namely, that the weaker the resident and the resident program, then the more difficulties would be encountered with a combined program." Additionally, two comments of interest read as follows: "The whole idea is almost a necessity, not only in this institution but in the country as a whole," and "This is an idea whose time has come better late than never."

I speak for greater cooperation of the complete team: the physician anesthetists and nurse anesthetists, the nurse technologist or any other nonphysician paramedical associate. There is, however, a certain fundamental preparation in the philosophy for team work that assumes the following:

(1) The finest educational standards; (2) the greatest independence for accreditation schools; (3) the finest teachers in independent nurse-taught nurse anesthesia schools that could theoretically be obtained; and

(4) complete examinations of candidates to reveal high quality candidates with equal technical and basic scientific knowledge to that of physician residents in training.

I would still hold that nurses trained in such an atmosphere in all probability will fail in three most important elements: (1) The ability to *receive* critical medical judgments and act upon them; (2) the ability to accept appropriate medical *learning*; (3) the ability to be a humble, cooperative member of a team.* Although nurses so trained would be an improvement in the communities where anesthesiologists are not available, this situation is in the minority in this nation, notwithstanding repetitive and unfounded claims to the contrary.

I therefore respectfully submit that this nation is best served when nurse anesthetists or anesthesia technologists, or any other definition of paramedical anesthetists, have been fully trained with physician direction, preferably as a team approach in an academic center consisting of members of the anesthesia care team representing all disciplines and subspecialties of the anesthesiology sphere of medical knowledge. Finally, I believe the end product, after appropriate certification, should be under medical direction in the administration of his or her paramedical services.

---

*N.B. "Mere dependency" vs. cooperative team member

REFERENCES

American Board of Anesthesiology: Quality anesthesia care: A model of future practice of anesthesiology. Anesthesiology, *47*:488–489, 1977.

Demographic study of nurse anesthetists, 1972, by ASA and AANA, under contract NIH 72–4269P, Figure 9.

Flagg, P. J.: The Art of Anaesthesia. 1st and 5th eds. Philadelphia, J. B. Lippincott, 1916 and 1932.

Greene, N. M.: Anesthesiology and the University. Philadelphia, J. B. Lippincott, 1975, pp. 144–145.

Gunn, I. P.: Preparing today's nurse anesthetists to meet contemporary needs. A philosophic and pragmatic approach. A.A.N.A.J., *42*:25–38, 1974.

Pandit, S. K., Brown, A. C. D., and Cohen, P. J.: Co-existence of resident and student nurse anesthetist training programs — Experience in the "team" concept. Annual Meeting of American Society of Anesthesiology, Inc., 1977.

by IRA P. GUNN

Council on Accreditation of Nurse Anesthesia Educational Programs

NURSE ANESTHETISTS SHOULD CONTROL THE TEACHING AND PRACTICE OF THEIR PROFESSION

The issue of domination of nurse anesthetists through control of education and practice is perhaps at the root of many of the interorganizational differences existing between the American Association of Nurse Anesthetists (AANA) and the American Society of Anesthesiologists (ASA). This issue is so clouded with socioeconomic, political, and egocentristic overtones that it cannot be viewed objectively or, at times, rationally by either anesthesiologists or nurse anesthetists. Neither can the issue be separated from the cultural influences that have patterned men and women, doctors and nurses, to react and interact in specific ways.

The changing social environment and requirements and the elevation of group consciousness, particularly among women and nurses, have made these groups more aggressive and their actions at times difficult to understand by those not experienced or those misunderstanding this phenomenon. The lack of understanding between many doctors and nurses is enhanced by the long-standing communication game that has been played in the doctor-nurse relationship, described and characterized by Stein (1967) as a transactional neurosis. This game has influenced not only how we communicate but also the actual language each profession uses. In describing the language difference between medicine and nursing, Lynaugh and Bates (1973) state that it is reflective of professional territoriality. I believe it is symptomatic of the doctor-nurse game, used to avoid overt territorial conflicts, hoping to moderate tension while allowing required contributions of nursing for accomplishment of mutual health goals without appearing to encroach on medicine's perceived territorial boundaries.

According to Lynaugh and Bates (1973),

When separate cultures are forced into close proximity, the dominant group seeks to control the others and to impose its own mores and values. Such a forced homogeneity is achieved only through the loss of variety and the intrinsic values of the less dominate systems. It is our belief that modern patient care requires the full contribution of many disciplines most frequently those of medicine and nursing. To maximize these contributions rather than block them, nurses and physicians may need to become bilingual, both in the words and in the understanding of each other's subcultures.

Many nurses, including nurse anesthetists, have tired of the doctor-nurse game and view it, as Stein does as inhibitory, stifling, and anti-intellectual (Stein, 1967). Perhaps the biggest detriment to the game is its continued promotion of an immature relationship characterized by reinforcement of an inappropriate and misleading attitudinal set pertaining to physician dominance and omniscience and nurse subservience and passivity. Thus, more and more nurses break the rules of the game and tensions rise, and will continue to do so until a more appropriate and mature relationship between medicine and nursing is developed and accepted. Interestingly enough, this is often not difficult on a one-to-one basis.

The resolution of organizational differences between ASA and AANA, or at least their acceptance and understanding by anesthesiologists and nurse anesthetists, has little chance to succeed in an environment in which the merit of traditional values and mores of each group cannot be discussed openly and honestly and then objectively evaluated in terms of today's reality. Resolution is further impeded when unilateral, misleading pronouncements are issued, heightening suspicion and mistrust and escalating polarization between the groups. Patients become the ultimate losers in this situation, as they would be by total domination of nurse anesthetists by anesthesiologists, nurses by doctors, or of all health care professionals by physicians. Such a situation leads to a lopsided professional and economic monopolization, with its inherent problems, and to denial or minimization of the unique contributions of each profession to patient care. Herein lies the basis for the philosophical differences between many anesthesiologists and nurse anesthetists, and indeed between the ASA and AANA, pertaining to who should control the education and practice of nurse anesthetists. Rather than perceiving doctors and nurses as unique professionals sharing certain responsibilities and functions, many physicians, including anesthesiologists, perceive all other health care workers, professional and otherwise, as extensions of themselves, having the responsibility as well as right to control the education and practice of all their extensions.

Nurses and many other health professionals find this unacceptable, believing that each professional group has a unique contribution to make separate and apart from medicine, although they recognize and accept role overlap. Each profession is expert in the area of its own uniqueness. Holding this view, I believe that the best chance for cooperation, collaboration, and achievement of our mutual goals for anesthesia care in this nation lies in the understanding, accepting, and maximizing of the unique practice attributes of both anesthesiologists and nurse anesthetists. Furthermore, I believe that maximizing the unique contribution nursing has to make to anesthesia requires that the responsibility for the education and practice of nurse anesthetists appropriately lies with nurse anesthetists and the profession to which they belong.

PROFESSIONAL UNIQUENESS

Professions are identified and differentiated on the basis of the existence of a central purpose for being. Dorothy Johnson has said the following about nursing:

> Whatever 'it' is, there is ample reason to believe 'it' does not change with age, or geographic setting, or medical diagnosis, anymore than law, medicine and teaching change with such variables. Certain activities may change; the problems encountered in practice may differ in degree or even in kind, but the central purpose of the profession and the reason for its being does not change with shifts in the location of patients, or the age group involved, or the category of disease. It is on the basis of the existence of a central purpose in being that professions are identified and differentiated and by virtue of which they endure over time. (Johnson, 1964)

If one accepts the thesis that the uniqueness of a profession is bound to its central purpose for being, then nursing and medicine can be differentiated on this basis. Medicine's central purpose for being is *cure;* nursing's central purpose for being is *care.* One must recognize that cure and care are not mutually exclusive, thus providing the area of role overlap and lack of differentiation so frequently the basis for confusion and conflict.

The description of nursing's central purpose for being as care contributes to confusion, since it is the nature of the care that provides for nursing's uniqueness. The word "care" in and of itself is nondifferentiating and can be appropriately utilized by most helping professions. The nature of care that is uniquely nursing is bound to the nurturing process, i.e. to providing that type and quality of health-oriented care (or assistance) needed to support the optimal achievement of growth, development, and independence and, in periods of disease or distress, that care or assistance required for recuperation, well being, and comfort. This type of care is analogous to that provided by the self or the family under usual and ordinary circumstances but owing to changed circumstances or magnitude of requirement mandates special and advanced knowledge and skill.

Medicine's central purpose for being, cure, is characterized best by the functions of diagnosis and treatment, words not unique to medicine but when used in reference to medicine having unique connotations. It is medicine's prerogative to make a medical or pathological diagnosis, i.e., to put an appropriate title on a syndrome of signs and symptoms and to prescribe or perform medical therapeutic actions aimed at curing or modifying the disease process.

Nurses, by virtue of their patient and surrogate family role, are the individuals who are in sustained contact with the patient and family, providing physical and emotional care of a helping, comforting, guiding, and protecting nature. This sustained presence affords nurses not only the opportunity but also the responsibility for continuous observation and identification of signs and symptoms, in light of their deviation from normal, and for implementation of appropriate nursing actions or available physician orders in an attempt to return the patient to normal or to achieve a state of comfort or status consistent with the patient's response capability. Sometimes it is appropriate to refer the patient to the physician with information that may necessitate the re-evaluation and revision of the medical regimen.

THE NATURE OF THE ANESTHESIA CARE PROCESS

The ASA appears to view the anesthetic process as a purely medical one, in contrast to the view held by most nurse anesthetists and the AANA. The purely medical view of the process has been presented most recently in the ASA document, "Differences in Services Provided by Anesthesiologists and Nurse Anesthetists" (ASA, 1977) and in an article entitled "Anesthesia Manpower in the United States: 1976" (Carron and Burney, 1976) furnished to the AMA Committee on Emerging Health Professions as part of the proposal for the recognition of anesthesiologist assistants as a new health occupation. To this author, Carron and Burney reflect a woeful lack of understanding of nursing education and practice as well as a limited view of clinical anesthesia. They state, "The rationale for nursing education prior to entrance into nurse anesthesia schools is doubtful. . . . Most nursing school curricula do not pertain to clinical anesthesia." (Carron, 1976)

These views may be consistent to the preparation, utilization, and supervision of a physician assistant but certainly are inappropriate with reference to a nurse specialist whose unique professional attributes have much to contribute to the practice of anesthesia.

I believe, as does the AANA, that anesthesia care is neither exclusively medical nor exclusively nursing in nature, as with psychiatric and pediatric health care. In fact, with the exception of diagnostic and therapeutic blocks, seldom is anesthesia provided solely for the purpose of diagnosis and treatment. To be sure, it creates the conditions in which selected diagnostic and therapeutic regimens can be effected, as well as on occasion creating untoward effects requiring diagnosis and therapy. In and of itself, however, anesthesia is usually not a diagnostic or therapeutic modality. Anesthesia is a process through which patients are rendered insensitive to pain with or without unconsciousness and are often paralyzed to facilitate other medical requirements. As a result of the process, the patient is usually rendered incapable of caring for himself because protective automatic internal reflexes are reduced or eliminated. Thus, the care component becomes critical to the process, mandating constant vigilance and monitoring, which are aimed at protecting the patient and detecting unanticipated changes that result in modification of the process in order to maintain the patient at near optimal status. This is a traditional nursing function.

Anesthesia care is intensive in nature and, for the most part, is similar to other intensive care situations, except that the anesthesia and the surgical procedure impose an additional requirement upon pre-existing disease. As in any intensive care setting, the patient undergoing anesthesia and operation is subject to many nursing judgments and actions that may not require physician intervention. Nurses are taught to care for patients unconscious from a broad spectrum of causes long before they learn to produce unconsciousness with anesthetic agents, imposing many of the same requirements for care as relate to cardiovascular, respiratory, neurological, and renal systems; fluid and nutritional balance; patient positioning; and protection from iatrogenic complications. They have learned to care for patients paralyzed from a variety of causes long before they paralyzed patients with local anesthetic agents and adjunctive drugs, again imposing similar requirements for care.

To be sure, there are situations with risks to patients in which medical diagnosis and treatment become necessary before, during, and after the anesthetic process as a result of either anesthesia management or pathophysiological conditions or as a consequence of the concomitant medical treatment. Although the ideal situation would be for qualified anesthesiologists to be available for required medical intervention, there is no legal requirement that this intervention be limited to anesthesiologists. The maldistribution of physician anesthetists precludes the achievement of this ideal. Fortunately, in the majority of these situations, the patient's attending physician is fully qualified to provide the needed intervention.

To objectively judge the validity of either the ASA or the AANA philosophy with regard to anesthesia care requires a better analysis of the anesthesia care process than has been offered to date, a multidisciplinary approach to judging the nature of the functions and tasks that make up the care of the anesthetized patient, and agreed upon definitions of medicine and nursing. Perhaps the most difficult of these to achieve is the last.

EDUCATION AND PRACTICE OF NURSE ANESTHETISTS

My view of the issue (who should control the education and practice of nurse anesthetists) evolves from a philosophical basis and from experience as a practicing nurse anesthetist; a nurse anesthesia educator, a consultant on nurse anesthesia affairs to the U.S. Army Surgeon General; and an educational consultant to the AANA, the Council on Accreditation of Educational Programs of Nurse Anesthesia, and schools and programs that prepare nurse anesthetists. To me, education and practice do not exist in a vacuum but co-exist and feed each other. With regard to professional education, it is the practice of anesthesia that determines the curricular content of the education, just as it is education that determines the entry competence and capability of the practitioner.

Traditionally, it has been the prerogative of individual professions to determine the educational standards by which new members gain entry into that profession. There are valid reasons for this, although such determination certainly should not be done in isolation or without input from interrelated disciplines. The validity of this traditional prerogative lies in the fact that each profession is expert in its own uniqueness, its role, what its members must know and be able to do to implement its role and be responsible for it, and how this can best be achieved within legal constraints. Furthermore, as in the case of any specialization, it is the particular specialist who knows what base of education is best for building the special competence and how to build on that base to achieve the desired educational outcomes. Consultation is at times needed and helpful.

I have come to believe in the validity of this traditional prerogative of professions, not from abstract reasoning but from a broad base of experience confirmed in study and in discussion with other professionals, including nurse anesthetists.

It has been my experience that some anesthesiologists, most often associated with academic health centers where anesthesiology residency programs are conducted, have somewhat different role expectations for nurse anesthetists than those generally held by most nurse anesthetists. These anesthesiologists often have a more restricted view of the role of nurse anesthetists, and perhaps this stems from their practice situation, where anesthesiologists are always available. As a result, I have observed and experienced some nurse anesthesia educational programs existing within these often prestigious facilities but not providing nurse anesthesia students with a comprehensive, complete education adequate for entering the practice of nurse anesthesia, particularly at outside facilities, where anesthesiologists are not available. Certainly this is not true of all academic health centers, but the problem had become of sufficient magnitude that, in the 1974 revision of the Educational Standards for Nurse Anesthesia Programs, an old principle implicit in previous standards was more explicitly stated, i.e., that nurse anesthesia educational programs must prepare the graduate to function competently in the absence of anesthesiologists. This had nothing to do with political motivations of AANA, nor was it an attempt by nurse anesthetists to usurp the role of anesthesiologists. It reflected practice reality because, despite agreement between the ASA and AANA that the ideal anesthesia practice system is one in which anesthesiologists and nurse anesthetists work together, both groups are fully aware that this ideal cannot be achieved now or in the foreseeable future (AANA, 1972). This is as true now as it was in 1972. Even in situations in which nurse anesthetists work with one anesthesiologist, he cannot always be available.

When nurse anesthetists function without anesthesiologists, they can do so safely and competently only when they have been adequately prepared for such conditions. This includes knowing when to proceed with anesthesia and when to defer and refer a patient to another facility or request the services of a consulting anesthesiologist, when the patient's condition or magnitude of surgical intervention so warrants. Nurse anesthetists, who are meeting the anesthesia needs of society in areas unattractive to anesthesiologists, have become expert in the utilization of attending physicians or consultants, so that patients needing such medical attention are not denied care. Their success is reflected in a survey reported in 1973 by Surgical Team in which many surgeons and anesthesiologists believed that remarkable competence was the rule rather than the exception when working with today's CRNA's (Surgical Team, 1973). Jenicek, reporting on the nurse anesthetist in Vietnam, stated, "Either as a member of or the leader of such a team (anesthesia team), the daily contribution of the nurse anesthetists to casualty survival has earned professional praise from military and civilian consultants." (Jenicek, 1967)

The success that nurse anesthetists have achieved in cooperation with many anesthesiologists in the education and preparation of nurse anesthetists, despite recent and I believe unsubstantiated allegations to the contrary by some ASA leaders (Ament, 1977), stems from several factors:

1. The nurse anesthetist is prepared to function as a nurse specialist and not as a physician assistant.

Until recently, it appeared that anesthesiologists and nurse anesthetists were in agreement that "all individuals administering anesthesia must at sometime exercise varying degrees of clinical judgment and responsibility and that this can be best exercised by individuals familiar with the process of rendering total patient care." (AANA, 1972) There is evidence today of a backing away from this belief by some of the hierarchy of the ASA and other anesthesiologists, as demonstrated by the ASA proposed revision of the ASA-AANA Joint Statement of 1972 (ASA, 1977) and by the anesthesiologist assistant movement. This group appears to believe that anesthesiologists should be prepared in the total patient care process but that it is unncessary for others who are prepared to administer anesthesia to have this type of patient care orientation and education.

In general, nurse anesthetists continue to believe that the education and experience acquired in total patient care is an essential prerequisite on which to build anesthesia education for the preparation of safe, competent practitioners regardless of whether they are physicians, nurses, or assistants who must administer anesthesia. The nurse anesthetist, particularly in the absence of anesthesiologists, using prior nursing knowledge and competence enhanced by appropriate anesthesia education and experience, must integrate the anesthetic process for a patient assigned to his care into that patient's total care process and, if necessary, utilize physicians, including the patient's attending physician, for necessary medical decisions. I believe that this combination of education and experience relating to total patient care and anesthesia specialization has provided the nurse anesthetist with the capability of functioning safely and competently when anesthesiologists are unavailable.

2. Nurse anesthetists, rather than anesthesiologists, are role models for nurse anesthesia students.

The importance of the role model in teaching lies in providing students with a model to emulate with reference to needed knowledge, skills, and values and how to implement the role for which the model is prepared. The physician is not an appropriate role model for the nurse; likewise, the anesthesiologist is not the appropriate role model for nurse anesthetists. Some physicians negate the importance of role models and feel that roles can be taught by definition. This is just about as successful as telling one's children "Don't do as I do, but do as I say."

A primary function of a role model is to demonstrate when and how to accept medical delegation and when to decline and bow out of unacceptable delegation without detriment to the patient. There is a tendency among physicians to believe, autocratically, that what they order, the nurse must perform. Such a situation would put the nurse in a tenuous legal position because the nurse is required by law to make judgments with regard to the legality and appropriateness of the order, the nurse's capability to perform the order, and the probable effect on the patient. As long as the law requires this of the nurse, the physician has a teammate to whom he may toss the ball but from whom he may get it back. He does not in essence control the nurse. No doubt what the nurse does with medical delegation is a function of what the physician is willing, desires, or needs to delegate. Thus the legally defined relationship between doctors and nurses, despite specific language or words in some practice acts, is essential to assure patient safety because it evokes a check and balance system of care despite the differing roles of the two, analogous to the check and balance system of branches of government, each having its own unique functions and responsibilities while sharing, hopefully, mutual goals.

3. Nurse anesthetist educators have neither adopted the philosophy of postgraduate medical education nor transferred it to nurse anesthesia education.

Not only is role expectation reflected in the curriculum but the philosophy of education is also reflected in both the curriculum and its implementation. One cannot transfer the traditional philosophy of postgraduate medical education to postnursing education with success even though there appears to be a tendency by physicians to attempt this.

A major form of anesthesiology residency training appears to center on self-directed study. Although it is the goal of nurse anesthesia educational programs to develop the capability for self-direction in their graduates, I believe there is a requirement for formalized, organized classes to enhance the basic science theory on which anesthesia is built.

Some nurse anesthetists believe that a traditional philosphy of postgraduate medical education, satirized as "see one, do one, teach one," is often a deficiency in anesthesiology residency programs. The tendency to "allow" the resident to get into problems in order to learn how to resolve such problems is another point of difference between some anesthesiologists and nurse anesthetist faculty members. Most nurse anesthetist faculty believe enough problems occur despite attempts to stay out of them, that adequate experience is available for their resolution. Learning to prevent the problem is the most effective means of ensuring it will not create difficulties for patients.

Nurse anesthetists are not the only ones who have challenged the philosophy of postgraduate medical education. Many medical residents are doing so today.

SUMMARY

For reason of length, I have limited my discussion of the role of the nurse anesthetist to its major component — anesthesia management. What is true for this aspect of practice, however, is also true of many of the other components of care that fall within this specialty, such as cardiopulmonary resuscitation and respiratory care.

It is my belief that the control of the education and practice of nurse anesthetists must rest with nurse anesthetists and the profession to which they belong for the following reasons:

1. To preserve the unique nursing contribution to the role of the nurse anesthetist, a critical component in the anesthesia care process.

2. To more appropriately design and implement the curricula reflective of the role of the nurse anesthetist as required by societal needs, building, and interfacing the specialty education on nursing education.

3. To afford role models appropriate to the nursing practice of anesthesia.

4. To ensure a type of practice consistent with societal needs, within specified legal constraints, affording all patients the availability of safe, competent, comprehensive anesthesia care.

In addition, recognizing that there is role overlap and a medical component to anesthesia care on many occasions delegated to nurse anesthetists, I believe that anesthesiologist participation in the education of nurse anesthetists is required.

I believe with Stein that many differences between physicians and nurses are transactional in nature (Stein, 1967). Resolution of these differences requires that a more mature relationship, reflecting today's reality and environment, be established betweeen these two groups, one in which open and honest dialogue is welcomed and understood, rather than the current game playing.

I further believe that patients have more to gain from an effective collegiate relationship between anesthesiologists and nurse anesthetists than from the paternalistic, autocratic relationship from which many of our differences and problems stem.

REFERENCES

Ament, R.: American Society of Anesthesiologists' oral presentation to the council on postsecondary accreditation, ref: AANA Council on Accreditation's Petition for initial recognition by COPA, October 12, 1977.

American Society of Anesthesiologists: Differences in services provided by anesthesiologists and nurse anesthetists. Hearings before the Subcommittee on Health of the Committee on Finance — United States Senate (95th Congress, First Session on S. 1470). Medicare-Medicaid Administrative and Reimbursement Reform Act. June 7–10, 1977, pp. 378–384.

Carron, H., and Burney, R. G.: Anesthesia manpower in the United States 1976. Unpublished paper provided to the AMA Committee on Emerging Health Professions with the proposal to recognize anesthesiologist assistants as a new health occupation, 1976.

The CRNA as a Member of the OR Team. The Surgical Team, 2:3, 1973.

Jenicek, J. A.: Vietnam — new challenge for the army nurse anesthetist. AANA Journal, 35:5, 1967.

Johnson, D. E.: Directions of graduate education for nursing and development of psychiatric-mental health programs. Report of work conference in graduate education, University of Pittsburgh School of Nursing, November 9–13, 1964, p. 51.

Joint Statement of the American Society of Anesthesiologists and the American Association of Nurse Anesthetists Concerning Qualifications of Individuals Administering Anesthetics. AANA Journal 40:1, 1972.

Lynaugh, J. E., and Bates, B.: The two languages of medicine and nursing. Am. J. Nurs. 73:66–69, 1973.

Proposed 1977 Joint Statement of the American Society of Anesthesiologists and the American Association of Nurse Anesthetists Concerning Qualifications of Individuals Administering Anesthetics. ASA proposal, ASA Newsletter, April 1977, p. 3

Stein, L. I.: The doctor-nurse game. Am. J. Nurs., 68:101–105, 1968; formerly published in Arch. Gen. Psychiatry, 16:699–703, 1967.

THE TRAINING AND SUPERVISION OF NURSE ANESTHETISTS

EDITORIAL COMMENT

For 50 years following the first public demonstration of ether anesthesia, the administration of anesthetics was not attractive to many American physicians as a full time specialty. Anesthesia was looked on as a service, requiring neither special training nor continued and thoughtful application. At the end of the 19th century, the assignment of nurses to the task of anesthetizing patients on a continuing basis was a significant advance. They were able to learn from their experiences and apply those experiences to subsequent patients. Nonetheless, they were under the supervision of the surgeon, who was not a student of the effects of anesthesia or anesthetics but was intent upon the surgical procedure at hand. As surgical procedures became more complex, there are ample references in the literature indicating that the training of surgeons and of nurse anesthetists was not equal to the task of caring for some patients. On this basis, physicians began to pay special attention to anesthesia. Although the rush to the specialty was not overwhelming, a few surgeons began to rely on the services of anesthesiologists, and several universities and medical centers accepted physicians as the logical leaders of training programs in anesthesia. Nurses continued to administer the majority of anesthetics, preferred by many surgeons, who did not want another physician overseeing activities in the operating room, and by hospital administrators, who looked on nurse anesthetists as a source of income to balance deficits incurred in other hospital departments. In the wake of World War II, an influx of physicians trained or partially trained in anesthesia and a burgeoning of training programs in anesthesiology set the stage for controversy between nurse anesthetists and anesthesiologists.

If one carefully follows the arguments of Gunn and Ditzler, it appears that they are not too far apart, but I am not sure. Ditzler doubts the ability of most surgeons or internists to make adequate anesthetic judgments when critical judgment is needed. Neither has the background or training to make these judgments. Gunn has more faith in the knowledge of surgeons and equates anesthesia administration with patient care, something that most anesthesiologists will find unacceptable. If one is not thoroughly versed in physiology, pathology, and pharmacology, how can one anticipate the ultimate action of

221

drugs? The editor is not sure of what is meant by the "uniqueness" of what a nurse anesthetist can offer versus what an anesthesiologist can provide. Nor can he decipher why nurses can provide unique or better training for nurse anesthetists!

Nonetheless, Gunn makes a point that some programs better prepare individuals to take care of the majority of reasonably healthy patients requiring routine surgical procedures. I cannot argue that some anesthesiology training programs may spend too much time in trying to make super specialists of their products, have diluted their operating room experience, and do not imbue them with the importance of superior anesthetic skill in routine procedures. Some anesthesiologists are bored with the administration of routine anesthesia and only want to be involved with the difficult or unusual. Others never realize the talents given them and allow themselves to become technicians. Some nurses, through study and experience, become equal to nearly any challenge presented to them and perform on a level of competence equal to most anesthesiologists in the operating room.

The administration of anesthetics and the care of the anesthetized patient is the practice of medicine. It is unlikely that there will ever be enough physicians to administer all anesthetics, and all anesthetics need not be administered by physicians. Both physicians and nurses can be involved in all training programs. When anesthesiologists are available, nurse anesthetists should look to them for anesthesiological advice, not to surgeons or to internists who, on the whole today, have minimal to no training in anesthesia. Anesthesiologists should also be willing to assist in nurse training programs and willingly help nurse anesthetists in the operating room.

To nurse anesthetists who may be offended by this stance, I might point out that my attitude to training and supervision for nurse anesthetists is parallel to that for training and supervision of family practitioners. Specialists should assist in the education of family practitioners and supervise them in practice where such supervision is required by lack of experience of the practitioner or complexity of the patient's disease.

Part 11

NURSE ANESTHETISTS AND REGIONAL ANESTHESIA

THE PROPOSITION:

> Nurse anesthetists should be taught to administer regional anesthesia and should be privileged to practice the technique in the absence of an anesthesiologist.

ALTERNATIVE POINTS OF VIEW

> By M. J. Mannino
>
> By M. T. Jenkins

EDITORIAL COMMENT

by MARY JEANETTE MANNINO

University of California, Irvine

NURSE ANESTHETISTS SHOULD ADMINISTER REGIONAL ANESTHESIA

A controversy exists regarding the administration of regional anesthesia by Certified Registered Nurse Anesthetists (CRNA's). Both CRNA's and anesthesiologists have presented heated arguments for and against this practice (Ament, 1977; Gunn, 1977). In their effort to gain recognition as practitioners of regional techniques, the members of the American Association of Nurse Anesthetists (AANA) devoted a clinical session to regional anesthesia at their 1977 annual meeting, and various articles on regional anesthesia, many written by CRNA's, have been published in the *AANA Journal* (Mannino, 1977; Reese, 1977).

The controversy surrounding CRNA administration of regional anesthesia raises many complex questions: Who currently administers anesthesia and under what circumstances? How are anesthesia personnel distributed? What are the projected shortages? Are CRNA's properly educated and technically capable of handling this technique? What role does regional anesthesia play in present day practice and would this be legal? Further ramifications include an evaluation and restructuring of educational and certification programs necessary to qualify these individuals to practice regional techniques.

Who administers anesthesia today? Currently, there are over 14,000 practicing CRNA's and 10,000 anesthesiologists in the United States (Gunn, 1977). A 1971 survey showed that CRNA's administered more than 50 per cent of the anesthesia in hospitals of less than 250 beds and more than 65 per cent in hospitals of less than 100 beds (Biggins et al., 1971). The availability of physician-administered anesthesia has been further affected by the demographic maldistribution of anesthesiologists. States with the highest population density have the highest ratio of anesthesiologists to population, but the number of nurse anesthetists is inversely proportional to the number of anesthesiologists (Carron, 1974; Supply, 1976).

Regardless of the cause of this maldistribution, the type and quality of anesthesia services available to the health care consumer are affected. For example, in a hospital of less than 250 beds, which is

225

usually in a rural or less populated area, the only person capable of giving an anesthetic may be a CRNA who is not permitted to use regional techniques. In this circumstance, the selection of the anesthetic for a particular patient is not determined by the patient's needs but rather by what is available. A regional may be the anesthetic of choice, yet optimal anesthesia is prevented owing to the limitations placed on CRNA's. Especially in this situation, to allow CRNA's to administer regional anesthesia would be to improve the quality of anesthesia care.

Demands on CRNA's from within the profession are increasing. In recent years, despite their increased numbers, anesthesiologists have extended their services outside the operating room to include respiratory care, pain clinics, acute care medicine, and research. This expansion places great responsibility on the CRNA, especially in management and monitoring of patients. An offshoot of this expansion, which has been frequently discussed, is the *team concept* of anesthesia, in which CRNA's and anesthesiologists work together. Many CRNA's who have functioned under such arrangements find it advantageous to have anesthesiologists available for consultation and advice.

Although the team concept may be the ideal, the actual and projected shortages of anesthesia personnel are real factors to be considered. The Department of Health, Education and Welfare booklet, "Supply, Need and Distribution of Anesthesiologists and Nurse Anesthetists in the U.S., 1972–1980," concludes that with a universal task delegation employing anesthesiologists and nurse anesthetists in a 1 to 2 team configuration, 12,750 anesthesiologists and 25,530 nurse anesthetists will be needed by 1980 (Supply, 1976).

The questioning of CRNA's technical capabilities often provides the focus for arguments against CRNA's administering regional anesthesia. These arguments tend to be highly emotional and lack supportive documentation. In a letter sent to members of the California Legislature by the president of the Union of American Physicians, scare tactics were even used: "We are also aware of the need for economy in medical care, but the preposterous nature of entrusting spinal anesthesia to anyone other than fully trained physicians is analogous to authorizing Do-It-Yourself Brain Surgery Kits — it is outside any consideration of reasonableness." (Marcus, 1977) In contrast to this point of view, Alon P. Winnie, a noted expert on regional anesthesia, strongly supports the administration of these procedures by CRNA's as an opportunity to improve anesthesia care (Winnie, 1977). In an editorial published by the Illinois Society of Anesthesiologists, Dr. Winnie questioned whether anesthesiologists fear that their own technical abilities in regional anesthesia may be exceeded by those of nurses.

Indeed, when CRNA's have been trained to perform regional anesthetics, they have proved to be technically adept. As with general anesthesia, the actual performance of a regional block is a technical procedure that can be mastered with sufficient instruction, supervision, and experience. In areas in which student nurse anesthetists and anesthesia residents were taught regional techniques, no statistically significant difference in the occurrence of sequelae or morbidity could be attributed to either category of practitioner (Rosenberg, 1973).

Further evidence suggesting that nurse anesthetists are technically capable of administering regional anesthesia can be found in military procedures when CRNA's are taught and practice regional anesthesia. In 1973, the United States Army recognized the limited availability of physician anesthesiologists for future years. Consequently, in the interests of total patient care, Army Nurse Corps anesthetists are now trained in selected regional techniques (Department of the Army, 1973). Similarly, the Navy requires its nurse anesthetists to become competent practitioners of regional anesthesia and places strong emphasis on these techniques in its education program.

In spite of CRNA's efforts to administer regional anesthesia, Bonica reported a marked decrease in the use of regional anesthesia for surgery (Bonica, 1969). Some of the reasons cited include greater information on the action of general anesthesia, the advent of muscle relaxants and intravenous anesthetics, the use of balanced anesthesia, and the neglect of this method of anesthesia. Even though some regional techniques have fallen into disuse and disfavor, there is a renewed enthusiasm for the techniques, as evidenced by the recently formed American Society of Regional Anesthesia. In a recent editorial in the society's journal, *Regional Anesthesia,* Philip Bridenbaugh discussed the current and future state of regional anesthesia (Bridenbaugh, 1977) and attributed some of the current lack of enthusiasm to "superstitions, half truths, prejudice, and even frank ignorance." He also noted that use of regional techniques is regaining popularity for relief of terminal pain and for obstetric anesthesia. For the future, he suggested that a statistical comparison of regional and general anesthesia relative to safety factors and untoward effects was in order.

Perhaps the largest group of advocates for the administration of regional anesthesia by CRNA's are obstetric anesthesiologists. Anesthesia is one of the four leading causes of maternal mortality, and 95 per cent of these deaths are preventable. In the past decade, the total anesthesia death rate decreased because fewer deaths were associated with spinal anesthesia. The death rate associated with inhalation of vomitus, however, remained the same (Greiss and Anderson, 1971). The Joint Commission of Accreditation of Hospitals (JCAH), because of their concern for maternal health, requires that ". . . the same competence of anesthesia personnel shall be available for obstetrical procedures as is available for elective procedures." (JCAH, 1976)

The obstetric anesthesiologists' support for the administration of spinal and epidural anesthetics by CRNA's is well founded. They want to increase the availability of regional anesthetics to their patients, improve overall patient care, and decrease maternal mortality. Frederick Hehre provided an unequivocal summation of the obstetric anesthesiologists' point of view when he stated rather dogmatically,

Why should any physician regardless of his training place a local anesthetic in the subarachnoid space and immediately turn the patient over to a nurse anesthetist for management. Complications caused by physiologic effects of spinal anesthesia are far more life threatening than the actual art of induction of the anesthetic itself . . . . It is more sensible to allow qualified individuals to make the decision to administer conduction anesthesia to an obstetrical patient with a known full stomach, than to risk the aspiration of vomitus with inhalation anesthesia which is the leading anesthetic cause of maternal death. (Hehre, 1974)

Although CRNA's do not administer the actual block, they are responsible for managing the complications and side effects of the anesthetic. In other words, the very people who are not permitted by tradition or law to insert the needle or anesthetic are expected to manage the patient after the block is performed by someone else.

Despite the fact that tradition has dictated that nurses not perform regional techniques in certain parts of the country, there are areas, particularly in the Midwest and West, where nurse anesthetists are educated in regional techniques. Because CRNA's are registered nurses, they have statutory authority to practice through nurse practice acts legislated by state governments. The California Supreme Court ruling in Chalmers-Francis vs. Nelson determined the legality of nurses' administering anesthesia. The Court stated, "A licensed registered nurse employed by a hospital will not be enjoined from administering general anesthesia in connection with surgical operations where the court finds upon ample evidence that everything done by the nurse generally in the administration of anesthesia is done under the immediate direction and supervision of the operating surgeon and his assistant." (Chalmers-Francis vs. Nelson, 1936) Because the Chalmers-Francis vs. Nelson decision specified general anesthesia, it served as the basis for the 1972 California Attorney General's opinion that nurses should not administer regional anesthesia. On the other hand, the Attorney General addressed other aspects of nurse anesthesia practice not covered in the Chalmers-Francis vs. Nelson decision. He indicated that any person licensed in the healing art, i.e., physician, osteopath, or dentist, may supervise nurse anesthetists and that nurse anesthetists may bill for freelance services (California Attorney General, 1972). In spite of the California Attorney General's opinion, most states recognize the dynamic aspects of nursing and grant nurses authority to perform more sophisticated patient care activities (California Business and Professions Code, 1974). Registered nurses are now performing such functions as arterial puncture, cardiac defibrillation, physical assessment of patients, and other procedures that were once performed only by physicians.

In addressing the subject of CRNA's administering regional anesthesia, it is necessary to consider the educational preparation for learning these techniques. It is unthinkable for anyone without proper instruction and supervision to administer regional anesthesia. It is in this area that CRNA's often fall short of the ideal.

For reasons previously mentioned, regional anesthetic techniques are not stressed in schools of nurse anesthesia and are not an educational requirement. If nurse anesthetists are sincerely interested in offering their patients this technique, emphasis on regional anesthesia should be made within the basic educational structure. Didactic instruction in anatomy, physiology, and pharmacology are as important as instruction in technique.

An even more difficult dilemma is faced by the practicing CRNA who wishes to include regional anesthesia as a part of his or her armamentarium. If they have not been trained in these techniques or have not actively practiced them, where do they go for instruction? Training centers for regional anesthesia should be developed, where CRNA's who are not adept could be certified in these techniques after completing a structured educational program. Because regional blocks have long been considered the domain of anesthesiologists, it would be proper and advisable to invite their active involvement in the education and certification of CRNA's in regional techniques.

Nurses have been administering anesthesia in this country since the turn of the century, when many surgeons trained their operating room nurses to administer open drop ether. Today, nurse anesthetists, after completing a registered nurse's program, receive formal anesthesia training in accredited programs. The AANA Council of Accreditation, the profession's monitor of these institutions, has set minimum requirements for curricula that include 365 hours of advanced didactic study and 450 clinical anesthetics administered (AANA, 1976). To be certified, the nurse anesthetists must also pass a qualifying exam. To maintain certification, he or she must be actively engaged in the practice of anesthesia. Recently, the AANA membership unanimously approved a mandatory continuing education program for recertification. Consequently, to be recertified biennially, a CRNA will have to show evidence of continuing education.

The controversy at hand involves the practice of nurses administering anesthesia, the present and future needs for anesthesia, as well as the original question of whether CRNA's should include regionals as part of the accepted technique of their practice. Since CRNA's perform and will continue to perform a vital role in the delivery of anesthesia services, should they not be able to administer all forms of anesthesia well? If allowed to administer regional anesthetics, CRNA's would then be able to tailor anesthetics to the needs of the individual patient and thereby provide optimal patient care.

REFERENCES

Ament, R.: ASA president expresses concern to AANA members. ASA Newsletter, 41(9):1, 1977.
American Association of Nurse Anesthetists, Council on Accreditation: Standards for Anesthesia Schools, 1976.
Biggins, D. E., Bakutis, A., Nelson, Y., and Petraitis, M.: Survey of anesthesia services, 1971. A.A.N.A.J., 10:371, 1971.
Bonica, J. J.: Regional anesthesia for surgery. Clin. Anesth., 2:123, 1969.
Bridenbaugh, P. O.: The future of regional anesthesia. Regional Anesthesia, 2:1, 1977.

California Attorney General: Opinion. CV72–106, Vol. 56, 1972.

California Business and Professions Code Sec. 2725, 1974.

Carron, H.: Anesthesia manpower in the United States. *In* P. Safar (ed.): Public Health Aspects of Critical Care Medicine in Anesthesiology. Vol. 10/3. Philadelphia, F. A. Davis Co., 1974.

Chalmers-Francis vs. Nelson, 6 CAL 2nd 402, 1936.

Department of the Army Technical Bulletin MED 43, 12 March 1973.

Greiss, F. C., and Anderson, S. G.: Elimination of maternal deaths from anesthesia. Obstet. Gynecol., *29*:677, 1971.

Gunn, I. P.: An apple is not an orange, but is good in its own right: A response to the professional conflict between ASA and AANA. A.A.N.A.J., *45*:584, 1977.

Hehre, F.: Observations, philosophical and opinionated on obstetric anesthesia coverage. *In* P. Safar (ed.): Public Health Aspects of Critical Care Medicine in Anesthesiology. Vol. 10/3. Philadelphia, F. A. Davis Co., 1974.

Joint Commission of Accreditation of Hospitals (JCAH): Accreditation Manual for Hospitals, 1976.

Mannino, M. J.: Conduction (regional) anesthesia and the CRNA: A philosophy. A.A.N.A.J., *45*:485, 1977.

Marcus, S. A.: Correspondence to California legislators, 7 April 1977.

Reese, C. A.: Conduction anesthesia of the upper extremity — a literature and technique review. A.A.N.A.J., *45*:267, 1977.

Rosenberg, H.: Spinal anesthesia by nurse anesthetists. A.A.N.A.J., *41*:330, 1973.

Supply, Need, and Distribution of Anesthesiologists and Nurse Anesthetists in the U.S., 1972 and 1980. PHS, DHEW Publication, 1976.

Winnie, A. P.: CRNA's and regional anesthesia: An opportunity to improve care. Illinois Society of Anesthesiologists Bulletin, *10*:1, 1977.

by M. T. JENKINS

University of Texas Southwestern Medical School

NURSE ANESTHETISTS SHOULD NOT ADMINISTER REGIONAL ANESTHESIA

Historically, there have not been enough trained physicians to administer all anesthetics given each year in the United States; therefore, the nurse anesthetist has fulfilled an important role in the conduct of anesthesia, theoretically under the direction and supervision of a physician. During the years this tradition was being established, training for the nurse anesthetist was entirely in general anesthesia, and surgeons placed faith and confidence in their management of anesthesia for the surgical patient even though supervision was loose or absent. As this tradition developed, surgeons performed regional procedures themselves when they were deemed appropriate and indicated. In the absence of anesthesiologists, the onus of selecting and performing regional procedures weighed heavily on surgeons, so that regional procedures were selected only after considerable thought and judgment. These circumstances tended to make surgeons solicitous of the patients' comfort and also of the preparedness of the nurse anesthetists given the responsibility for monitoring the patient's vital signs while the surgeon performed the operation.

Today, nurse anesthetists who either allege or actually have had experience in performing regional techniques may find that surgeons feel exempt from the obligation of weighing the indications, contraindications, limitations, and risks when specifying regional anesthetic procedures. Having relieved themselves of a comparative selection, surgeons also may lack compunction for doing everything possible to make the procedure successful and may, through lack of specific knowledge of anesthesia and its consequences, ascribe any intraoperative and postoperative complication to the anesthesia and the nurse anesthetist.

The felicitous simile, "captain of the ship," applied to surgeons has been used to express different and sometimes contradictory ideas, so that in one instance surgeons assume the entire medical and legal obligation for regional procedures performed by nurse anesthetists and in other circumstances, perhaps depending upon state laws, they declare the legal responsibility to be solely that of the nurse anesthetist.

I do not believe that the basic training and later practice of nurse anesthetists should include regional anesthesia techniques; they should be neither requested nor expected to perform spinal, epidural, or block anesthesia. Furthermore, surgeons should not be put in the untenable position of accepting medical, ethical, moral, and legal responsibilities for regional anesthesia performed by nurse anesthetists. This stand is not based on whether the techniques can be learned; of course skill can be acquired by the dedicated and intelligent medical or paramedical individuals possessing technical dexterity, just as basic surgical maneuvers or the unqualified steps in flying airplanes can be learned in time by nonsurgeons or nonpilots *if specific judgmental decisions are not required.*

The curricula for nursing students leading to bachelors degrees or registered nurse status, or both, have undergone great changes in recent years. In many schools, the curriculum for student nurses develops and emphasizes managerial skills and places emphasis on social and economic aspects of illness. The emphasis on preventive medicine and health care is at the expense of time for hands-on, direct responsibility for nursing care of individual patients. Thus, nurse student anesthetists do not begin anesthesia training with a sufficiently broad background to allow the full scope of anesthesia to be acquired.

Modern practice of anesthesia encompasses new and increasingly sophisticated technology, including blood gas analysis, electronic monitoring, and computers. I believe the minimum base for nonphysician anesthetists should be college level chemistry, physics, biology, and mathematics. Nurses with diplomas or associate degrees seldom have this background. Considering the great emphasis upon psychosocial aspects of disease and health restoration in four-year nursing schools, the science background of baccalaureate degree nurses may also provide an inadequate base for nurses entering anesthesia training.

The two-year training program for nurse student anesthetists is already too crowded and too short to allow mastery of anatomy, pharmacology, physiology, pathology, neurology, indications, contraindications, and limitations implicitly required for conduct of general anesthesia. To dilute this time by incorporating instruction and practice in regional techniques insures inadequate preparation for all aspects of future anesthesia practice.

Considering subsequent years to be devoted to anesthesia following formal schooling, can the nurse anesthetist defer learning and practicing regional anesthesia techniques and reasonably expect to build on what I have described as an inadequate background? A corollary question is, should the nurse anesthetist be expected to gain experience in trying clinical surgical circumstances, where adequate academic supervision is absent? I believe experience in regional techniques at this stage will not substitute for a deficient background and at best could create and reinforce prejudices at the expense of safety in patient care.

Psychologically, it is inopportune for nurse anesthetists to be learning totally new techniques with new sets of criteria when no longer bona fide students in an anesthesia teaching program. A few successful regional procedures could lull a nurse anesthetist, as well as the operating surgeon, into believing that regional techniques are easy, without hazard, and applicable to all patients and consequently require indifferent care. This is not different from the general practitioner who successfully completes a few abdominal operations, then believes he is on par with surgeons who have devoted years to training. Such soothing justifications will be periodically dispelled by major complications that could and should have been prevented.

Why is the background acquired in medical school of importance, especially when much of it does not seem to apply directly to anesthesia and its techniques? A medical school education reflects extensive knowledge acquired from a broad spectrum of inter-related subjects over a period of years. For example, in at least 10 major courses, a medical student learns anatomy, physiology, pharmacology, and pathology of the autonomic nervous system and its responses, which are important in the conduct of anesthesia. This still does not provide a medical student with all of the information needed for a knowledgeable practice of anesthesia, but it does provide a store of information that can be recalled, correlated, and built upon, then applied to the anesthetized patient with deranged physiology.

In contrast, an anesthetist without a medical school background learns the salient technical points in a cookbook style of do's and don'ts whose value is lost by shadings of physiology and disease. One's perspectives and decisions as a technician become based upon prejudice or even hearsay in these circumstances. Applying a technique, agent, and dose that work well for a healthy patient to a sick and debilitated patient can easily result in complications, not only harmful to the patient but also prejudicial to the technician's further utilization of the method. The problem may also go unrecognized. Lasting opinions based on the responses of a single patient are common regardless of illuminating statistics pointing to different conclusions for a larger cohort of patients.

In my opinion, teaching for nurse student anesthetists should remain in conduction of general anesthesia under direction of anesthesiologists. Of necessity, this puts emphasis on airway control and resuscitation, primary skills needed for the care of patients comatose from whatever cause.

Maintenance of patients during general anesthesia requires a wide range of knowledge, skills, and experience. This includes the pharmacology of anesthetic agents and adjuvants and responses to these under conditions of a variety of diseases and surgical requirements. Resuscitation is a secondary important skill learned during the conduct of general anesthesia. Resuscitation may be defined as getting out of trouble caused by the patient's disease, surgical interference, and the inescapable effects of the anesthetic necessary to allow pain-free operations. The period of schooling for nurse student anesthetists is too short to acquire knowledge beyond an abridged cookbook version of general anesthesia. If there is insufficient time for training in general anesthesia, then let us not transgress further by instruction in regional anesthesia.

While in training, the nurse student anesthetist will monitor the vital signs and psychological responses of patients being operated on using spinal, epidural, or regional block anesthesia. This is a necessary part of training in anesthesia, since on occasion during regional anesthesia patients may need sedation even to the point of conversion to general anesthesia. In some circumstances during regional anesthesia, patients will need resuscitation by tracheal intubation and controlled ventilation. Technical skills in regional anesthesia and detailed knowledge of the local anesthetic process are not essential for nurse student anesthetists to monitor and perform resuscitative maneuvers. Drugs, such as those needed to correct hypotension, may be administered by the nurse student anesthetist but under the direction and prescription of the physician who has produced the regional anesthesia and bears the ethical, medical, moral, and legal responsibilities.

There are other reasons I believe nurse anesthetists should not be requested or required to perform regional anesthesia, even if under the direction of anesthesiologists. If an anesthesiologist performs a spinal tap and injects the agent, for example, then psychologically the sense of responsibility of that anesthesiologist is greater than if a nurse anesthetist had performed it.

If a surgeon had requested spinal anesthesia for a particular patient, the anesthesiologist can and should exercise medical judgment before agreeing that spinal anesthesia is the best, or even an acceptable, technique. By contrast, if the surgeon scheduled the patient for spinal anesthesia to be performed by a nurse anesthetist, the possibilities for medical judgmental review are reduced. The supervising anesthesiologist, if there is one, with more than one anesthetic to oversee, will feel less responsibility and will, in fact, have less legal responsibility than does the surgeon. Consequently, limitations in the technique and even contraindications may be overlooked.

In hospitals where anesthesiologists are unavailable, a surgeon may judge spinal or epidural anesthesia proper for a specific patient and operation. With background information to reach this decision, the surgeon should be able to perform the procedure and monitor with the nurse anesthetist the patient's responses until they are stable and the desired level of anesthesia is achieved. To turn over monitoring completely to the nurse anesthetist earlier is to abandon medical and legal responsibility.

A specious argument is often put forth that nurse anesthetists in the military services must learn regional anesthesia techniques in preparation for assignment where anesthesiologists are unavailable. In my opinion, if physicians at a military base have the capability to designate regional anesthesia and to perform the operation, then they should be able to perform regional techniques. Otherwise, I question whether surgical operations should be done at that particular military installation, especially considering the rapid transportation available today to move patients to adequately staffed hospitals. The same comments are equally or more applicable to small civilian hospitals viewed in the present medical and legal climates.

What about a dire emergency, the life-or-death situation, in which there is insufficient time to transfer a patient from an inadequately staffed military facility or a small civilian hospital? In general, the greater an emergency, the greater the indication for judicious general anesthesia with high oxygen administration and assisted or controlled ventilation, therefore the less the indication for spinal or epidural anesthesia.

Should nurse anesthetists be trained in regional procedures so these techniques can be employed when postanesthesia recovery rooms are unavailable? No! Operations should never be performed today unless skilled postoperative observation can be provided. The patient needs concerned attention following spinal or epidural anesthesia no less than that required after general anesthesia. To suggest that a patient after any type of anesthesia needs less than optimum postanesthesia care is unacceptable.

There are tangential reasons why nurse anesthetists should not be taught or be expected to perform regional anesthesia procedures. Historically, it is not a part of the education and practice of nurse anesthetists, it has not established a tradition, and it is not considered customary throughout the United States. Therefore, its legal acceptance has not been established. Even in communities where the practice may have become "customary" recently, I believe it will be difficult for a surgeon and nearly impossible for a "supervising" anesthesiologist to defend it legally or ethically.

Anesthesiologists, including residents in training, should administer regional anesthesia, when regional procedures are the best choices, to maintain and sharpen their skills. Usually, if anesthesiologists are available in an operating suite, little or no time would be saved by turning the regional procedures over to nurse anesthetists who should be supervised. Even if time were saved, saving time between operations is neither a legal nor an ethical factor in patient care.

In 1978, more anesthesiology residents are training in the United States than at any time in our history, just as there are more medical students than any time in the past. I predict that increasing numbers of students will apply to anesthesia residency programs as they discover the spectacular relationships of the basic sciences to the clinical practice of anesthesiology. Greater numbers of anesthesiologists will further decrease the needs for and opportunities of nurse anesthetists to perform regional anesthetic procedures.

In conclusion, from all viewpoints, I believe that regional anesthesia should not be taught to the nurse anesthetist and that nurse anesthetists should confine their anesthesia practices to techniques in general anesthesia.

NURSE ANESTHETISTS AND REGIONAL ANESTHESIA

EDITORIAL COMMENT

Long before physicians became continuously involved with the administration of anesthetics, nurses were asked to perform this function under the direction of the surgeon. The choice among anesthetics was minimal, in the United States principally confined to diethyl ether. Surgical procedures were brief (by today's standards), respiration was sustained throughout the operation, and the critically ill or extremes of life were not considered suitable surgical candidates. The nurse anesthetists were taught how to monitor the vital signs and to inform the surgeon if there was deviation from the anticipated. Without a doubt, a thoughtful nurse anesthetist learned more over a period of years about care of the anesthetized patient than a surgeon ever perceived, but unfortunately for us, few ever committed their observations to paper. Surgeons were intent on the surgical task, expected to be warned if vital signs changed, and, as is typical of the surgical personality, if trouble did arise made a prompt judgment and expected an equally prompt response. Furthermore, if the outcome was an anesthetic morbidity or mortality, surgeons did not shirk their responsibility.

The introduction of spinal anesthesia was within the surgical domain. By injecting a local anesthetic into the subarachnoid space, the surgeon could produce optimal conditions of analgesia and relaxation and the anesthetist would do the same thing as before — monitor the vital signs. The judgment of whether to use ether or a spinal remained the surgeon's, as did the responsibility. As operations became more complex and as sicker patients were operated on, surgeons became concerned. More training was required for the person at the head of the table. Anesthesiologists began to appear; a few surgeons perceived the need decades before others. The introduction of ethylene, cyclopropane, thiopental, and curare and the need for assisted and controlled ventilation moved anesthesia beyond the training of most surgeons. The editor lived through an era when the surgeons he worked with were reluctant to give up unsupplemented spinal anesthesia for cholecystectomy, choledochostomy, and gastric resection but eventually did so, bowing reluctantly to physician anesthetic judgment and experience. Today, few surgeons will accept the legal responsibility for dictating anesthetic techniques and patient safety during anesthesia. Herein is the basis of this controversy.

The technical performance of regional anesthesia can be mastered readily by the dedicated nonphysician. The questions at hand are whether or not the nurse has sufficient background to apply the judgment required as to when to use the technique; whether the surgeon with minimal training in anesthesia is willing to listen to the advice of an experienced nurse anesthetist; whether the nurse is sufficiently trained to adequately perceive impending complication during regional anesthesia; and whether the surgeon will accept responsibility should morbidity and mortality result.

Mannino conceives the techniques as not being extraordinarily difficult; therefore, nurses should be trained in their use and should be permitted to use them. I agree. Jenkins is concerned about judgment in application of the technique, sufficient depth of training for detection of impending complication, and unwillingness of surgeons or anesthesiologists to accept the responsibility. I also agree. I find no fault with training nurses to do regional anesthesia so long as the indications, contraindications, and management of regional techniques are taught by physicians as supplements to existing nurse training programs. At the same time, were I a nurse anesthetist prepared to do regional anesthesia, I would want an agreement with the surgeon that my judgment will be respected and that should trouble arise, he or she and I are equally responsible. I doubt many programs are going to accept the first suggestion and suspect that few surgeons will acquiesce to the second.

Part 12

INTERMITTENT POSITIVE PRESSURE BREATHING

THE PROPOSITION:

Intermittent Positive Pressure Breathing should be used routinely in surgical patients with pulmonary disease.

ALTERNATIVE POINTS OF VIEW

By Barry A. Shapiro
By Robert H. Bartlett

EDITORIAL COMMENT

by BARRY A. SHAPIRO

Northwestern University Medical School

IPPB THERAPY IS INDICATED PREOPERATIVELY AND POSTOPERATIVELY IN SOME PATIENTS WITH PULMONARY DISEASE

Until the mid-20th century, pulmonary physiology was limited to considerations of gas exchange. Although there can be no challenge to the concept that the prime function of the pulmonary system is to allow atmospheric gases to exchange with blood, a clear tracheobronchial tree must be maintained to adequately accomplish this function. Prior to 1955, there was little concern for *nonrespiratory* functions of the pulmonary system. Even though the past 20 years have resulted in a wealth of information concerning these functions, clinical medicine has been slow to appreciate their importance. Much of this hesitancy may be attributed to the fact that the pulmonary system is mechanical; therefore many of the therapeutic modalities applicable to its care and maintenance are not pharmacologic. For example, medicine has paid great attention to the bronchospastic elements of pulmonary disease because bronchospasm is common and readily reversible pharmacologically. In hospitalized patients, retained secretions probably occur with greater frequency than does bronchospasm, yet there has been great hesitancy to accept the techniques and modalities for preventing and treating retained secretions.

The progress of clinical respiratory care over the last decade has erased any legitimacy to the question: Is bronchial hygiene necessary? Today the question is: How should bronchial hygiene be applied and how do we evaluate its effectiveness? The technique of concern is intermittent positive pressure breathing (IPPB), a single technique of bronchial hygiene that has been misused, abused, and overused. The fact that physicians are now concerned with this overuse is legitimate and welcome; however, the conclusion that IPPB is of no benefit under any circumstances is one that is not only erroneous but also of significant potential detriment in the care of certain surgical patients. To understand the rationale for appropriate use of IPPB therapy, it is necessary to review the normal bronchial hygiene and pulmonary defense mechanisms.

THE MUCOUS BLANKET

The pulmonary epithelium contains numerous serous and mucous glands whose secretions form a continuous, uninterrupted covering of the epithelium known as the *mucous blanket* (Fig. 1). Submucosal glands produce bronchial secretions in the healthy adult estimated at approximately 100 ml. per day. The composition of normal mucus is 95 per cent water, 2 per cent glycoprotein, 1 per cent carbohydrate, and trace amounts of lipid and DNA, in addition to cellular debris and other foreign elements. This mucus is constantly produced and extruded onto the surface of the pulmonary epithelium and has very specific hydration, pH, electrolyte balance, and numerous other factors that ensure proper mucokinesis. The surface goblet cells react readily to irritation by becoming enlarged and chronically inflamed; their abnormal secretions under these circumstances play a great role in malfunction of the mucous blanket.

There is a progressive decrease in the water content of mucus from its formation point at the mucosal surface toward the inner luminal surface. These layers have been arbitrarily subdivided into a *sol* layer (adjacent to the mucosal surface) and a more viscous *gel* layer (Fig. 1). The gel layer is very viscous and normally flows continuously toward the larynx as a result of ciliary action.

The cilia lie almost entirely within the fluid sol layer. The ciliary control mechanisms are unknown, but their "beating" action has been well studied. The forward movement of cilia makes the upper end of the hairlike projection extend into the viscous gel layer and pulls it forward. During its backward motion, the cilia folds up on itself. Thus, the backward motion is entirely within the sol layer and has little backward pull on the mucous blanket. Because of the viscous and elastic properties of the gel layer, this intermittent ciliary "pull" is transformed into a continuous movement toward the larynx. The normal mucous blanket moves at a reasonably rapid rate (1–2 cm./min.) and can completely cleanse the normal adult lung in less than 20 minutes (Slonim and Hamilton, 1971). Mucus abnormalities cause slowing of the blanket, resulting in retained secretions. Almost any physiologic stress may result in abnormal ciliary function, and a multiplicity of factors may cause abnormalities in mucus production, e.g., pulmonary epithelial inflammation, abnormality of the mucous and serous glands, or, in fact, almost any disease process that involves the tracheobronchial tree.

In summary, normal bronchial hygiene is dependent on normal

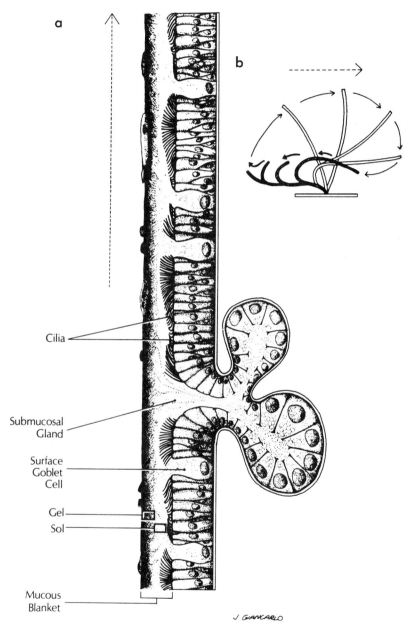

a

b

Cilia

Submucosal
Gland

Surface
Goblet
Cell

Gel

Sol

Mucous
Blanket

J GIANCARLO

Figure 1. *A,* The mucociliary escalator. *B,* A conceptual scheme of ciliary movement, allowing forward motion to move viscous gel layer and backward motion to take place entirely within more fluid sol layer. (From Shapiro, B. A., Harrison, R. A., and Trout, C. A.: Clinical Application of Respiratory Care. Copyright © 1975 by Year Book Medical Publishers, Inc., Chicago. Used by permission.)

mucus production and ciliary function. Any disease process, but especially one involving the pulmonary system, may result in abnormal mucokinesis, which will lead to retained secretions. Although investigations into the details of mucus production and ciliary motion continue, there is more than enough evidence to substantiate these generalizations.

THE COUGH MECHANISM

When malfunction of the mucociliary escalator occurs, the primary defense mechanism is a cough. There is little evidence that coughing is a necessary component of normal pulmonary hygiene; rather, it functions as the primary defense mechanism in the presence of abnormalities, such as copious, dry, or thick mucus; poor ciliary activity; and diseased pulmonary epithelium. The adequacy of the cough mechanism is dependent on numerous factors but primarily on an adequate inspiratory volume (Shapiro, et al., 1975). Coughing without adequate inspiration is usually ineffective. Various investigators have attempted to quantitate the minimum adequate inspiratory volume for an effective cough, and most agree that an inspiratory capacity of at least 75 per cent of normal is necessary (Slonim and Hamilton, 1971). Others have found that less than three times a predicted tidal volume or a vital capacity below 20 ml. per kg. provides an ineffective cough (Bendixen, et al., 1965). Regardless of the specific guidelines applied, the principle that a patient must have the mechanical capacity to breathe deeply for an effective cough cannot be ignored.

The purpose of the cough is to produce a high velocity air flow from the pulmonary tree that will mobilize mucus. Obviously, the more fluid and continuous the mucous blanket, the greater will be the degree of mobilization. It must be appreciated that no matter how effective the cough may be mechanically, it must have a reasonably intact mucous blanket to mobilize.

THE SURGICAL PATIENT AND BRONCHIAL HYGIENE

Surgical and anesthetic stress produce transient depression of ciliary activity and usually decreased production of mucus (Slonim and Hamilton, 1971). Thus, postoperative retention of pulmonary secretions is to be expected even when pulmonary mechanics remain adequate. Such retained secretions lead to atelectasis and infection — the most common postoperative complications.

Postoperative pulmonary complication is a difficult area to investigate because surgical technique and postoperative procedures vary significantly from institution to institution. In addition, the definition of postoperative pulmonary complication is by no means universally accepted — its diagnosis varies from fever of unknown origin to chest x-ray evidence of atelectasis or pneumonia. The most reasonable approach is to take the data from intrainstitutional studies and compare the incidence of postoperative pulmonary complications with various factors, as shown in Table 1. A reasonable conclusion is that the preoperative forced expiratory spirogram (screening pulmonary function study) is the most available and least expensive means of effectively delineating the patient at high risk for postoperative pulmonary complications. Thus, preoperative pulmonary function screening will alert us to the high-risk patient and also quantitate the vital capacity so that the significance of postoperative decreases may be anticipated.

The limitations to breathing mechanics secondary to surgical intervention are reproducible. Abdominal and thoracic surgery results in a transient restrictive pulmonary disease typified by significant decreases in vital capacity. For example, an upper abdominal procedure usually results in a 75 per cent decrease in preoperative vital capacity within the first 24 hours; a lower abdominal or thoracic procedure (not involving sternal splitting) will usually result in a 50 per cent decrease in preoperative vital capacity within the first 24 hours (Churchill, et al., 1927; Honatt, et al., 1962). The major restrictive insult usually occurs within the first 24 hours postoperatively and then improves dramatically over the next several days if complications do not arise (Bendixen, et al., 1965).

IPPB THERAPY

IPPB therapy is generally defined as the therapeutic application of inspiratory positive pressure to the airway (usually via mask or mouthpiece) by a competent therapist or technician. The efficacy of any therapy depends on the therapist! In the absence of an appropriately trained therapist working with the patient, all bronchial hygiene therapy will be limited in its effectiveness — IPPB being no exception.

To appropriately study the efficacy of treatment regimens, an attempt must be made to ensure that the administration is appropriate and standardized. This is relatively easy to accomplish in pharmacologic studies but difficult in mechanical or manipulative regimens. Those who demand specific physiologic evidence to test the qualitative and quantitative benefits of IPPB must be reminded that therapist ap-

Table 1.   Incidence of Postoperative Pulmonary
Complication in Relation to Various Factors

Abnormal pulmonary function study/Normal	23/1
Abdominal operation/Non-abdominal	4/1
Smoking history/Non-smoker	4/1
Above 60 years/Under 60 years	3/1
Overweight (20%)/Not overweight	2/1

plication is difficult to standardize. On the other hand, those who believe IPPB therapy is effective must be reminded that unsubstantiated clinical impression and dogma is far from irrefutable fact. Most clinical studies of IPPB have failed to make clear distinction between methodology and equipment, positive pressure breathing and bronchodilator, acute disease and chronic, or pulmonary function improvement and clinical improvement. If objectivity is to exist in the support or nonsupport of IPPB therapy, reasonable and practical therapeutic goals must be clearly stated.

There are five documented physiologic effects of intermittent positive pressure breathing: (1) An increase in mean airway and intrathoracic pressure (Cournand, et al., 1948; Price, Conner, and Dripps, 1954; Werkö, 1947), (2) an increase in inspiratory mechanical bronchodilation (Bates, Macklem, and Christie, 1971), (3) a decrease in the work of breathing (Noehren, et al., 1958), (4) manipulation of inspiratory to expiratory ratios (Wilson, Farber, and Collins, 1957), and (5) an increase in tidal volume (Noehren, 1970; Ziment, 1973; Noehren, et al., 1958; Wilson, Farber, and Collins, 1957).

The significant advantage of IPPB for the surgical patient is that at physiologically advantageous inspiratory to expiratory patterns a deeper breath may be provided than the patient *can or will* produce spontaneously. In my opinion, this is the therapeutic rationale for the application of IPPB to the surgical patient for bronchial hygiene purposes.

Since it is reasonable to predict that the abdominal and thoracic surgical patient will be severely limited in his inspiratory capacity for several days postoperatively, it is reasonable to predict that the ability to cough effectively will be significantly compromised during this period. By no means does this intimate that all abdominal and surgical patients need postoperative IPPB therapy — such misinterpretation has contributed to the widespread misuse and abuse of IPPB. If the patient's *preoperative* pulmonary status is significantly limited, however, IPPB therapy may well be indicated to avoid the high incidence of postoperative pulmonary complication.

PREOPERATIVE PULMONARY DISEASE

The most prevalent serious pulmonary problem in our population today is chronic obstructive pulmonary disease (COPD) (U.S. Dept. of HEW). Patients with COPD have been the subject of numerous studies to attempt to delineate the effectiveness of bronchial hygiene therapy — IPPB therapy in particular (Cherniack, 1974; Lefcoe and Carter, 1970; Pierce and Saltzmann, 1974; Murray, 1974). The pathophysiology of COPD clearly delineates the need for augmented bronchial hygiene as a chronic therapy (Mayock, 1974; Shapiro, et al., 1975). Recent studies of the effectiveness of bronchial hygiene modalities (including IPPB therapy) have shown profound benefits (Shapiro, et al., 1977); however, contrary studies exist (Cherniack and Svanhill, 1976) — therefore the question remains an open debate.

The vast majority of COPD patients have significant decreases in vital capacity as well as in expiratory flow rates and thus are at high risk for postoperative complications. Since the majority will have vital capacities significantly below 20 ml. per kg. for several days postoperatively, cough augmentation with IPPB therapy is indicated for that period of time. Since the efficacy of IPPB therapy depends on both the therapist and the patient, preoperative training in IPPB therapy is useful for those patients needing the therapy postoperatively.

CONCLUSION

Aggressive postoperative respiratory therapy (IPPB, aerosol, chest physical therapy) has been the "vogue" for the last 20 years and has been overused, misused, and abused. Neither nursing staffs nor physicians have the time or training to effectively apply bronchial hygiene regimens to "high-risk" patients, however; the expense and personnel time involved in the proper administration of aggressive respiratory therapy cannot be justified for *all* patients. The answer lies in the ability to preoperatively identify the "high-risk" patient for pulmonary complications and appropriately apply respiratory therapy in the preoperative and postoperative periods.

In order to cough and deep breathe adequately, the vital capacity must exceed 20 ml. per kg., and the patient must be alert and cooperative and have a hydrated mucous blanket. The postoperative patient not meeting these minimal requirements runs a higher risk of pulmonary complication. This may be avoided in many instances by applying appropriate respiratory therapy techniques.

I believe screening pulmonary function testing (forced expiratory spirogram) should be performed preoperatively on all patients for abdominal and thoracic operations. Those manifesting preoperative vital capacities of less than 40 ml. per kg. will potentially benefit from IPPB therapy for several days postoperatively. In addition, COPD patients in this group will benefit from several days of preoperative respiratory therapy including IPPB.

Common sense dictates that the least costly and least time-consuming effective methods for bronchial hygiene should be used for each patient. This automatically rules out IPPB as a routine modality for most patients. I have no disagreement with the concept that simple "stir up" regimens and incentive spirometry are preferable for most surgical patients; my disagreement is with those who claim those regimens are effective for *all* surgical patients! In my opinion, IPPB therapy is indicated and effective in those patients transiently requiring augmented inspiratory volumes for effective coughing.

REFERENCES

Bates, D. V., MacKlem, P. T., and Christie, R. V.: Respiratory Function in Disease. 2nd ed. Philadelphia, W. B. Saunders Company, 1971.

Bendixen, H. H., Egbert, L. D., Hedley-Whyte, J., Laver, M. B., and Pontoppidan, H.: Respiratory Care. St. Louis, The C. V. Mosby Company, 1965.

Cherniack, R. M.: Intermittent positive pressure breathing in management of chronic obstructive disease: current state of the art. Am. Rev. Resp. Dis., *110*:188–192, 1974.

Cherniack, R. M., and Svanhill, E.: Long-term use of intermittent positive-pressure breathing (IPPB) in chronic obstructive pulmonary disease. Am. Rev. Resp. Dis., *113*:721–728, 1976.

Churchill, E., and McNeil, D.: The reduction in vital capacity following operation. Surg. Gynecol. Obstet., *44*:483, 1927.

Cournand, A., Motley, H. L., Werko, L., and Richards, D. W., Jr.: Physiological studies of effects of intermittent positive pressure breathing on cardiac output in man. Am. J. Physiol., *152*:162–174, 1948.

Howatt, W. F., Talner, N. S., Sloan, H., and DeMuth, G. R.: Pulmonary function changes following repair of heart lesions with the aid of extracorporeal circulation. J. Thorac. Cardiovasc. Surg., *43*:649, 1962.

Lefcoe, N. M., and Carter, P.: Intermittent positive-pressure breathing in chronic obstructive pulmonary disease. Can. Med. Assoc. J., *103*:279–281, 1970.

Mayock, R. L.: IPPB is a useful modality in the treatment of chronic obstructive lung disease. In Ingelfinger, F. J., Ebert, R. V., Finland, M., and Relman, A. S. (eds.): Controversy in Internal Medicine II. Philadelphia, W. B. Saunders Company, 1974.

Murray, J. F.: Review of the state of the art of intermittent positive pressure breathing therapy. Am. Rev. Resp. Dis., *110*:193–199, 1974.

Noehren, T. H.: Is positive pressure breathing overrated? Chest, 57:507–509, 1970.

Noehren, T. H., Lasry, J. E., and Legters, L. J.: Intermittent positive pressure breathing (IPPB/I) for the prevention and management of postoperative pulmonary complication. Surgery, *43*:658, 1958.

Pierce, A. K., and Saltzman, H. A.: Conference on the scientific basis of respiratory therapy. Am. Rev. Resp. Dis., *110*:1–3, 1974.

Price, H. L., Conner, E. H., and Dripps, R. D.: Some respiratory and circulatory effects of mechanical respirators. J. Appl. Physiol., *6*:517–530, 1954.

Shapiro, B. A., Harrison, R. A., and Trout, C. A.: Clinical Application of Respiratory Care. Chicago, Year Book Medical Publishers, Inc., 1975.

Shapiro, B. A., Vostinak-Foley, E., Hamilton, B. B., and Buehler, J. H.: Rehabilitation in chronic obstructive pulmonary disease: A two year prospective study. Resp. Care, *22*:1045, 1977.

Slonim, N. B., and Hamilton, L. H.: Respiratory Physiology. 2nd ed. St. Louis, The C. V. Mosby Company, 1971.

U.S. Department of Health, Education, and Welfare, National Center for Health Statistics, 1950–1969.

Werkö, L.: Influence of positive pressure breathing on circulation in man. Acta Med. Scand. [Suppl.], *193*:1–125, 1947.

Wilson, R. H. L., Farber, S. M., and Collins, J. E.: Intermittent positive pressure breathing: a clinical evaluation of its use in certain respiratory diseases. Calif. Med., 87:161–165, 1957.

Ziment, I.: Why are they saying bad things about IPPB? Resp. Care, *18*:677, 1973.

by ROBERT H. BARTLETT

University of California, Irvine

IPPB SHOULD NOT BE ROUTINE PULMONARY PROPHYLAXIS

Pulmonary complications remain a major cause of morbidity and mortality after surgical operations. Surgeons, anesthesiologists, respiratory therapists, and nurses spend time and effort to prevent this problem, usually by exhorting patients to carry out various respiratory maneuvers, often with the aid of machines, gimmicks, and gadgets. In the 1960's this well-intentioned activity led to general acceptance and use of mechanically assisted ventilation "treatment" with a pressure limited ventilator (IPPB). "IPPB, 5 min qid" became a standard postoperative order. Every hospital purchased portable pressure-driven ventilators. Respiratory therapy departments blossomed. Publications (without data) appeared (Noehren, Lasry, and Legters, 1958; Rudy and Crepeau, 1958), extolling the virtues of IPPB. Is this a worthwhile expenditure of energy?

To assess the value of any maneuver designed to prevent postoperative respiratory complications, we must understand the pathogenesis of this syndrome and the physiology of the maneuvers designed to prevent it.

DEFINITION OF POSTOPERATIVE PULMONARY COMPLICATIONS

A complex of signs, symptoms, and clinical events are usually lumped together under the heading of "postoperative pulmonary complications." These usually include tachypnea, tachycardia, sometimes dyspnea, fever, rales or ronchi, no cough followed by nonproductive cough followed by thick sputum production, and the findings of atelectasis or consolidation, or both, on chest x-ray examination. Direct measurement usually discloses decreased functional residual capacity (FRC) and associated decreased compliance. Hypoxemia is pres-

249

ent, caused primarily by ventilation perfusion imbalance and a 10 to 15 per cent transpulmonary shunt. This complex can occur at any time but most commonly 48 to 72 hours following operation. It can occur after any type of operation or anesthesia but is most common (50 per cent) after thoracotomy or operations on the upper abdomen (25 per cent) (Hamilton, et al., 1964; Zikria, 1971). It is less common (10 per cent or less) following pelvic or extremity operations. The incidence increases with advancing age, history of smoking, and history of pre-existing lung disease.

CAUSES OF POSTOPERATIVE PULMONARY COMPLICATIONS

Normal humans inhale to total lung capacity at least once each hour in the course of talking, eating, yawning, or simply as spontaneous deep breathing. Postoperative patients have a normal tidal volume and normal minute volume but lack the periodic variation in the pattern of breathing (Bartlett, 1971; Okinaka, 1965). This may be due to voluntary and involuntary splinting, pain reflexes, anesthetics, narcotics, or a combination of these factors. The lack of spontaneous deep breaths for a few hours, even in healthy subjects, results in significant alveolar atelectasis (Caro, Butler, and DuBois, 1960; Ferris and Pollard, 1960). This can be readily reversed by a few deep breaths, but without deep breathing, segmental and lobar atelectasis can follow rapidly. Mucus pools in the bronchi leading to the atelectatic areas, probably because of the loss of air flow. This sequence of events occurs in all patients after operations on the chest or abdomen (Lee, et al., 1969). Usually the patient returns to a normal pattern of breathing, collapsed alveoli open spontaneously, and clinical symptoms never result. In some patients, however, the clinical symptoms listed above become obvious on the first or second day following operation, an x-ray is taken, and the patient is declared to have pulmonary complications (or atelectasis or early pneumonia). Patients with a pre-existing decreased FRC or small airway disease start from a compromised baseline. They will present clinical symptoms sooner, more often, and with increased severity.

Patients who develop "pulmonary complications" are usually treated with measures designed to remove the collected mucus, since that is the most visible problem. Coughing, endotracheal suctioning, chest physical therapy, and bronchoscopy are used (usually with good results in clearing mucus from the tracheobronchial tree). Although the emphasis is on expiratory maneuvers, somewhere in the course of this exercise the patient inhales vigorously, opens the areas of collapsed alveoli, and returns to normal function. If the pathogenesis of this syndrome starts with lack of spontaneous deep breathing, however, efforts intended to prevent it should be focused on maximal lung inflation, not expiration.

A COMPARISON OF RESPIRATORY MANEUVERS

Various inspiratory and expiratory maneuvers have been proposed to prevent postoperative pulmonary complications. These maneuvers are reviewed in detail elsewhere (Bartlett, Gazzariga, and Gerghty, 1973). Sustained maximal inspiration is the only maneuver with any solid rationale for the reasons outlined above. This can be accomplished by spontaneous inspiratory effort or by use of a positive pressure mechanical ventilator. Although some would argue that spontaneous diaphragmatic breathing provides better ventilation to the lower lobes than passive positive pressure via the airway, inflation to total lung capacity should be possible with either approach. It is essential that postoperative maneuvers be taught *pre*operatively to all patients to establish the baseline maximal inspiratory capacity and to accustom the patient to the technique when free of pain and narcosis.

IPPB AS A ROUTINE PROPHYLACTIC MANEUVER

Although both of these methods of maximal inflation should produce the same results, IPPB has proved to be of little or no value as a routine prophylactic maneuver in all postoperative patients. Four controlled studies of IPPB as routine prophylaxis have been reported (Anderson, Dossett, and Hamilton, 1963; Baxter and Levine, 1969; Becker et al., 1960; Sands et al., 1961); when the groups were comparable, the incidence of pulmonary complications was the same or slightly higher in the IPPB-treated groups. This would seem to contradict the hypothesis of an abnormal breathing pattern causing postoperative pulmonary complications, but the reasons for failure of IPPB lie not in the theory but in the practice. The maximum possible inhaled volume must be ensured with each maneuver, and maximal inspiration should be performed at least every hour to be effective. IPPB was commonly administered only four times a day or less, and pressure-limited ventilators were used without concomitant measurement of volume. Since the FRC was already decreased and patients tended to resist the inspiratory flow because of pain, the inspiratory pressure cutoff was reached at a low tidal volume. Thus, sustained maximum inspiration was never achieved. Some patients involuntarily swallow during IPPB, leading to gastric dilation and the possibility for increase risk of pulmonary complications with the use of that device.

The futility of routine IPPB and the difficulty of quantitating spontaneous breathing exercises led to the development of the incentive spirometer (Bartlett et al., 1973). This device simply encourages patients to do sustained maximal inspiratory maneuvers, requires inhalation of a preset volume, and records the frequency with which the maneuvers are done. The patient is told to inhale the desired volume at least 10 times each hour, thus providing an incentive and measurement technique for deep breathing exercises. The use of deep breathing exercises in association with chest physical therapy (Brattström, 1954) or with the use of an incentive spirometer (Bartlett et al., 1973; McConnell, Maloney, and Buckberg, 1974; Van de Water et al., 1972) has been shown to reverse atelectasis and transpulmonary shunting and to decrease the incidence of postoperative pulmonary complications. Compared to IPPB, the technique is not only effective but also inexpensive (van de Water, 1972). Finally, it emphasizes the role of nursing and patient participation in postoperative pulmonary prophylaxis, freeing the respiratory therapist for more important responsibilities with ventilator patients. If IPPB were used every hour, with guaranteed volume rather than pressure, it would probably be effective in preventing postoperative pulmonary complications. Since easier, less expensive, more satisfactory alternatives exist, however, there is no place for routine IPPB in postoperative care.

PROPER USE OF IPPB

IPPB was originally proposed as a method for delivering nebulized drugs into the lower airway. In fact, its use for anything else has never been actively advocated by the manufacturers of the devices. The technique does provide an excellent method of delivering nebulized drugs. It *is* useful as a postoperative prophylactic maneuver in patients who are too old, feeble, scared, or uncooperative to carry out spontaneous deep breathing exercise. It is also extremely useful as an adjunct to the treatment of established atelectasis or consolidation (with or without attempts at airway cleaning). In both of these circumstances, the ventilator should be left at the bedside. The patient should be instructed in its use and a spirometer attached for measurement of exhaled volume. The patient should be instructed to inhale to a maximal predetermined volume using the device several times each hour. After the initial set-up, this course of treatment is a nursing responsibility.

IPPB is also helpful in the postoperative management of patients with pre-existing lung disease who are accustomed to using IPPB regularly. Such patients are often psychologically dependent on IPPB, as well as profiting from the physiologic benefits of delivery of bronchodilator and broncholytic drugs.

PREOPERATIVE PREPARATION

Many factors are important in *pre*operative pulmonary preparation, including cessation of smoking, elective weight loss, general conditioning and exercise, and teaching and practice of sustained maximal inspriatory maneuvers. Patients with existing pulmonary disease should be vigorously treated and proved to be in the best possible pulmonary condition prior to elective operations. This includes treating chronic bronchitis with culture-specific antibiotics, treating asthma until the patient is free of bronchospasm if possible, and treating emphysema with whatever combination of broncholytic and bronchodilator drugs is most effective for the patient. IPPB is a useful adjunct in these patients, both to deliver nebulized drugs and to familiarize the patient with hourly large volume inflation, which may be necessary following operation.

REFERENCES

Anderson, W. H., Dossett, B. E., Jr., and Hamiliton, G. L.: Prevention of postoperative pulmonary complications. J.A.M.A., *186*:763–766, 1963.

Bartlett, R. H.: Post traumatic pulmonary insufficiency. *In* Cooper, P., and Nyhus, L. (eds.): Surgery Annual 1971. New York, Appleton-Century-Crofts, 1971.

Bartlett, R. H., Gazzaniga, A. B., and Geraghty, T. R.: Respiratory maneuvers to prevent pulmonary complications: a critical review. J.A.M.A., *224*:1017, 1973.

Bartlett, R. H., Gazzaniga, A. B., Brennan, M., and Hanson, E. L.: Studies in pathogenesis and prevention of postoperative pulmonary complications. Surg. Gynecol. Obstet., *108*:814, 1973.

Baxter, W. D., and Levine, R. S.: An evaluation of intermittent positive pressure breathing in the prevention of postoperative pulmonary complications. Arch. Surg., *98*:795, 1969.

Becker, A., Barak, S., Braun, E., and Meyers, M. P.: The treatment of postoperative pulmonary atelectasis with intermittent positive pressure breathing. Surg. Gynecol. Obstet., *111*:517, 1960.

Brattström, S.: Postoperative . . . . Acta Chir. Scand. [Suppl.], 105, 1954.

Caro, C. G., Butler, J., and DuBois, A. B.: Some effects of restriction of chest cage expansion on pulmonary function in man: an experimental study. J. Clin. Invest., *39*:573, 1960.

Ferris, B. G., Jr., and Pollard, D. S.: Effect of deep and quiet breathing on pulmonary compliance in man. J. Clin. Invest., *39*:143, 1960.

Hamilton, W. K., McDonald, J. S.,

Fischer, H. W., et al.: Postoperative respiratory complications; a comparison of arterial gas tensions, radiographs and physical examination. Anesthesiology, *25*:607, 1964.

Lee, A. B., Kinney, J. M., Turino, G., and Gump, F.: Effects of abdominal operation on ventilation and gas exchange. J. Natl. Med. Assoc., *61*:164, 1969.

McConnell, D. H., Maloney, J. V., Jr., and Buckberg, G. D.: Postoperative intermittent positive-pressure breathing treatments. Physiological considerations. J. Thorac. Cardiovasc. Surg., *68*(6):944, 1974.

Noehren, T. H., Lasry, J. E., and Legters, L. J.: Intermittent positive pressure (IPPB/I) for the prevention and management of postoperative pulmonary complications. Surgery, *43*:658, 1958.

Okinaka, A. J.: Closure of pulmonary air spaces following abdominal surgery. Surg. Gynecol. Obstet., *121*:1282, 1965.

Rudy, N. E., and Crepeau, J.: Role of intermittent positive pressure breathing postoperatively. J.A.M.A., *167*:1093, 1958.

Sands, J. H., Cypert, C., Armstrong, R., et al.: A controlled study using routine intermittent positive pressure breathing in the post-surgical patient. Dis. Chest, *40*:128, 1961.

Van de Water, J. M., Watring, W. G., Linton, L. A., et al.: Prevention of postoperative pulmonary complications. Surg. Gynecol. Obstet., *135*:229, 1972.

Zikria, B. A., Spencer, J. L., Michailoff, T., et al.: Breathing patterns in preoperative, postoperative, and critically ill patients. Surg. Forum, *22*:40, 1971.

INTERMITTENT POSITIVE PRESSURE BREATHING

```
┌─────────────────────────────────────────────────────────┐
│                                                           │
└─────────────────────────────────────────────────────────┘
```

EDITORIAL COMMENT

Respiratory care has come a long way from the days of the old oxygen tent, in which the patient was likely being treated in a hypoxic environment, or of the humidifier, in which oxygen was bubbled through contaminated water, resulting in no humidification, some drying, and occasional pulmonary infection. Once improved techniques became available and men like Julius Comroe began to publish books on clinical pulmonary physiology, there was a rush to treat the respiratory tract of all hospitalized patients, particularly those on a surgical service. For a while, the indiscriminate use of "inhalational therapy" became absurd and without factual basis. Even today, one might question the routine use of face hoods with humidified oxygen for every patient admitted to a recovery room.

Shapiro and Bartlett both decry the extensive use of IPPB for the past 20 years, with Shapiro claiming the technique has been "overused, misused, and abused." Bartlett would prefer breathing exercises and use of an incentive spirometer, reserving IPPB for patients "who are too old, feeble, scared, or uncooperative" or for those addicted to IPPB. He denies that IPPB does any better and points to four controlled studies to verify his stand. Shapiro advocates the routine use of IPPB in patients with COPD, claiming profound benefit from his own experiences but acknowledging that others have not confirmed his results. He lays the failure of benefit to accrue to improper selection of patients and faulty application of the technique.

IPPB is costly, much more so than voluntary pulmonary exercising and incentive spirometry. A controlled study should not be that difficult to devise and carry out in multiple institutions to obtain a large patient population. This controversy has gone on too long. Why can't it be settled quickly?

Part 13

INTRA-ARTERIAL MONITORING

THE PROPOSITION:

Intra-arterial monitoring is a safe and routine procedure for major surgical procedures.

ALTERNATIVE POINTS OF VIEW

By Malcolm G. Miller, John Hedley-Whyte
By Jay Jacoby

EDITORIAL COMMENT

Part D

INTRA-ARTERIAL
MONITORING

by MALCOLM G. MILLER

JOHN HEDLEY-WHYTE
Harvard Medical School

INTRA-ARTERIAL MONITORING: A ROUTINE AND SAFE PROCEDURE

If we were to undergo a major surgical procedure, we would want intra-arterial monitoring. Percutaneous cannulation of superficial vessels can be accomplished with minimal discomfort using local anesthesia. Continuous intra-arterial pressure monitoring and intermittent arterial blood gas analysis afford early recognition of deviation from the desired normal and correction of the abnormality before irreversible damage occurs. The configuration of the arterial wave form and whether it fluctuates with respiration provide early information regarding the blood volume before hypotension ensues.

INDUCTION OF ANESTHESIA

The hemodynamic consequences of induction, laryngoscopy, and tracheal intubation can be rapid and profound (Fig. 1) (Prys-Roberts et al., 1973). The sequence of myocardial depression and hypotension consequent upon most induction agents and the hypertension and tachycardia associated with laryngoscopy and tracheal intubation can cause serious myocardial ischemia. These hemodynamic changes can be recognized immediately if intra-arterial monitoring is established before induction of anesthesia. If dangerous hypertension and tachycardia are provoked by the laryngoscopy, instrumentation can be interrupted and measures can be taken to block these sympathetic responses. Topical anesthesia is only marginally useful. An incremental dose of the intravenous induction agent or deepening of inhalational anesthesia may allow a subsequent, less traumatic, laryngoscopy to be performed. A reduction in systemic vascular resistance by intravenous

257

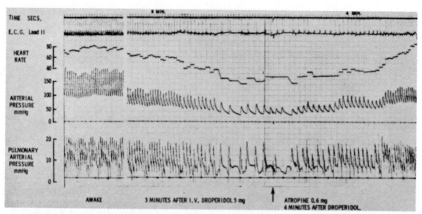

Figure 1. Circulatory changes occurring during and after laryngoscopy and tracheal intubation. Arterial hypertension occurred within 15 seconds of laryngoscopy, despite having fallen to 100/50 mm. Hg after induction. Tracheal intubation was accompanied by prolonged ventricular bigeminy and further systemic hypertension. Pulmonary hypertension also occurred and persisted into maintenance anesthesia. Depression of the S-T segment and T-wave inversion also persisted into maintenance anesthesia, indicating myocardial ischemia in association with the low arterial pressures. (From Prys-Roberts, C., Green, L. T., Meloche, R., and Foex, P.: Studies of anesthesia in relation to hypertension. II. Haemodynamic consequences of induction and endotracheal intubation. Br. J. Anaesth., 43:531, 1973.)

infusion of nitroprusside, nitroglycerin, or trimethaphan is an alternative. Sublingual administration of nitroglycerin is also effective. Adrenergic beta-blockade can also be used. A suitable short-acting beta-blocker is not yet available, and if propranolol is used, the duration of its action should be taken into account once the stress of the laryngoscopy and tracheal intubation is passed (Prys-Roberts et al., 1973; Siedlecki, 1975).

Patients who especially require these precautions are those with hypertension, especially if untreated or if medication has been withdrawn, and patients with coronary artery disease (Prys-Roberts, Meloche, and Foëx, 1971).

Oxygenation

Increased intrapulmonary shunting and arterial hypoxemia have been observed during anesthesia and operation. These increases occur especially in those with cardiorespiratory disease and during upper abdominal surgical procedures. Arterial oxygen tension measurements during nitrous oxide-oxygen anesthesia in patients with cardiac or pulmonary disease who were undergoing upper abdominal, lower abdominal, and peripheral surgery, respectively revealed that suboptimal oxygenation occurred frequently (Slater et al., 1965) (Figs. 2 and 3). In fact, in one fourth of patients having upper abdominal surgical

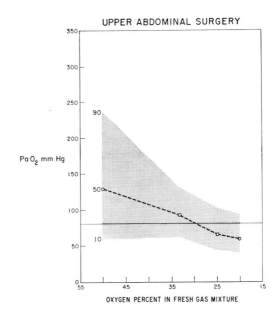

Figure 2. Relationship of inspired oxygen concentration in nitrous oxide and the arterial oxygen tension (PaO_2) during upper abdominal surgery. The figures 10, 50, and 90 mark the 10th, 50th (median), and 90th percentiles of the PaO_2 measurements. In a quarter of the patients having upper abdominal surgery even 50 per cent oxygen did not provide a PaO_2 of over 80 mm. Hg. (From Slater, E. M., Nilsson, S. E., Leake, D. L., Parry, W. L., Laver, M. B., Hedley-Whyte, J., and Bendixen, H. H.: Arterial oxygen tension measurements during nitrous oxide-oxygen anesthesia. Anesthesiology, *26*: 642, 1965.)

procedures, even 50 per cent oxygen did not provide an arterial oxygen tension of more than 80 mm. Hg (Fig. 2). Intrapulmonary shunting is increased by intra-abdominal packing and retraction. In the absence of cardiorespiratory disease, no increase in hypoxemia is caused by prolonged anesthesia with tidal volume of over 10 ml. per kg. body weight.

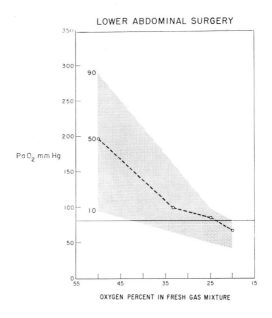

Figure 3. Relationship of inspired oxygen concentration in nitrous oxide and the arterial oxygen tension (PaO_2) during lower abdominal surgery. The oxygen tensions are higher than during upper abdominal surgery but lower than during peripheral surgery. (From Slater, E. M., Nilsson, S. E., Leake, D. L., Parry, W. L., Laver, M. B., Hedley-Whyte, J., and Bendixen, H. H.: Arterial oxygen tension measurements during nitrous oxide-oxygen anesthesia. Anesthesiology, *26*:642, 1965.)

BLOOD GAS ABNORMALITIES AND ORGAN DYSFUNCTION

Brain

The brain is the organ least able to tolerate inadequate oxygenation, and varying degrees of neurologic dysfunction will ensue after a hypoxic insult. The fact that a patient awakens from anesthesia after a hypoxic episode can be falsely reassuring, since coma and death can occur after a "lucid interval." The regions that are especially vulnerable to ischemic damage are layers 3, 5, and 6 of the cerebral cortex, the hippocampus, the central and basolateral portions of the amygdaloid nucleus, the Purkinje and basket cells of the cerebellum, and certain sensory nuclei in the brain stem. The spinal cord is most resistant; involvement of the thalamus, striatum, pallidum, and subthalamic nucleus is variable. The reasons for the pattern of selective vulnerability are unclear at present (Brierley, Meldrum, and Brown, 1973). Cerebrovascular resistance decreases with reduction of arterial oxygen tension and results in an increase in cerebral blood flow, which tends to minimize the cerebral hypoxia. If the decrease in arterial oxygen tension is accompanied by hyperventilation and a reduction in arterial carbon dioxide tension, cerebrovascular resistance rises, blood flow falls, and hypoxia is enhanced.

Heart

The heart, although relatively sensitive to hypoxia as compared with most structures of the body, is less sensitive than the nervous system. Consequently, in the absence of severe coronary artery disease, serious manifestations of cardiac impairment do not commonly occur when there is generalized hypoxia. Neurologic manifestations dominate. Diminished oxygen tension in any tissue except the lungs results in local vasodilation, and, in generalized hypoxia, diffuse vasodilation often results in an elevation of cardiac output. In patients with pre-existing heart disease, particularly coronary artery disease, the combination of hypoxia and the requirements of the peripheral tissues for an increase of cardiac output may precipitate congestive heart failure.

Kidney

With arterial oxygen saturation of less than 70 per cent, the glomerular filtration rate and clearance of para-aminohippuric acid is decreased and renovascular resistance is increased. The systemic administration of phenoxybenzamine for denervation of the kidneys attenuates these changes, suggesting that they are caused by neuro-sympathetically induced renal vasoconstriction. Some studies, however, suggest that renal perfusion is unaltered or even increased during hypoxia. The contradictory findings are often a result of a failure to monitor and control the changes in arterial carbon dioxide tension and pH that are known to occur with hypoxia during spontaneous ventilation (Hall and Steinman, 1976). General anesthesia also profoundly affects the reflex circulatory regulation to stress that may be imposed on the kidney (Vatner and Braunwald, 1975).

Liver

Profound hypoxemia may also affect hepatic function. The inhalation of 10 per cent oxygen in man impairs sulfobromophthalein (BSP) clearance. Acute, severe hypoxia in normothermic, unanesthetized, newborn guinea pigs and adult mice impairs hepatic transport of radioactively labeled sulfobromophthalein and rose bengal at the excretory step between liver cells and canalicular bile, a defect that is abolished by the inhalation of 5 per cent carbon dioxide (Shorey, Schenker, and Combes, 1969). Portal venous flow is reduced by 30 to 60 per cent during intermittent positive pressure ventilation. When dogs are ventilated with tidal volumes of 40 ml. per kg. body weight, there is an increase in hepatic venous pressure, portal venous pressure, and mesenteric vascular resistance, as well as a decrease in blood flow in the portal vein. These changes are the same during hypocapnia and normocapnia (Fig. 4) (Hedley-Whyte et al., 1976); Johnson, 1975).

Figure 4. Effect of hyperventilation on hepatic and mesenteric hemodynamics in two groups of seven dogs each. Normocapnia was maintained in one group by using a mixture of compressed air and carbon dioxide. During hyperventilation [tidal volume (V_T) = 40 ml./kg.] there is an increase in hepatic venous pressure (P_{HV}), portal venous pressure (P_{PV}), and mesenteric vascular resistance (R_{MES}) and a decrease in portal venous blood flow (F_{PV}) during normocapnia and respiratory alkalosis. (From Johnson, E. E.: Splanchnic hemodynamic response to passive hyperventilation. J. Appl. Physiol., 38:156, 1975.)

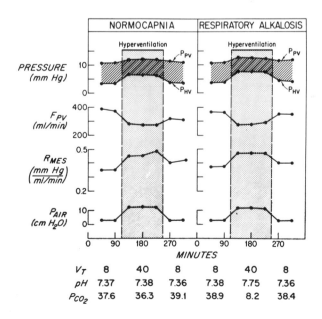

SAFETY OF INTRA-ARTERIAL MONITORING

Percutaneous cannulation of the radial artery has fewer vascular complications than does catheterization of the brachial and femoral arteries, even in patients with arteriosclerosis of the arteries of the arm. Major ischemic complication is avoided if ulnar artery patency is demonstrated by the modified Allen's test, which should be performed as follows. While the patient makes a tight fist, both radial and ulnar arteries are occluded. The patient then opens the hand and pressure over the ulnar artery is released. Ulnar artery patency is indicated by the immediate appearance of an erythematous blush over the entire palmar surface of the hand and fingers. Ulnar artery filling is judged to be slow when 7 to 15 seconds pass before the blush is apparent. Radial artery cannulation has been done safely in patients with slow ulnar artery filling, but when the hand remains blanched for longer than 15 seconds, the radial artery of that hand should not be catheterized.

A study of 105 percutaneous radial artery cannulations in 100 patients utilizing physical examination and Doppler flow measurements attests to the safety of this technique. No major ischemic complication was observed in any patient despite the fact that 40 of the 105 cannulations (38 per cent) resulted in radial artery thrombosis. The incidence of thrombosis increases with the duration of cannulation to 40 hours. Cannulae in place for 2 hours did not cause thrombosis, and the incidence of thrombosis did not increase beyond 38 per cent when cannulation lasted beyond 40 hours. The onset of thrombosis was often delayed for some days following decannulation. Of the 40 patients who developed radial artery occlusion, four had some distal vascular insufficiency in the form of a pale, cold, thenar eminence. Two other patients each had cold, purple, tender tips of their index fingers, indicating peripheral embolization. These findings cleared within seven days. No difference in incidence of thrombosis could be related to the patient's ages, catheter size, degree of trauma during cannulation, volume of flush solution infused, or the type of flush mechanism employed (Bedford and Wollman, 1973).

In a study of 32 patients who had their radial arteries percutaneously catheterized 35 times, 20-gauge nontapered catheters were used 11 times, 18-gauge nontapered catheters were used 14 times, and 18-gauge tapered catheters were used 10 times. Arteriography was performed with 1 to 3 ml. of a radiopaque solution that went through the catheters shortly after insertion and daily thereafter. Arterial occlusion did not occur with the 20-gauge nontapered catheters. Arterial occlusion occurred 4 out of 14 times with the 18-gauge nontapered catheters and 9 out of 10 times with the 18-gauge tapered catheters. Thrombus formation occurred regardless of the catheter employed. The extent of thrombus formation was greatest with the 18-gauge tapered catheters and least with the 20-gauge nontapered catheters (Downs et al., 1973).

The dorsalis pedis or superficial temporal arteries may be catheterized percutaneously when the radial artery cannot be catheterized due to inadequate ulnar artery flow, as evidenced by the hand remaining blanched for longer than 15 seconds after pressure on the ulnar artery is released. When continuing monitoring is considered mandatory for optimal care, flow in a thrombosed radial artery can be restored by thrombectomy using a #3 French embolectomy catheter. The same radial artery has been used on five occasions in four patients for continued monitoring without any ischemic complications (Fig. 5) (Feeley, 1977).

When a patient cannot cooperate to perform the modified Allen's test or is already anesthetized, ulnar artery flow can be assessed by either of the following methods. The arm is elevated and the fist passively clenched; pressure is then applied to both radial and ulnar arteries. The latter is then released and the time noted that it takes for the entire palmar surface of the hand to flush. Ulnar artery flow may also be assessed by applying a finger-pulse transducer to the thumb, obliterating the finger pulse by compression of both radial and ulnar arteries, and then releasing the ulnar artery (the Brodsky test). If the finger pulse is not promptly restored, cannulation of the radial artery of that hand is contraindicated (Fig. 6) (Brodsky, 1975).

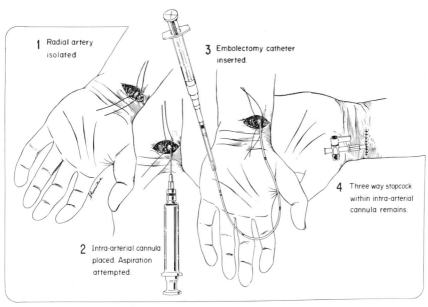

1 Radial artery isolated

2 Intra-arterial cannula placed. Aspiration attempted.

3 Embolectomy catheter inserted.

4 Three way stopcock within intra-arterial cannula remains.

Figure 5. Technique of catheter thrombectomy of the radial artery. The radial artery is isolated at the wrist by cutdown, and ligatures are placed around it proximal and distal to the proposed puncture site (1). An 18-gauge Angiocath is inserted into the artery, the catheter needle is removed and an attempt is made to aspirate blood (2). If no blood can be aspirated the Angiocath is removed and a #3 French embolectomy catheter is inserted through the arteriotomy made by the Angiocath (3). The catheter is advanced proximally about 25 cm., the balloon inflated, and the catheter slowly withdrawn to remove thrombotic material. When flow is re-established the 18-gauge Angiocath is reintroduced into the vessel and a three-way stopcock is attached. The distal ligature is removed. The proximal ligature may be removed or tied if necessary to control bleeding from the arteriotomy site. The skin is then closed (4). (From Feeley, T. W.: Re-establishment of radial-artery patency for arterial monitoring. Anesthesiology, *46*:73, 1977.)

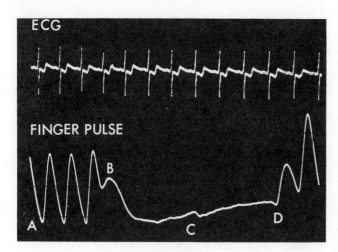

Figure 6. Assessment of ulnar artery flow by placement of a finger-pulse transducer on the thumb. Compression of both radial and ulnar arteries abolishes the finger pulse, A, as shown in the lower tracing at point B. Release of the ulnar artery, C, causes no change in the abolished finger pulse, indicating inadequate ulnar artery flow. Release of the radial artery, D, restores the finger pulse. Radial artery cannulation is contraindicated in this patient. (From Brodsky, J. B.: A simple method to determine patency of the ulnar artery intraoperatively prior to radial-artery cannulation. Anesthesiology, 42:626, 1975.)

In critically ill patients with impaired tissue perfusion and a hypercoagulable state, peripheral arterial cannulation may cause severe ischemia and necrosis of an extremity despite testing for adequate collateral circulation and the use of smaller, nontapered catheters.

SUMMARY

We know that arterial oxygenation is dangerously unpredictable, especially during upper abdominal surgical procedures, and that blood gas abnormalities cause dysfunction of the central nervous system, heart, kidneys, and liver. Intra-arterial monitoring, when employed with certain safeguards, contributes to the optimal care of patients. If we require major surgery, we insist on it.

REFERENCES

Bedford, R. F., and Wollman, H.: Complications of percutaneous radial-artery cannulation: an objective prospective study in man. Anesthesiology, 38:228, 1973.

Brierley, J. B., Meldrum, B. S., and Brown, A. W.: The threshold and neuropathology of cerebral "anoxic-ischemic" cell change. Arch. Neurol., 29:367, 1973.

Brodsky, J. B.: A simple method to determine patency of the ulnar artery intraoperatively prior to radial-artery cannulation. Anesthesiology, 42:626, 1975.

Downs, J. B., Rackstein, A. D., Klein, E. F., Jr., and Hawkins, L. F., Jr.: Hazards of radial-artery catheterization. Anesthesiology, 38:283, 1973.

Feeley, T. W.: Re-establishment of radial-artery patency for arterial monitoring. Anesthesiology, 46:73, 1977.

Hall, S. V., and Steinman, T. I.: Alterations in renal function during acute respiratory failure. Int. Anesthesiol. Clin., 14(1):179, 1976.

Hedley-Whyte, J., Burgess, G. E., III, Feeley, T. W., and Miller, M. G.: Applied Physiology of Respiratory Care. Boston, Little, Brown and Company 1976.

Johnson, E. E.: Splanchnic hemodynamic response to passive hyperventilation. J. Appl. Physiol., *38*:156, 1975.

Prys-Roberts, C., Foëx, P., Biro, G. P., and Roberts, J. G.: Studies of anaesthesia in relation to hypertension. V. Adrenergic beta-receptor blockade. Br. J. Anaesth., *45*:671, 1973.

Prys-Roberts, C., Green, L. T., Meloche, R., and Foëx, P.: Studies of anaesthesia in relation to hypertension. II. Haemodynamic consequences of induction and endotracheal intubation. Br. J. Anaesth., *43*:531, 1973.

Prys-Roberts, C., Meloche, R., and Foëx, P.: Studies of anesthesia in relation to hypertension. I. Cardiovascular responses of treated and untreated patients. Br. J. Anaesth., *43*:122, 1971.

Shorey, J., Schenker, S., and Combes, B.: Effect of acute hypoxia on hepatic excretory function. Am. J. Physiol., *216*:1441, 1969.

Siedlecki, J.: Disturbances in the function of cardiovascular system in patients following endotracheal intubation and attempts at their prevention by pharmacological blockade of sympathetic system. Anaesth. Resusc. Intensive Ther., *3*:107, 1975.

Slater, E. M., Nilsson, S. E., Leake, D. L., Parry, W. L., Laver, M. B., Hedley-Whyte, J., and Bendixen, H. H.: Arterial oxygen tension measurements during nitrous oxide-oxygen anesthesia. Anesthesiology, *26*:642, 1965.

15. Vatner, S. F., and Braunwald, E.: Cardiovascular control mechanisms in the conscious state. N. Engl. J. Med., *293*:970, 1975.

by JAY JACOBY

Jefferson Medical College

┌───┐
└───┘

INTRA-ARTERIAL MONITORING IS NOT A ROUTINE PROCEDURE

In the practice of medicine generally, and in the practice of anesthesiology in particular, the physician must adhere to the principle "primum non nocere."

The contemporary physician and his patient are beneficiaries of the most dramatic expansion of medical capability in the long history of our art. But the rapid proliferation of medical knowledge has not been entirely benign. Our reverses have been minor when contrasted to our advances, but negative effects cannot be ignored or derogated. This discussion involves one aspect of the problem — the emergence of what I have called "diseases of medical progress." (Mosner, 1969)

At the 1977 meeting of the American Society of Anesthesiologists, the question of invasive monitoring was discussed. H. Barrie Fairley stated that "invasive monitoring comes at a cost." He described professional "mesmerism" by invasive monitoring devices. "It is really possible to believe that the single variable that you are monitoring is *the* variable and that the patient's life depends on it." (Fairley, 1977)

Among the causes of iatrogenic complications, invasive procedures are important; arterial cannulation is invasive. No one will deny that certain benefits may accrue to a patient because of arterial monitoring, but the complications that may result receive insufficient attention. Before considering these complications, let us review why it is used. The two principal reasons are to measure blood pressure and to have easy access for the withdrawal of arterial blood samples for gas analysis.

The measurement of blood pressure utilizing an arterial catheter is usually accurate and continuous, and a written record is easily made. This item readily fits in the category of professional mesmerism.

Serial sampling of arterial blood, if really necessary for patient care, is a good reason to insert an arterial catheter that will remain for several days and is preferable to doing multiple individual punctures that might cause more trauma than the arterial catheter.

266

The drawbacks and complications of any procedure must be considered as they appear not in the hands of superexperts but in those of the average person who does the procedure. The complications of arterial cannulation may be denied or minimized by a superexpert, but the average individual does experience them. Of course, after a while, the average individual might become a superexpert, but a trail of complications marks his progress. The following is an incomplete list of complications from arterial cannulation that are common knowledge or that are verified by publications:

1. *Technical difficulty and loss of time.* There may be difficulty in the insertion and connection of an arterial catheter. Repeated attempts may be needed to penetrate the artery and insert the catheter properly. The delay in starting an urgent operation may reduce the patient's chance to survive. The pain involved in multiple efforts at cannulation, in spite of the use of local anesthesia, may cause the patient anguish. The time lost may try the patience of everyone waiting to proceed with the operation. (Bedford and Wollman, 1973)

2. *Ligation of the artery.* If one is unable to perform arterial cannulation by the percutaneous technique, then cannulation must be done by cutdown. Ordinarily in this procedure, the distal end of the artery is ligated. This may result in difficulties for the patient, in spite of a satisfactory Allen's test. Instead of ligation, a plastic operation may be done on the artery in an effort to maintain patency. A better procedure is to thrust the catheter needle into the artery under direct vision, without incision or ligation. (Samaan, 1971)

3. *Hematoma.* Each time an artery is pierced by a needle, hematoma formation is a possibility. Pressure should be maintained over the puncture wound for a minimum of five minutes. If one attempts to insert a catheter and thrusts the catheter through both walls of the artery, impaling it, and then withdraws the catheter, there is leakage from two puncture wounds rather than one. Frequently, pressure is not applied for five minutes because of anxiety to complete the procedure. The catheter is withdrawn and additional thrusts are made in an effort to place it properly. While additional thrusts are being made and afterward, blood continues to leak from the arterial puncture wounds. The hematoma is not only unsightly and painful postoperatively but it may also impair the circulation in the extremity because of tissue compression, requiring incision for drainage, release of the pressure, and restoration of adequate circulation. If this is not done, the patient might develop Volkman's contracture. Carpal tunnel syndrome also occurs as a postcannulation complication. (Bedford and Wollman, 1973; Fleming and Bowen, 1974; Linscheid, Peterson and Juergens, 1967; Matsen and Clawson, 1972)

4. *Pathologic changes.* Injury of an artery may result in a mycotic aneurysm, dissecting aneurysm, pseudoaneurysm, arteriovenous fistula, or atheromatous emboli. (Gabow et al., 1976; Kumar, Trivedi, and Smith, 1975; Ritland and Butterfield, 1973; Samaan, 1971)

5. *Malfunction and false information.* After the catheter is properly placed, it may not function well because of kinking, thrombus forma-

tion, or defect in the attached equipment. If the catheter is being used for sampling, it simply fails to function; if it is being used for blood pressure readings, the observer may be misled, since the patient's actual blood pressure may be different from that indicated by the instrument. The clue to the latter is damping of oscillations, but this is not always recognized. By failing to function properly, the arterial monitor may give false information, leading to improper treatment, a possibility that leads us to apply a standard blood pressure cuff as a back-up measuring device.

6. *Distraction.* If the anesthesiologist recognizes a malfunction of the measuring equipment, an attempt is made to correct it, causing distraction from care of the patient. The anesthesiologist becomes a doctor for the machine, and he may miss some critical need of the patient.

7. *Catheter embolism.* An attempt may be made to clear the catheter and re-establish the lumen by passing the starter needle through it again. If the catheter is kinked or bent, the needle can pierce its wall, producing a weak area at which the catheter may break off in the patient's artery, forming an embolus. The catheter also may break because of an inherent defect or if subjected to mechanical strains. (Samaan, 1971) (Fig. 1)

8. *Thromboembolism.* The blood vessel within which the catheter is located may develop a thrombus that occludes the lumen. When a thrombus forms around the outer walls of the catheter, this thrombus is wiped off into the arterial stream as the catheter is withdrawn, and

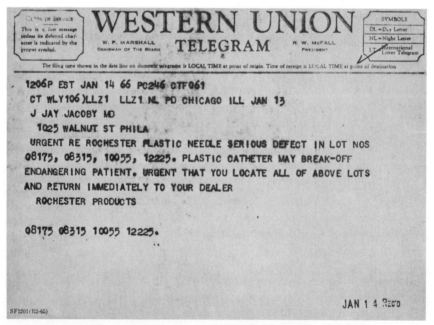

Figure 1. Similar telegrams were sent to all purchasers. How many cases were reported before this notice was sent? How many broken catheters were not reported?

it becomes an embolus. Vascular spasm may also be present, facilitating retention of a thrombus that may extend proximally or distally. The shape, diameter, and material of which the catheter is made and the diameter of the vessel are important influences on the incidence of this complication. (Bedford, 1975; Bedford and Wollman, 1973; Bell, 1963; Downs et al., 1973; Formanek, French and Amplatz, 1970; Matthews and Gibbon, 1971)

9. *Necrosis and gangrene.* Before arterial cannulation, Allen's test should be carried out, supplemented by use of a Doppler instrument, if possible. Although this is a good means for preventing trouble, it is not infallible and it may not be done properly, or even worse, not done at all. In any event, impaired blood flow to an extremity, uncompensated by another artery, may be followed by changes in sensation, motor power, and viability of the tissue; gangrene may occur. If recognized early, serious complications might be avoided by instituting a variety of treatments, including arteriotomy and thrombectomy. (Johnson, 1974; Samaan, 1971)

10. *Infection.* Cellulitis has occurred at the site of catheter insertion and in the soft tissues. The infection may involve the blood vessel itself, and generalized sepsis may develop. Any indwelling catheter must be viewed with suspicion in patients who develop signs of septicemia. (Samaan, 1971)

11. *Osler's nodes.* Defined by Dorland's Medical Dictionary as "small, raised, swollen tender areas, about the size of a pea, characteristically bluish but sometimes pink or red, and sometimes having a blanched center, occurring most commonly in the pads of the fingers or toes, in the thenar or hypothenar eminences, or the soles of the feet; they are practically pathognomonic of subacute bacterial endocarditis." These nodes have been described as complications of arterial cannulation. (Michaelson and Walsh, 1970)

12. *Splinter hemorrhages.* Defined by Dorland's Medical Dictionary as "linear hemorrhages beneath the nail; when located near the base of the nail they are characteristic of subacute bacterial endocarditis." These hemorrhages have also been noted after use of arterial catheters. (Matthews and Gibbon, 1971)

13. *Improper injections.* After several vascular catheters have been inserted and the patient has been covered by surgical drapes, it is easy to confuse which tube leads to which catheter. Given several potential injection sites in the plastic tubes, there is a possibility of injecting substances into the artery. Some drugs are unsuitable for intra-arterial injection. The consequences of arterial injury by chemicals have been described repeatedly. (Hawkins, Lischer, and Sweeney, 1973; Maxwell, Olcott, and Blaisdell, 1972; Samaan, 1971)

14. *Air embolism.* The flushing fluids used to clear arterial catheters periodically must be free of air, and the container should be a collapsible plastic bag or air embolism may occur. (Samaan, 1971)

15. *Cerebral embolization.* This complication has resulted from rapid irrigation of arterial catheters with large volumes of fluid, sweeping thrombi, or plaques into the central circulation. (Lowenstein, Little, and Lo, 1971)

16. *Exsanguination and death.* If the monitoring equipment becomes disconnected from the arterial catheter, serious bleeding may occur. Unbelievable though it may seem, such a catastrophe has happened. One might believe this could happen only in an institution with poor nursing care, a substandard institution, but that is not the case. I have been asked to consult in a lawsuit involving a hospital of national repute, where a patient in the intensive care unit, presumably receiving the best care possible, bled to death in bed because the disconnection of an arterial catheter went unrecognized. How do you explain this to a jury and a judge, to the family, or to your own conscience? I am willing to grant that the frequency of such complications must be very small, but considering the fact that the procedure is judgmental to begin with, and perhaps more for the benefit of the doctors than the patient, there is a real problem of justification.

The excellent study by Mortensen (1967) reported major complications in 4.4 per cent and minor complications in 14.3 per cent of cases of percutaneous catheterization; 3193 cases of arterial entry (needle, catheter, and cutdown) were studied. Complications included 4 deaths, 14 arterial obstructions requiring surgery, 12 major hemorrhages, 12 false aneurysms, 10 massive ecchymoses requiring surgical treatment, and 2 amputations. Thirty-three operations were required for the 66 major complications.

We are all aware that every complication is not reported in the literature. It is safe to assume that physicians do not publicize the complications they have had unless they are professionally secure, retired, or out of reach of a malpractice lawyer. It is also safe to assume that for every complication reported, many more have occurred, perhaps some types that have never been reported. I refrain from providing a multitude of gruesome photographs.

Recognizing that these complications occur, does the benefit of arterial cannulation warrant the risk?

Why should we want an accurate, continuous, and written record of the patient's blood pressure? I have questioned many anesthesiologists and conclude that their attitudes toward arterial catheter blood pressure monitoring resemble those of a child with a security blanket: "I wouldn't want to be without it." Or, "I would be afraid to be without it." These responses did not refer to every routine major operation but only to special cases.

I believe that arterial cannulation for measuring blood pressure should be carried out only for certain cases in which the benefits outweigh the risks: (1) open heart surgery, in which standard measurement is impossible; (2) induced hypothermia, in which vascular constriction may make noninvasive measurement difficult; and (3) induced hypotension, in which accurate control of the degree of hypotension is critical for the patient's welfare. If the pressure is unduly reduced, there may be impairment of blood flow to major organs, with catastrophic results. A blood pressure of 70 torr systolic is safer than a blood pressure of 60 torr, and it is worthwhile to take some risk to be able to determine this precisely. Accuracy and continuity are important, and a written record helps to ensure absence of an interval of serious hypotension.

In other situations in which arterial cannulation for blood pressure monitoring seems to be most popular, I believe it is unnecessary. In major vascular operations, I see no significant benefit from having an accurate, continuous, and written record of the blood pressure. I believe that the anesthesiologist could manage a case of this kind with crude measurement of blood pressure, and, if necessary, without any measurement of blood pressure at all. Proper management of patients having operations in which there may be massive blood loss requires close attention to the quantity of blood lost; treat the patient with appropriate fluids before hypotension develops. In a properly managed operation and anesthesia, hypotension should not develop.

Rather than rely on intra-arterial monitoring to trigger a late alarm, the anesthesiologist should be alert to early subtle clues: Blood loss that requires energetic therapy is often manifested to the anesthesiologist by his hearing the surgeon exclaim "Oops" followed by a string of four-letter words, the gurgling of suction, and the splatter of soaked sponges hitting the floor. At this point, the anesthesiologist should be pumping blood through two or three intravenous lines. There is no need to await information regarding the quantity of blood loss by weighing sponges, measuring suction bottles, or determining the hemoglobin level of wash water; these take time. Instead, a quick estimate of blood loss should be made from the appearance of the operative site, the sponges, and the receptacles. To await arterial blood pressure changes is to delay effective therapy and allow the patient to develop hemorrhagic shock. Then the measurement reveals how bad things are. The prudent anesthesiologist does not permit them to become bad in the first place.

In considering aortic aneurysm surgery, other factors should be mentioned: the possibility of hypertension when the clamp is placed on the aorta above the lesion. No one should claim inability to determine a rise in blood pressure under these circumstances. We also know that hypotension at the time the clamp is removed from the aorta must be anticipated, as blood is allowed to surge through the graft into the lower extremities. The prudent anesthesiologist takes steps to prevent serious hypotension a few moments before the clamp is removed. Again, it is unnecessary and undesirable to refer to the written record of hypotension when the aim should be to prevent the blood pressure fall.

Hypotension may occur in nonvascular cases because of the patient's disease or problems with the operation or the anesthetic. In such instances, is it necessary to have an accurate, continuous written record? I believe not. One of the characteristics of low blood pressure is difficulty of measurement. One may have to use palpation of the pulse to help determine the blood pressure, and indeed, the pulse may become weak or thready or disappear. This is not an indication for more accurate measurement but for more prompt and vigorous therapy. It is not necessary for me to know whether the patient's mean blood pressure is 70, 50, or 30 torr. It is adequate for me to know that the blood pressure is below normal and has become difficult or impossible to obtain. This tells me that I must do something quickly and effectively. When the patient's condition improves, the blood pressure will again become easy to measure. Later, it may be of prognostic value to know the severity and duration of the hypotension.

As mentioned before, let us not forget that misinformation may also come from the arterial catheter. When there is a kink, a clot, or a thrombus, the instruments may indicate a blood pressure unrelated to the patient's actual pressure. Observing the patient is far more important than observing any machine or monitors connected to him. This brings to mind the cartoon in which the anesthetist is intently observing a multitude of instruments after the patient has been disconnected and is being wheeled from the room.

We must address the question of whether, in the operating room, we are acting as physicians for the patient's benefit or as research scientists whose aim is to get accurate information. We seem driven to obtain numbers with an accuracy of two decimal places when all we may need is information of a 10 percentile change.

Are multiple blood gas determinations required for every major operation? Indeed, are any blood gas determinations required for most major operations? At Jefferson Hospital, most major operations are done without blood gas determinations. I do not believe that our patients get substandard care and am willing to compare morbidity and mortality with any institution.

I believe that serial blood gas determinations should be reserved for patients with severe lung disease or those threatened with respiratory failure because of critical illness or operation. For these patients, an arterial catheter should be inserted. For patients receiving ventilatory care who need only occasional blood gas determination, the use of a catheter is unwarranted. In the near future, technologic advances should permit noninvasive blood gas determinations.

My indications for arterial cannulation therefore are to monitor blood pressure for open heart operations and when induced hypotension or hypothermia is to be used and to facilitate the drawing of serial arterial blood samples when indicated. An examination of the surgical schedule for one month at Jefferson Hospital, a medical school general hospital where tertiary care is provided, reveals that only 53 operations were in the categories in which arterial cannulation was needed as defined above. In the remaining 1000 cases, arterial cannulation was not indicated, and to the best of my knowledge no patient suffered morbidity or mortality because arterial cannulation was not performed.

Having presented a case against routine cannulation, I wish to mention one use for arterial cannulation that most people have forgotten or never heard about, namely arterial blood transfusion. At one time, arterial transfusion was highly recommended for resuscitation. The rationale is that blood pumped into an artery distends the arterial tree and raises the arterial pressure almost instantly, flowing in a retrograde direction. If the blood is oxygenated before administration, the perfusion of vital organs is immediately enhanced and function improved, especially that of the heart. In contrast, blood pumped into the venous system may be pooled in distended veins and capillaries without greatly improving the patient's condition. In an exsanguinated subject, equal volumes of blood are dramatically more effective when administered into an artery. (Negovskii, 1962)

SUMMARY AND CONCLUSIONS

The reasons why arterial catheters are ordinarily inserted and the technical problems and complications of arterial cannulation have been reviewed. I have stated my estimate of the proper indications for arterial cannulation, with satisfactory risk:benefit ratio. For other situations, less hazardous alternatives are available that provide the clinician with the information needed in a timely fashion and with adequate accuracy. The alternative to arterial cannulation for monitoring blood pressure is a standard blood pressure cuff and stethoscope, a cuff and a Doppler, a cuff and palpation, or a noninvasive automatic device. Other personnel may also be called on to perform the chore of measuring the blood pressure in critical situations. If the blood pressure becomes difficult to measure, it is too low. It really does not matter what the pressure is in numbers; treat the patient and get the blood pressure back up to where it becomes easy to measure.

The alternative to arterial cannulation for the purpose of drawing blood samples is to avoid drawing such samples unless there is a compelling reason to do so, other than mere curiosity. Or use individual needle punctures for this purpose, since needle punctures appear less hazardous than cannulation. In some cases, there is no suitable alternative.

Arterial cannulation should not be regarded as a procedure so safe that it should be routinely utilized for all major cases. It should be viewed with great respect. It is not in the same category as an intravenous infusion. Arterial cannulation should be undertaken only if there is a specific, real value for which no other procedure offers an adequate substitute.

REFERENCES

Bedford, R. F.: Percutaneous radial-artery cannulation — increased safety using teflon catheters. Anesthesiology, 42:219–222, 1975.

Bedford, R. F., and Wollman, H.: Complications of percutaneous radial-artery cannulation: an objective prospective study in man. Anesthesiology, 38:228–236, 1973.

Bell, J. W.: Treatment of post-catheterization arterial injuries: use of survey plethysmography. Ann. Surg., 155:591–598, 1962.

Downs, J. B., Rackstein, A. D., Klein, E. F., Jr., and Hawkins, I. F., Jr.: Hazards of radial-artery catheterization. Anesthesiology, 38:283–286, 1973.

Fairley, H. B.: Invasive monitoring. Anesthesiology News. Nov./Dec.:1, 1977.

Fleming, W. H., and Bowen, J. C.: Complications of arterial puncture. Milit. Med., *139*:307–308, 1974.

Formanek, G., French, R. S., and Amplatz, K. S.: Arterial thrombus formation during clinical percutaneous catheterization. Circulation, *41*:833–839, 1970.

Gabow, P., deTorrente, A., Holt, S., and Kelly, G. L.: Arteriovenous fistula from drug abuse. J.A.M.A., *235*:2220–2221, 1976.

Hawkins, L. G., Lischer, C. G., and Sweeney, M.: The main line accidental intra-arterial drug injection. Clin. Orthop., *94*:268–274, 1973.

Johnson, R. W.: A complication of radial-artery cannulation. Anesthesiology, *40*:598–600, 1974.

Kumar, S., Trivedi, H. L., and Smith, E. K. M.: Carpal-tunnel syndrome: a complication of arteriovenous fistula in hemodialysis patients. Can. Med. Assoc. J., *113*:1070–1072, 1975.

Linschied, R. L., Peterson, L. F. A., and Juergens, J. L.: Carpal tunnel syndrome associated with vasospasm. J. Bone Joint Surg. [Amer.], *49*:1141–1146, 1967.

Lowenstein, E., Little, J. W., III, and Lo, H. H.: Prevention of cerebral embolization from flushing radial artery cannulas. N. Engl. J. Med., *285*:1414–1416, 1971.

Matsen, F. A., and Clawson, D. K.: Symposium on compartmental syndromes. Clin. Orthop., 113, Nov. 1975.

Matthews, J. I., and Gibbon, R. B.: Embolization complicating radial-artery puncture. Ann. Intern. Med., *75*:87–88, 1971.

Maxwell, T. M., Olcott, C., IV, and Blaisdell, F. W.: Vascular complications of drug abuse. Arch Surg., *105*:875–882, 1972.

Michaelson, E. D., and Walsh, R. E.: Osler's node — complication of prolonged arterial cannulation. N. Engl. J. Med., *283*:472–473, 1970.

Mortensen, J. D.: Clinical sequelae from arterial needle puncture, cannulation, and incision. Circulation, *35*:1118–1123, 1967.

Moser, R. H.: Diseases of Medical Progress — A Study of Iatrogenic Disease. Springfield, Illinois, Charles C Thomas, 1969.

Negovskii, V. A.: Resuscitation and Artificial Hypothermia. New York, Consultants Bureau Enterprises, Inc., 1962.

Ritland, D., and Butterfield, W.: Extremity complications of drug abuse. Am. J. Surg., *126*:639–648, 1973.

Samaan, H. A.: The hazards of radial artery pressure monitoring. J. Cardiovasc. Surg., *12*:342–347, 1971.

INTRA-ARTERIAL
MONITORING

EDITORIAL COMMENT

Intra-arterial monitoring for both pressure and blood gas measurements first appeared for research purposes. It arose from investigators attempting to obtain definitive data on the effects of drugs and diseases in normal and sick human beings; one could not be certain that observations made in laboratory animals were applicable to patients. As data began to accumulate and familiarity with monitoring techniques was gained, the natural question arose, "Why only for research?" "Wouldn't patient care be facilitated, especially in the critically ill?" Originally confined to academic medical centers, intra-arterial monitoring is now commonplace in hospitals, perhaps available in a majority of them. Some centers do use intra-arterial catheters for routine procedures, in fact many of our current surgical and anesthesiologic trainees have not seen certain procedures done without intra-arterial monitoring.

Miller and Hedley-Whyte point out the consequences of hypotension, hypertension, and hypoxia on various organ systems, outline certain safeguards concerning intra-arterial cannulation, and present statistics from their own experience. They do not ignore the existence of complications but conclude by saying that they would want this technique used were they to have a major surgical procedure.

Jacoby emphasizes the complications of intra-arterial catheters and outlines the severity of complications that have been reported. He also impresses the thought that changes in blood pressure or blood gases are not usually the first signs of impending trouble and implies that physicians often get a false sense of security by the presence of intra-arterial monitors, sometimes ignoring the patient as a whole. He pleads for matching risk against value and advises the technique only when the value of the information obtained outweighs the risk.

There is little question that as technology has improved, sophisticated procedures and equipment are used more and more for routine surgical and anesthetic care under the guise that it *may* be of help or that substandard medical care is implied if not used. Often young physicians ignore the complications of these techniques because they have not had enough personal experience to appreciate them. Some hospitals simply are not geared to sophisticated techniques and do not

275

have the personnel to provide continual supervision. And then, the courts have been involved in ruling malpractice if certain monitors are not utilized — often without justification.

Given the proper setting, the experienced personnel, and the gain exceeding the risk, intra-arterial monitoring is valuable. In the absence of experience, understanding of the risks, or justifiable need, the technique should be excluded. Obviously, the real goal is noninvasive monitoring that could eliminate most intra-arterial catheters.

Part 14

THE DIRECTION OF PATIENT CARE IN INTENSIVE CARE UNITS

THE PROPOSITION:

> Specially trained physicians should direct the care of all patients in an intensive care unit.

ALTERNATIVE POINTS OF VIEW

> By Peter Safar, Ake Grenvik
> By Lawrence L. Michaelis

EDITORIAL COMMENT

by PETER SAFAR

AKE GRENVIK
University of Pittsburgh School of Medicine

INTENSIVE CARE UNIT PATIENT CARE: A RESPONSIBILITY OF CRITICAL CARE MEDICINE PHYSICIANS*

We consider critical care medicine (CCM) to be the triad of resuscitation, emergency care for life threatening conditions, and intensive care (Safar and Grenvik, 1977; Safar, 1974; Safar et al., 1974; Society of Critical Care Medicine, 1972, 1973). Others have used a more physician-oriented geographic definition, equating CCM only with "intensive care," i.e., the management of patients in intensive care units (ICU) (Kinney, 1966; Petty, 1971, 1976; Safar et al., 1974; Shoemaker, 1975; Weil and Shubin, 1971). The latter definition equates the CCM physician with the intensivist (Safar, 1965) and is predicated on the assumption that all patients admitted to ICUs should be critically ill or injured, whereas only 2 to 5 per cent of those seen in emergency departments of general hospitals in the United States are in critical condition (Safar, 1974).

The development of modern life-support techniques in the form of respiratory care, arrhythmia control, and treatment of shock led to the application of these techniques to an ever-widening patient population. This trend, together with increasingly extensive surgical proce-

*Dr. Nancy Caroline made valuable suggestions and helped in the writing of these comments and recommendations. More than 100 CCM physician fellows, staff, and alumni of the Pittsburgh program helped shape these views. Supported in part by the department of anesthesiology and critical care medicine and by the Resuscitation Research Center, University of Pittsburgh and the Emergency Health Services Division, Commonwealth of Pennsylvania.

279

dures on critically ill and injured patients, inevitably entailed concentration of special personnel and equipment and collection of the critically ill and injured patients scattered throughout the hospital to locations where they could be watched more closely and treated more effectively by nurses and physicians.

ICUs developed from postanesthetic-postsurgical recovery rooms (for neurologic surgery since the 1920s, for cardiothoracic surgery since the 1940s), respiratory ICUs in Scandinavia (Eckenhoff and Dam, 1956; Ibsen, 1954) and multidisciplinary adult (Safar et al., 1961) and pediatric (Bachman et al., 1967; Kampschulte and Safar, 1973) ICUs with full-time physician staff. Cardiac care units introduced in the 1960s provided a unique life-saving potential of arrhythmia control. What began merely as a geographic convenience took on new dimensions as increasingly sophisticated measures for patient monitoring and long-term resuscitation ("titrated" management) were developed. Concomitantly came the recognition that mere surveillance by nurses was insufficient for this patient population, which requires the skills and insights of physicians specially trained in management of the critically ill (Safar, 1965). It soon became apparent that such skills were not the province of one medical specialty but cut broadly across many disciplines (Society of Critical Care Medicine, 1972, 1973).

Anesthesiologists dominated the initiation of combined medical-surgical ICUs and ICU organization in the 1950s and 1960s (Bachman et al., 1967; Safar and Grenvik, 1977; Safar et al., 1961). Intensive care, however, requires not only the expertise in respiratory support and resuscitation of anesthesiologists but also the systems orientation and broad concept of pathophysiology of internists and pediatricians and the action-oriented approach of surgeons. The physician caring for the critically ill or injured has to master not only physiology but also areas of bioengineering in order to wisely use and understand the tools that enable translation of the language of the body into algorithms and equations. This physician also has to be capable of making rapid decisions and carrying out the appropriate actions based on monitored physiologic variables and collected information.

THE CHALLENGE OF A NEW FIELD

Life-support of patients with multiple organ failure requires a variety of skills, knowledge, and experiences encompassing airway control, oxygenation, artificial ventilation, arrhythmia control, assisted circulation, cardiopulmonary resuscitation, fluid and electrolyte and acid-base balances, treatment of a variety of shock and intoxication states, extracorporeal circulation and oxygenation, hemodialysis, detoxification ("hemoperfusion"), and more recently, brain resuscitation and management of central nervous system failure. Life support, in addition, includes the use of an array of pharmacologic agents with dose administration, frequently by continuous intravenous infusion, adjusted by the pharmacokinetic influence of renal or hepatic failure and various degrees of shock, as well as many minor surgical interventions (cutdown, placement of chest tubes, tracheotomy, insertion of intracranial pressure monitoring devices). Clearly, this calls for a breed of physician not represented by one traditional discipline.

The development of this new breed followed *two avenues*: (a) creation of a new subspecialist, the "critical care physician," born of the union of several traditional disciplines (Safar, 1965; Safar and Grenvik, 1977; Society of Critical Care Medicine, 1973) and (b) development of the multidisciplinary amalgam, a *team* of physicians from various specialties whose combined knowledge and skills encompassed the unique contingencies of critical care (Safar and Grenvik, 1977; Safar et al., 1974; Shoemaker, 1975; Weil and Shubin, 1971). Both approaches have merits and drawbacks and are not mutually exclusive; indeed, the optimal implementation of intensive care requires both.

Physicians specially trained in critical care are needed to orchestrate the total management of the patient critically ill with multiple vital organ failure and to coordinate and reconcile the diverse and sometimes conflicting therapeutic efforts of all involved in the patient's care. A single physician cannot master the whole of all primary disciplines. The skills and expertise of many others are needed in order to accomplish the various therapeutic interventions that may be necessary in any given case. Thus, the intensive care physician must be part of a *team* of specialists.

We and others fully appreciate the need for the patient's primary physician's and the operating surgeon's persistent involvement during the patient's stay in the ICU. They continue to perform the care in which they are specially trained and experienced, provided they can remain with the patient to carry out this duty. There is considerable difference between a "consultant" and an "obligatory team member" in intensive care, however. The consultant is involved only when the primary physician or surgeon realizes that help is needed and is willing to seek it. Both are often not the case. Furthermore, critically ill patients need more than opinions. They need life-support expertise, just as critically ill surgical patients in the operating room need the anesthesiologist's involvement as a team member to render continuous life support. Therefore, physicians who have developed interest and expertise in emergency and long-term resuscitation, i.e., intensive care, should be involved in ICUs at least as "obligatory team members," not merely as consultants.

The lack of reliable patient care evaluation methods makes it difficult to document the life-saving and morbidity-reducing impact that ICU patient care responsibility by specially trained CCM physicians might have. Nevertheless, published mortality data support the value of ICUs and their staffing not only by specially trained nurses but also full-time ICU physicians (Safar, 1974). For example, at the University Health Center of Pittsburgh, mortality of adult ICU patients since the mid-1960s remained the same, while the proportion of desperately ill patients (those requiring prolonged mechanical ventilation) increased; mortality in the pediatric ICU decreased. These improvements in both ICUs occurred when there was a steady increase in full-time ICU staff physicians and fellows (Kampschulte and Safar, 1973; Safar and Grenvik, 1977; Safar, 1974). Mortality data supporting multidisciplinary compared to departmental ICUs are scarce, but in one university hospital, when specialty ICUs were replaced with one multidisciplinary ICU (both staffed by physician specialists), mortality from respiratory insufficiency decreased from 30 to 10 per cent and mortality from myocardial infarction from 30 to 15 per cent.*

PROBLEMS AND OBSTACLES

Titrated Care

ICU experiences over two decades have shown that in both community hospitals and teaching hospitals the concept of treating critically ill patients by "rounding and prescribing" is incapable of making maximal use of modern medicine. The critically ill patient is unstable. Subtle changes in vital organ function must be recognized and dealt with swiftly to avoid dangerous complications. Thus, the care of critically ill patients requires the constant presence at the patient's bedside of a physician skilled in monitoring and appropriate therapeutic interventions, management by "titration." The importance of the difference between management by rounding and prescription and management by titration has been appreciated by physiologists and pharmacologists in the laboratory, by surgeons and anesthesiologists in the operating room, and by internists and pediatricians during cardiac catheterization and treatment of shock. In intensive care, this titration may have to be continued for weeks in some cases.

The primary physician or surgeon who admits the patient to the ICU cannot possibly fulfill this role. There are responsibilities elsewhere — on the wards, in the operating room, in the office — that prevent constant attendance at the patient's side. The visits to the ICU must, of necessity, be sporadic, a few minutes borrowed here and there from other obligations. In addition, appearances on the ICU cannot be expected to coincide with the urgent needs of the patient; emergencies do not wait for convenient moments. Indeed, many reasonably minor and easily manageable problems evolve into catastrophes through delay in intervention, a fact long recognized by our surgical colleagues. Furthermore, even when present, the primary physician may lack the skills required for modern life support.

The situation is compounded by the contingencies of night and weekend call. The patient's primary physician is not, cannot, and should not be present in-house 24 hours a day, 7 days a week. During absences, responsibility for the patients is turned over to colleagues

---

*D. Kassebaum: Personal communication. University of Oregon, 1973.

who cannot know the details of the patient's case as thoroughly as does the primary physician. Under these circumstances, care becomes fragmented and discontinuous. But this need not be the case. The ICU physician team offers a built-in mechanism for continuity of intensive care, since all members of the team are constantly involved in the surveillance of a small number of patients, and each team member is intimately familiar with all ICU patients' current conditions. When one team member goes home for the night, there is another present equally conversant with the patients on the unit and with the overall plans for their management. If responsibility for care were vested in the ICU physician team, the primary admitting physician and the house officer might go home for the evening with assurance that their patient's management would proceed according to the plan worked out between the physician and the ICU team members. Plans of management should not change merely because one shift leaves and another takes over.

The operating surgeon, who often possessively wants to control patients remotely, usually does not take or have the time to "babysit" the patient. Therefore, a reluctance to delegate life support to colleagues of any disciplines who have decided to devote themselves to "babysitting" the critically ill is not understandable, even if the surgeon were well trained and experienced in caring for critically ill patients. Unfortunately, that is often not the case. Many American surgical residency programs are not presently able to include needed mandatory assigned anesthesiology and ICU rotations in their already too thinly manned rotations. Through experience in anesthesiology and intensive care, surgical residents can learn, under controlled conditions, techniques and concepts of life support, ranging from airway control and artificial ventilation to the treatment of shock, dysrhythmias and other vital organ systems malfunctions in a titrated fashion. Likewise, each anesthesiology resident needs some surgical training to learn about surgical concepts, techniques, and complications.

Care Fragmentation by Multiple Consultants

There is a well-known fable about a group of blind men asked to describe an elephant. One blind man, groping about the elephant's hind leg announced that an elephant was like a tree trunk. Another, palpating the trunk, described the pachyderm as resembling a garden hose. A third, running his hands across the beast's flank, declared that the elephant was a wall. Each report lacked perspective of the total picture.

This fable has relevance to the situation of the critically ill patient as evaluated and managed by consultant specialists, each of whom sees the patient in terms of a particular concern. Patient care is fragmented when groups of physicians separately concern themselves with the lungs, kidneys, cardiovascular system, and so on. Someone must look at the whole patient, who is more than the sum of his parts. One physician, or physician team, preferably that most familiar with the patient and most in contact with him, must orchestrate the therapeutic effort, with a view to the interaction of all organ systems involved. Most ICU organizations today fall short of this concept. Orders for respiratory care may be written by one physician, while other physicians write orders for fluids and medications, often without cognizance of the overall implications of these orders. It scarcely benefits the patient for the ICU physician to adjust the ventilator to improve oxygenation when that oxygenation is being impaired by injudicious fluid management under another physician's control. Isolating respiratory care orders from total management is intolerable. For instance, PaO_2 control is impossible without adjustments of blood volume, oncotic pressure, fluid-electrolyte balance and drug therapy. Likewise, brain homeostasis is impossible if the ICU physician adjusts the ventilator, the admitting house officer adjusts the mannitol infusion, and the nurse monitors intracranial pressure. Patients have been hurt by such irrational, uncoordinated management.

The Inverse Hierarchy Principle

It is a peculiarity of our system of physician education in American university hospitals that most of the nonoperative management of patients is conducted primarily by those least prepared for this task. The more skilled and knowledgeable one becomes in medicine, the more removed from direct patient management. Thus, an intern, inexperienced and uncertain, directs the patient's care, guided by advice from a junior resident, who in turn looks to a senior resident, with the progressively dilute sequence of consultation finally ending with an attending, whose years of experience and practice may or may not be ultimately reflected in the patient's treatment.

This inverse hierarchy was developed in the interests of providing the most junior trainee with experiences that might rapidly increase skills and self-assurance — the trial-by-fire philosophy of education. This assumes that some learning will be derived from errors, from mistakes in judgment, discussed, reviewed, and atoned. In medicine, in which one's vocation involves custody of human lives, the margin for error is not large, and in critical care medicine, in which the patient is delicately poised between irrevocable alternatives, the margin for error is very narrow indeed.

It may not, therefore, be appropriate to extend the inverse hierarchy principle of patient control to the care of the critically ill. Instead, this should be similarly organized to the situation in the operating room, where a surgical resident does not perform his or her first operation of a special kind without direct supervision by an experienced surgeon. As presently organized in most university hospitals, intensive care is in the hands of junior house officers of admitting services, who remain in charge of total patient management in the ICUs without training in modern life support techniques. ICU staff physicians and fellows, Board-eligible or certified in Anesthesiology, Medicine, Surgery, or Pediatrics, are often barred from effective participation in patient management in spite of many years of experience in management of the critically ill.

With each admitting house officer running his own show, the introduction of guidelines or protocols for patient care as well as for clinical research is impossible. Even when a consistent plan of management is generally agreed on for a patient, changing personnel on a rotating shift may make major alterations in therapy without full appreciation of the overall plan. Furthermore, the junior house staff who control patient management are frequently unaware of recent advances in this field. Their management often reflects concepts and regimens of textbooks that may be outdated before publication; as another extreme, they quote recent journal articles out of context and brush aside the years of their tutor's experience. This is undesirable in institutions that foster scholarly activities and innovations that call for an ability for immediate change and progress.

Training Specialists in Intensive (Critical) Care

The Joint Commission on Accreditation of Hospitals (JCAH), the Society of Critical Care Medicine (SCCM), the American Society of Anesthesiologists, the American Hospital Association, and other national organizations have recommended that ICUs be directed by physician specialists with competence and interest in critical care (Safar, 1974; Society of Critical Care Medicine, 1972). Ever since the creation of the first CCM (intensivist) fellowship training program in the U.S. in 1963 (Safar, 1965), anesthesiologists, and later an increasing number of internists, pediatricians and occasional surgeons, have sought training in CCM (ICU) educational programs, in addition to their base specialty training. Individuals so trained, usually in a one to two year fellowship program together with the "grandfathers" of the movement (involved in resuscitation and intensive care since the 1950s) formed the Society of Critical Care Medicine (SCCM) founded in 1970 (Safar, 1974; Shoemaker, 1975; Weil and Shubin, 1971). This society established guidelines for ICU organization (Society of Critical Care Medicine, 1972) and physician education in CCM (Society of Critical Care Medicine, 1973), which led in 1978 to a firm commitment by the Primary Boards of Anesthesiology, Medicine, Pediatrics and Surgery, in conjunction with the American Board of Medical Specialties (ABMS), to create sub-specialty status for CCM, parallel to traditional sub-specialties of Medicine, such as cardiology and pulmonary medicine, or sub-specialties of surgery (Grenvik, 1978). These Boards, in cooperation with the SCCM and the ABMS, are in the process of developing certification of special competence in CCM, available to Board Certified anesthesiologists, surgeons, internists, pediatricians, and other specialists, after approved fellowship training in CCM.

There is an estimated need for 4000 ICU Directors and Co-directors with special competence in CCM to staff the nation's general ICUs in approximately 1500 general hospitals with over 250 beds. The membership of SCCM, which has made competence, commitment, and involvement, rather than specific specialty affiliation, criteria for membership, has increased from 28 founders in 1970 to over 1000 in 1979. Approximately 35 per cent are anesthesiologists, 24 per cent internists, 5 per cent pediatricians, 14 per cent surgeons, and 22 per cent others (scientists, nonphysician health professionals, and overseas members). In spite of this startling growth, primarily through the enthusiasm and commitment of scholarly individuals of various disciplines, recruitment has been impaired by the frustrations and limitations imposed by our system. Highly qualified candidates for CCM fellowship training have shied away from this endeavor because of the absence of patient care responsibilities and national recognition of this branch of medicine. Highly trained and qualified physicians do not wish to work in environments where their skills, experience, and commitment are underutilized. To reverse this trend, conditions must be created that are more conducive to fellowship training by extending responsibility for ICU coverage to a greater number of physicians and by giving CCM fellowship trainees authority commensurate with the level of training.

If we are to approach the estimated manpower requirement in the next 10 years, we must produce at least 300 CCM physicians per year, a figure beyond the output of the existing 33 programs with about 102 fellowship positions in 1978. Of these training programs, about 15 are administratively under anesthesiology departments; 10 are under departments of medicine, pediatrics, or surgery; and 8 are multidisciplinary. Twenty-five of the 33 programs seem to conform to SCCM guidelines. Clinical research is available in most programs.

The Need to Train Generalists

Life support education obviously should start with medical students. To provide enough ICU physicians for teaching and community hospitals, we must, in addition to expanding CCM fellowship programs, also train residents and staff physicians of traditional disciplines in resuscitation and life support sufficiently so that they can share 24-hour, 7 days a week coverage. This might be possible through modification of existing residency programs, which must include a truly multidisciplinary faculty.

First-hand guided experience in CCM should be provided for residents in anesthesiology, medicine, surgery, and pediatrics by short-term block rotations through ICUs, where they are trained as team members guided by CCM staff and fellows. They must assume their rightful roles as members of the intensive care team. Experience cannot be adequately gained by caring for patients in ICUs, in addition to those on the wards, through visitations. Remaining constantly at the bedside of a critically ill patient may be one of the most valuable learning experiences of any physician, because the bedside vigil en-

genders a depth of commitment and concern not duplicated elsewhere in medicine in terms of techniques, concepts, and humanizing
experiences that add up to the unique combination of art and science
inherent in medicine.

RECOMMENDATIONS

The Team Approach

Traditional specialty boundaries have organized the delivery of
health care according to the skills and interests of physicians rather
than to the needs of patients; i.e., the organizational pattern is phy-
sician-centered or "iatrocentric." This is undesirable on philosophic
and logical grounds. Our present system is structured so that the patient is fragmented into organs and specialties. In the management of
minor and chronic illnesses, we get by, somehow, with this iatrocentric
system. For the critically ill, however, this system breaks down, since a
whole patient approach is crucial for a successful outcome.

Ideally, the critically ill or injured patient should be managed by a
Renaissance (know-it-all) physician, i.e., an individual who has mastered the principles and skills of all the many disciplines that must be
brought to bear and who, traditionally, can be constantly at the patient's side. Such a Renaissance physician does not exist, however; nor
is it likely, with the increase in depth and complexity of specialties,
that he or she ever will.

Realistically, the Renaissance physician is replaced by a team,
which permits pooling of resources and talents. The patient must resume a rightful place at the center of the team's efforts. The team
must be integrated and as much interdependent as the multisystem
we call a human being. We must recognize our limitations as individual physicians, as well as our potentials.

The coordinator, not dictator, of the team (who should be the
full-time CCM [ICU] physician) should be selected on the basis of
competence, interest, availability, and commitment. The primary physician or surgeon who admits the patient to the ICU should be part of
the team, with special contribution to the patient's overall care. The
remainder of the team should comprise those skilled in life support
and able to maintain the constant bedside vigil necessary in managing
the critically ill, and selected consultants.

Governance of ICUs and Teaching Programs

In agreement with the authors' experience and national guidelines, ICU medical directors should be chosen on the basis of competence, interest, and availability rather than specialty affiliation (Safar,
1974; Shoemaker, 1975; Society of Critical Care Medicine, 1972, 1973;

Weil and Shubin, 1971). They should have completed residency training in a clinical discipline of importance to intensive care and have
acquired advanced skills and knowledge in life support techniques.
The ICU director and his designates should not be administrative fig-
ureheads but should approve all admissions and discharges and be
responsible for monitoring, resuscitation, and life support, at least as
obligatory team members, on all ICU patients, preferably as the coordinating physicians. In either role, they should insure that the care of
patients in need of multiple services is coordinated.

Depending on the work load, the ICU director should have at
least one full or part-time associate director to always have one of them
available during day hours and for night and weekend on-call coverage. Additional ICU block–assigned house staff or staff physicians already trained in intensive care must be provided to share 24-hour
in-house coverage in advanced medical-surgical ICUs (Type I ICUs),
which are recommended for Category I hospitals, and in-house coverage, not necessarily full-time in the ICU, in basic medical-surgical
ICUs (Type II ICUs) recommended for Category II hospitals. ICUs
recommended for Category III hospitals are not required to have full-
time physician coverage; they are continuously covered by nurses, respiratory therapists, and other nonphysicians, with the admitting physician remaining in charge of primary care. They should have a part-
time or full-time ICU director providing administration, consultation,
and teaching. It has, however, proved feasible also for community
hospitals without house-staff to develop Type II ICUs, where staff
anesthesiologists, emergency department physicians, and other interested colleagues, with appropriate training or experience in CCM,
share ICU coverage (Ersoz, in Safar, 1974). Ideally, staff coverage
should be by ICU directors and co-directors, who jointly represent the
major clinical disciplines of anesthesiology, medicine, surgery, and pediatrics, as indicated.

In large medical centers, particularly teaching hospitals, independent ICU (CCM) programs could be created, having their own medical
directors, advisory boards, and budgets separate from those of clinical
departments. These programs could be concerned primarily with the
service, teaching, and clinical research activities associated with multidisciplinary medical, surgical, and pediatric ICUs. The program
should closely cooperate with a cardiac care unit, neonatal ICU, and
hemodialysis unit, which are among those functioning well in most
hospitals under the governance of a traditional department or division. The establishment of separate respiratory ICUs (Petty, 1976) is
ill-advised, since almost all critically ill or injured patients have respiratory insufficiency, and respiratory failure patients frequently develop other vital organ failure.

Responsibility for the coordination of an ICU program encompassing several general, medical or surgical ICUs would rest with a program director who should be identified by a multidisciplinary search
committee, approved by the hospital's medical staff, and appointed by
the board of trustees. The ICU directors of these individual general

ICUs in large medical centers should have input into the selection of the program director, who may wish simultaneously to be director of one of the ICUs. Many of these arrangements have to be dealt with at the local level according to circumstances. Ideally, the program and ICU directors should have joint faculty and staff appointments in anesthesiology, medicine, pediatrics, or surgery, as indicated. In university hospitals, the program director could be academically responsible to the dean of the medical school or the vice chancellor of health professions.

Guidance of the program should come from a multidepartmental advisory board, which should serve as a forum for exchange of views among the disciplines, with the aim of continually upgrading service, teaching, and clinical research components of all ICUs involved.

The responsibilities of the program director and individual ICU directors would include: (1) establishing standards of care and supporting services, such as ICU laboratories; (2) leading, coordinating, and participating in teaching activities of all types of block-assigned trainees; (3) recruiting and appointing CCM fellows, staff associates, ICU head nurses, and special nonphysician personnel; (4) promoting and guiding clinical research in the ICU; (5) monitoring the quality of care and teaching; and (6) administering funds.

Departmental Versus Interdisciplinary ICUs

Surgical patients have medical problems and vice versa. The multidisciplinary ICU provides a unique setting in which a team representing the best of each discipline can address itself to the whole patient, an entity much advertised but seldom cared for.

Therefore, concentrating critically ill but potentially salvageable patients who have multiple organ failures in interdisciplinary medical-surgical ICUs or CCM centers, i.e., combinations of adjacent medical, surgical, and cardiac ICUs, has not only patient care but also economic advantages over purely department-specialty-organ-oriented ICUs (Weil and Shubin, 1971). National recommendations state that hospitals needing more than 8 to 10 beds for medical-surgical intensive care should create several 8 to 10 bed clusters located side-by-side for the sharing of staff, equipment, and ancillary facilities. Although in community hospitals, multidisciplinary ICU clusters have become increasingly popular, in large teaching hospitals, unfortunately, geographic and administrative separation into medical, surgical, and other specialty ICUs is commonplace, enhanced by departmental fragmentation in these university centers. Physical separation of medical and surgical ICU beds into geographically remote, separate units is unwise for the following reasons: (1) additional funding and manpower would be required; (2) the fluctuating occupancy rate of ICUs would be worsened; (3) the multidisciplinary concept of intensive care would be eroded; and (4) support services would suffer decreased efficiency and increased cost of operation. Thus, we recommend that separate ICUs be grouped into CCM centers.

A possible advantage of administratively separate medical and surgical ICUs in university centers is inherent in our present "political" situation, since ICU physicians who are "owned" by a base specialty department chairman are more likely to obtain primary patient care responsibility.

Physician Staffing and Responsibility

In addition to the ICU director and co-director, house staff or staff physicians are needed for in-house coverage, preferably full-time in-ICU coverage to make the care rendered truly intensive medical care. Participation by several departments is needed to provide such coverage. Residents should receive ICU training in a systematic block-assigned way and from those devoted to teaching this aspect of care and should share in-ICU coverage in the process. These assignments should be obligatory and full-time. Elective rotations are possible but less desirable, since an elective implies that this clinical area is regarded as having less importance.

In institutions with ICU fellowships, the SCCM guidelines should be used (Society of Critical Care Medicine, 1973). Fellows should be involved in ICU coverage as well as clinical research, and optionally laboratory research, in two-year programs.

The extent of ICU physician patient care responsibility will depend on local circumstances and should be expressed in the hospital's ICU policy. If obligatory block-assigned rotations through the ICU for house staff of the major disciplines is accomplished, the house officer should be given responsibility for titrated care — following a general plan agreed on for each patient by the attending physician and the ICU staff physicians.

Ideally, ICU physician staff and trainees should have primary patient care responsibility, as has been the practice in Canada and European countries for general ICUs, but in the USA, only in some specialty ICUs. If this is unacceptable, the following would be a *compromise*: In a multidisciplinary medical (or pediatric)-surgical ICU, residents of the main clinical departments should be block-assigned to the ICU under the direction of the ICU staff physicians. These residents should coordinate the recommendations of (a) the primary physician who remains in charge of general care while the patient is in the ICU; (b) the ICU staff physicians who, as obligatory team members, are responsible for the standards of life support (monitoring and support of vital organs); and (c) consultants called in by primary or ICU physicians. The admitting (attending) physician can, if desired, overrule the ICU physicians' decisions, but outside house staff should not be given this priority. If the ICU physicians, on the other hand, believe that a major error in therapy is being undertaken by the primary physician, recourse could be had to the chairman of the department under the auspices of which the patient is admitted to the ICU.

This system, in spite of its on-and-off frustrations, has proved feasible and, as an educationally desirable compromise, advantageous to house staff training of all departments concerned (Safar and Grenvik, 1977, Shoemaker, 1975; Weil and Shubin, 1971). The patient's principal house officer in the ICU, who takes over from the house officer on the ward, is the block-assigned resident of the same base discipline; house officers block-assigned to the ICU from other disciplines, share the responsibility for 24-hour coverage. During the patient's stay in the ICU, the admitting house officer becomes a team member, channeling input through the ICU house officer, who coordinates the orders. While the patient is in the ICU, the attending physician in charge of general care remains the same, the house staff changes, and the ICU staff physician remains responsible, as an obligatory team member, for resuscitation and life support, administration, and teaching. The attending-admitting physician may, in spite of the retention of authority over patient care, turn primary care responsibility over to the ICU staff physician for specific critical periods of the patient's course, which temporarily changes the compromise back to the ideal.

CONCLUSIONS

The goal of CCM is to improve care for acute life threatening illnesses and injuries, leading to increased salvage of lives with maintained human mentation and to a reduction of permanent disability. Personal experiences and published data suggest that titrated therapy with primary care responsibility by those competent and interested in resuscitation and prolonged life support, remaining at the patient's bedside, has advantages in terms of patient outcome and education over intensive nursing care with the primary physician or surgeon rounding, prescribing, and leaving for other duties. All anesthesiologists should be educated to the capability of functioning as consultants in resuscitation and respiratory intensive care. Their full-time or most-time involvement as team members or, ideally, as team coordinators in charge of primary care during the patient's ICU stay will depend on each individual's competence, interest, availability, and financial considerations. The present trend for CCM to become a subspecialty of anesthesiology, medicine, pediatrics, and surgery is most viable.

REFERENCES

Bachman, L., Downes, J.J., Richards, C.C., et al.: Organization and function of an intensive care unit in a children's hospital. Anesth. Analg., *46*:570–574, 1967.

Eckenhoff, J.E., and Dam, W.: The

treatment of barbiturate poisoning with or without analeptics. Am. J. Med., *20*:6, 1956.

Grenvik, A.: Certification of special competence in critical care medicine as a new subspecialty. A status report. Crit. Care Med., 6:355–359, 1978.

Ibsen, B.: The anesthetist's viewpoint on treatment of respiratory complications in poliomyelitis during the epidemic in Copenhagen, 1952. Proc. R. Soc. Med., 47:72–74, 1954.

Kampschulte, S., and Safar, P.: Development of multidisciplinary pediatric intensive care unit. Crit. Care Med., 1:308–315, 1973.

Kinney, J.M.: The intensive care unit. Bull. Am. Coll. Surg., 51:201–356, 1966.

Petty, T.L.: (a) Respiratory care is mod! Chest, 59:475–476, 1971; (b) Who should supervise respiratory ICUs? Chest, 70:323–324, 1976.

Safar, P., and Grenvik, A.: Organization and physician education in critical care medicine. Anesthesiology, 47:82–95, 1977.

Safar, P.: Critical care medicine — Quo vadis? Crit. Care Med., 2:1–5, 1974.

Safar, P., DeKornfeld, T., Pearson, J., et al.: Intensive care unit. Anaesthesia, 16:275–284, 1961.

Safar, P. (ed.): Public Health Aspects of Critical Care Medicine and Anesthesiology. (Clinical Anesthesia Series) Philadelphia, F.A. Davis, 1974, Vol. 10, No. 3. Chapters 3, 4, and 5.

Safar, P. (editor), Weil, M.H., Shubin, H.S., Petty, T.L., and Ersoz, C.J.: Critical care medicine — is it just another fad? Symp. Med. Opinion, et al. 3/10:18–50, 1974.

Safar, P.: The anesthesiologist as intensivist. In Eckenhoff, J. (ed.): Science and Practice in Anesthesia. Philadelphia, J.B. Lippincott, 1965.

Shoemaker, W.C.: Interdisciplinary medicine: Accommodation or integration? Crit. Care Med., 3:1–4, 1975.

Society of Critical Care Medicine: Guidelines for organization of critical care units. J.A.M.A., 222:1532–1535, 1972.

Society of Critical Care Medicine: Guidelines for physician education in critical care medicine. Crit. Care Med., 1:39–42, 1973.

Weil, M.H., and Shubin, H.: Symposium on care of the critically ill. Mod. Med., 39:83–137, 1971.

by LAWRENCE L. MICHAELIS

Northwestern University Medical School

THE ATTENDING SURGEON SHOULD RETAIN CONTROL OF SURGICAL PATIENTS IN THE INTENSIVE CARE UNIT

This article will defend the position that the attending surgeon should be responsible for surgical patients in the intensive care unit. The term "surgical patient" herein includes patients recovering from any operative procedure as well as those suffering from trauma and burns. It also includes patients who need observation in an intensive care environment prior to an anticipated surgical procedure (owing to gastrointestinal bleeding, cardiogenic shock, gas gangrene, and the like). The author agrees with Francis D. Moore, who stated, "The practice of surgery is the assumption of complete responsibility for the welfare of the patient suffering from these (surgical) diseases." (Moore, 1959)

In order to appreciate fully the surgeon's concern with surgical intensive care, a review of the development of the concept of intensive care and the contribution of surgeons to this field is appropriate. The modern surgical intensive care unit is an amalgamation of the postoperative recovery room, the trauma unit, and the special nursing units bred by complex surgical procedures. The evolution of intensive care units has been described in detail by Hilberman (1975), and it is quite evident that surgeons have been in the forefront as advocates of and innovators in this concept of patient care.

Walter Dandy of the Johns Hopkins Hospital and Martin Kirschner in Germany were proponents of surgical intensive care in the 1920's and 1930's. The 1940's saw the introduction of burn units, trauma hospitals, shock wards, and thoracic surgical units, for the most part because of World War II. In that decade, recovery rooms were intro-

293

duced by surgeons and anesthesiologists at the Mayo Clinic, Strong Memorial Hospital, the New York Hospital, and the Ochsner Clinic.

Perhaps the greatest stimulus to sophisticated care of the surgical patient was the development of cardiace surgery in the 1950's and 1960's. Suddenly, in the recovery rooms of major medical centers, a large number of patients appeared with central venous and arterial lines, temporary pacemakers, urinary catheters for continuous measurement of urinary output, and continuous ECG monitoring. Most of these patients required long-term ventilatory support, and many were receiving various cardiotonic and vasoactive drugs. Surgeons and surgical residents learned how to administer drugs that were formerly used principally by cardiologists, anesthesiologists, or pharmacologists.

In 1959, Francis D. Moore published a milestone in surgical literature, *The Metabolic Care of The Surgical Patient*. Surgeons responded by becoming apprised of the biochemical and nutritional needs of postoperative and traumatized patients. No longer were we primarily concerned with the technical details of an operative procedure; improved results after complex general, thoracic, and cardiovascular surgery depended on improvements in preoperative and postoperative care, and surgeons became proficient in implementing these improvements.

The 1970's have seen further sophistication in the application of intensive care units to specific medical and surgical conditions, and with it has come the development of the "intensivist," a physician trained particularly in the delivery of intensive care. These physicians, with basic training in medicine, anesthesiology, pediatrics, or surgery, spend 6 to 24 months of additional training in critical care medicine (Weil and Shubin, 1976), and now we hear that all patients transferred to the intensive care area should be under their supervision. Imagine the response of surgeons to this suggestion! For the last 40 years, surgeons have evolved the concept of total patient care with emphasis on proper selection, complete preoperative preparation, refinement of intraoperative techniques, and the type of postoperative care outlined previously. Now we are told that we should withdraw as the primary physician when the patient needs complex postoperative or post-traumatic care. Some of these "armchair philosophies," handed down by the intensivists, have been clouded by such statements as "the team approach" or "a consortium of care." There is, however, in my opinion, one irrefutable dictum that applies to the care of the critically ill patient — ultimately someone must be in charge. Good patient care cannot be provided by committee decision.

Why cannot a consortium work? Complex patient care requires an understanding of the whole physiologic system and of the priorities in the delivery of patient care. Difficulties invariably arise when specialists of different backgrounds treat an individual patient (Shoemaker, 1975). Consider these simplified examples:

1. The patient with pulmonary edema and low urinary output following a complex urologic procedure. A nephrologist or urologist thinks about forcing fluids to protect the kidneys and post-renal struc-

tures, whereas the internist is primarily concerned about withholding fluids in order to reverse the pulmonary edema.

2. A mechanically ventilated patient with low cardiac output following aortic valve replacement. The cardiologist may be adamant about digitalization, whereas the anesthesiologist might properly be concerned about an alkalosis present in the patient and hence reluctant to administer the drug.

3. The postgastrectomy patient who has aspirated during extubation. The anesthesiologist wants to give a steroid because it may prevent pneumonitis. The surgeon on the other hand may believe that steroids are of questionable value in this condition and that they can only increase the patient's other problems, such as inhibiting wound healing.

These three examples could well be in Dr. Safar's article, because they demonstrate that only one person can make the final decision in the care of the critically ill surgical patient. Responsibility must rest with a physician who has a broad overview of that particular patient's disease process. This physician must have an adequate understanding of respiratory, renal, cardiovascular, and gastrointestinal physiology in order to consider all of these aspects of patient care. I do not debate that the anesthesiologist may be better equipped than the surgeon to deal with pulmonary insufficiency in all instances; my contention is that we must train surgeons to deal with the routine problems in postoperative surgical patients and to recognize those situations for which the anesthesiologist should be called in consultation. The same applies for the surgeon's relationship with the nephrologist, cardiologist, neurologist, and specialist in infectious disease.

It is important to remember that intensive care, just like any other medical discipline, is not a strict science; it incorporates the art of medicine as well. Each physician must find a system of patient care that fits into his or her knowledge of physiology and pharmacology, philosophy of patient care, and technical expertise and that has been proved through experience to work. Only a surgeon can deliver this kind of care to a surgical patient.

As an example of why surgeons are reluctant to accept the intensivist's direction, I will hypothesize a surgical intensive care unit under the direction of an intensivist. This hypothetical intensive care unit is in a hospital that has a residency program in surgery; it is a large and fully equipped facility with the latest in computerized monitoring systems. The intensivist is an anesthesiologist who has had additional training in critical care medicine. All patients admitted to the surgical intensive care unit are automatically under the intensivist's supervision. There is a tacit understanding that surgical patients will be seen regularly by their attending surgeon, who will make recommendations to the intensivist appropriate to specific postoperative needs and potential complications that might arise in specific surgical conditions. I will now review objections, real and imagined, to this arrangement as seen through the eyes of a surgeon. Many of these situations have occurred; all could occur should the surgeon lose control of the patient.

The attending surgeon and the surgical resident are *not* going to be participating in minute-to-minute patient care if they are not in charge. Few will argue that in dealing with postoperative patients, a direct knowledge of the surgical procedure is vitally important to the specific care of the individual patient. Familiarity with the location of an intestinal anastomosis, the drainage of the retroperitoneal space, the quality of a bronchial stump closure, or the anatomy of the vascular system at the site of an anastomosis is important should a catastrophe occur. The intensivist assures us that we have a team approach; the surgeon will see the patient daily and will be available for any emergency. This is contrary to human nature. If a physician is not responsible for a patient, then that physician and the house staff on the service are not continually available. It is especially easy for the surgical house staff, who are frequently busy in the operating room, to delegate all responsibility to the intensivist; considerations of a specific operative procedure are lost in the transition of authority.

The hypothetical situation outlined before is also distasteful to surgeons because of our responsibility to the patient and the patient's family. Suddenly, a patient on whom we have operated is transferred to the care of a physician the patient and family have never met. The intensivist in our hypothetical situation is not even a surgeon and has neither seen the patient prior to the surgical procedure nor discussed the operative procedure with the patient or the patient's family. The intensivist is ill-equipped to handle specific emotional needs with which the attending surgeon may be quite familiar (Stahl, 1972). Finally, there are obvious legal implications involved in this sort of transfer of the postoperative surgical patient to the care of another physician that are beyond the scope of this article. Suffice it to say that if the patient dies or has a serious complication, the family is not going to blame the intensivist!

Most surgeons believe that education of the surgical house staff suffers in this environment. In addition to training residents in an environment in which abdication of responsibility for the patient's care following a surgical procedure is commonplace, the surgical resident is deprived of learning intensive care techniques. The intensivist responds that surgical residents will spend a three- to six-month rotation on the service in order to learn critical care, but in this situation, the surgical resident will always be short-changed, especially since the intensivist is not a surgeon. The intensivist in our hypothetical unit is an anesthesiologist by training and will have a natural tendency, if there are anesthesia, medical, and surgical residents rotating simultaneously through the intensive care unit, to give priority in such techniques as tracheal intubation, adjustment of ventilators, and procedures classically in the field of anesthesia to the anesthesia resident. The surgical resident is in a "Catch-22" situation, being taught postoperative surgical care by a nonsurgeon who believes surgeons should not be responsible for postoperative intensive care.

It is my opinion, and one shared by many other surgeons, that the greatest objection to the intensivist concept is the attitude of many critical care physicians. Continuous involvement with critical care medicine breeds a type of physician more interested in numbers than in the patient as a whole. Too often I have asked, "How is the patient doing?" and have heard the reply, "Her PO_2 is 56." A surgical colleague refers to the "blue-arm syndrome," which occurs when nonsurgical house officers are engaged in critical care; a patient is seen who has had a brachial artery cannula inserted and the arm becomes ischemic and dusky in color. The surgeon (or any experienced physician) immediately removes the cannula in order to restore circulation to the hand and arm while the nonsurgeon in charge of the patient's critical care may only reply, "How on earth are we going to collect samples for blood gas analysis?" I am personally repulsed when I see attending and staff rounds on ICU patients being held in a conference room with the staff reading flow sheets, rather than at the bedside looking at the patient. These outlandish examples demonstrate the tendency to think in terms of numbers rather than in terms of the whole patient. It occurs easily in critical care medicine because of the constant emphasis on measured data. Preoperative contact with the patient and patient's family and an awareness of the long-term outcome of specific diseases and operations help in combating this attitude.

The final objection to our hypothetical unit is the cost of intensive care. The era of subspecialization to the point at which a physician becomes more and more of an authority on fewer and fewer things is upon us (Shoemaker, 1975). When one has only a very narrow sphere in which to operate, there is a tendency to learn more about it and to use more sophisticated equipment. No one has yet demonstrated that the proliferation of computerized monitoring equipment has actually improved patient care. In fact, recently in a small hospital, no significant difference in surgical mortality rates could be demonstrated after a surgical intensive care unit was provided (Tagge et al., 1975). The intensivists are fond of expounding on the complexities of intensive care. I believe that to some extent they are perpetrating a hoax. Good postoperative intensive care, in most instances, is not difficult to learn and need not be expensive. Another cost consideration in this hypothetical intensive care unit has to do with bed occupancy. There is a constant temptation to keep patients in the intensive care unit if all beds are not occupied. This looks good on the books of the director of the intensive care unit and keeps the intensivist in contact with patients — whether or not a patient need remain there.

All of these situations, which can or do occur when surgical intensive care patients come under the direction of a nonsurgical intensivist, are distasteful to most surgeons. How do surgeons respond? The simple solution is not to send patients to the intensive care unit. Our hypothetical intensive care unit could well be "all dressed up with no place to go" because surgeons may refuse to admit their patients to such a unit. In the long run, everyone suffers.

What is the answer to this controversy? It is obvious that surgical intensive care units are here to stay; no reasonable person will refute the need for some surgical patients to be cared for in a critical care unit. Certainly there is a definite role for the intensivist. An intensive care unit must have a director (Walt and Wilson, 1975) and an intensivist is well suited for this role. Someone must be responsible for bed allotment, the financial condition of the unit, the direction of the nursing and paramedical personnel, and infection surveillance. In fact, many surgeons would be pleased to hand over these duties to an intensivist.

Some surgeons may want to place their patients under the supervision of another physician specially trained in critical care medicine. Many surgical subspecialists are not equipped to manage patients with multisystem failure and are eager to transfer these patients to an intensivist. Some general surgeons, trained prior to the development of the concept of intensive surgical care or in institutions in which this training was not provided, are in the same situation. The gist of my argument is that the surgeon must have the *option* of deciding whether or not to transfer a patient to the care of an intensivist. Most general, thoracic, and cardiovascular surgeons are adept in this specialized form of patient management, and they should be allowed to control their patient in the surgical intensive care unit. They are usually pleased to have an intensivist (in this situation probably someone with special competence in respiratory care) available for consultation in complex situations. In the vast majority of instances, however, well-trained surgeons will have little or no difficulty in caring for the postoperative thoracic, cardiovascular, or general surgical patient, as well as those with multiple trauma.

I believe therefore that the solution is to give the attending surgeon the prerogative of transferring patients to the care of the intensivist. At the same time, the surgeon must retain the privilege of regaining control of the patient whenever desired. This will prevent most of the controversies and mishaps described above. If the intensivist is diplomatic, seeks and implements advice from the referring surgeon, and generally follows the outlines of appropriate postoperative considerations in specific surgical problems, then the critical care program will flourish as will a referral practice. If the intensivist is more concerned with data from a computer sheet than with actual patient care, patients will not be referred and there will be no problem to solve.

There is a role for the subspecialist in critical care medicine. I believe that surgeons should encourage, to some extent, the development of this specialty. It is mandatory, however, that an intensivist in the surgical intensive care unit be a *fully trained surgeon* with additional training in critical care medicine. Hopefully, such a surgical intensivist would continue to perform in the operating room and hence not lose an overview of the practice of surgery. In the final analysis, perhaps Shoemaker (1975) was correct when he stated: "Unfortunately, there has been too much emphasis on who is in charge and too little emphasis on what is wrong with the system."

To insist that every surgical patient entering the intensive care unit automatically comes under the control of an intensivist is foolhardy. Patients and their families will not like it; the public cannot afford it; and surgeons will not permit it.

REFERENCES

Hilberman, M.: The evolution of intensive care units. Crit. Care Med., 3:159, 1975.

Moore, F. D.: Metabolic Care of The Surgical Patient. 1st ed. Philadelphia, W. B. Saunders Company, 1959.

Shoemaker, W. C.: Interdisciplinary medicine: Accommodation or integration? Crit. Care Med., 3:1, 1975.

Stahl, W. M.: Supportive Care of The Surgical Patient. 1st ed. New York, Grune and Stratton Company, 1972.

Tagge, G. F., Salness, G., Thoms, J., Wipple, G. H., and Shoemaker, W. C.: Experience with a multidisciplinary critical care center in a community hospital. Crit. Care Med., 3:231, 1975.

Walt, A. J., and Wilson, R. F.: Management of Trauma: Pitfalls and Practice. 1st ed. Philadelphia, Lea and Febiger Company, 1975.

Weil, M. H., and Shubin, H.: Critical Care Medicine: Current Principles and Practices. 1st ed. Hagerstown, Harper and Row Publishers, 1976.

THE DIRECTION OF PATIENT CARE IN INTENSIVE CARE UNITS

EDITORIAL COMMENT

Traditionally, when a physician admitted a patient to hospital, the responsibility for the patient's care rested solely with that physician unless the care was formally transferred to someone else. The physician's office might be remote from the hospital, the patient likely seen once daily, perhaps twice for the critically ill, and contact was retained through either housestaff or nurses. Those of us familiar with hospitals 40 years ago know that some patients died for lack of reasonably constant care and availability of adequately trained professional help. As Safar, Grenvik, and Michaelis point out, recovery rooms and intensive care units came into being first to bring together the patients and equipment needed to care for the injured, recently operated on, or critically ill and second to provide skilled individuals who could care for the patients. It all made sense; it was economical of equipment and personnel and was life-saving for many patients. The principal burden was placed on the nursing staff who had to be trained to detect danger signals and carry out therapeutic regimens while housestaff and attending physicians moved in and out according to their own schedules. With an expanding and aging population, surgical attack on diseases of the extremes of life, and attempts to salvage patients from diseases previously thought fatal, it became apparent that constant physician attendance was mandatory. The present controversy acknowledges that physicians must be present but disputes who should be in charge of the patients in the ICU.

Safar and Grenvik, champions of a subspecialty of critical care medicine, plead for special training in the care of patients in intensive care units, for the constant presence of physicians with such training, and for the direction and coordination of the units by physicians so trained. Michaelis wants to retain direction of his own patients even though, as he admits, he and his housestaff may be busy in the office or operating room — or in another hospital. He is unconvinced of the team effort, is fearful that his housestaff may not get the training due them, and apparently is not sure that his input concerning his own patients will be respected.

I suspect that Michaelis is fighting a losing battle and that the standards of medical care will preclude absentee direction. It harkens back to Beal's chapter on the demise of the captain-of-the-ship doctrine. In my estimation, the problem is one of cooperation, coordination, communication, and mutual respect. If a surgeon is not able to communicate with a director of an intensive care unit and does not respect his abilities, no proposed organization will work. Similarly, if the intensivist will not listen to the patient's surgeon and short changes residents from the surgical service, longevity in the position is apt to be short. The problems are most apt to come into focus in the early morning hours when the junior intensivist and the junior surgeon "have at" each other.

INDEX

Note: Page numbers in italics refer to illustrations. Page numbers followed by (t) refer to tables.

Isosorbide dinitrate, use of to combat hypertension during coronary by-pass operations, 150

Jaundice, unexplained occurrence of after administration of halothane, 33

Kidney, blood flow and oxygen require-ments of, 109–110
effects of hypoxia on, 260

Labor, pregnancy and, physiologic changes related to, 117–118
Laryngoscope(s), contamination of during use, 80
Larynx, infant, anatomy of, 165
Limb(s), phantom, painful sensations of, spinal anesthesia as cause of, 16
Liver, effects of hypoxemia on, 261
halothane-induced damage to, 33–34
Lumbar puncture, traumatic, avoid-ance of minimization of possibility of, 11
results of, 10–11
Lungs, complications in, as major cause of morbidity and mortality follow-ing surgery, 249
postoperative, 75, 244
causes of, 250
definition of, 249–250
incidence of in relation to various factors, 245(t)
respiratory maneuvers for, com-parison of, 251
preparation of prior to surgery, factors important in, 252–253

Mandatory, definition of in reference to endotracheal tube, 123
Medical practice, basic principle of, 73
Medicine, critical care, challenge of, 280–282
definition of, 279
physicians specializing in, direction of ICU and, 279–291
team approach to, 287
training specialists in, 285–286
traditional Chinese, 184–187
Medicolegal insult, fear of following deliberate hypotension, 112
Mendelson's syndrome, use of oral antacids to reduce risk of in par-turients, 119
Meningitis, abscess and, contaminated equipment as cause of, prevention of, 76
epidural abscess and, as complications of spinal anesthesia, 11

Methoxyflurane, development of post-anesthetic hepatic necrosis due to, 7–8
Miscarriage, incidence of in anesthesia department personnel, 51–52
Monitoring, intra-arterial. See *Intra-arterial monitoring.*
Morbidity, mortality and, deliberate hypotension as cause of, 102–103
Morphine, anesthesia with, cardiac surgery and, cardiovascular parameters during, 140, *141*
disadvantages of, 142
increased need for blood with, 151
release of catecholamines during, 140
use of for coronary bypass opera-tion, 138–142
balanced anesthetic technique and, 149–151
association of with hypotension, 149
benefits of in cardiac surgery, 149
deleterious circulatory effects of, 138
effects of, on coronary blood flow, 140
on ventricular function and periph-eral circulation, 139, *139*
incidence of hypotension with vs. in-halation anesthetics, 149
mechanism of action of on cardio-vascular system, 139
patients receiving, blood requirements of during coronary bypass opera-tions, 142
principal contribution of to anesthetic state, 149
use of, history of, 149
in balanced anesthetic technique for coronary bypass operations, 149–151
Mortality, maternal, aspiration as cause of, incidence of, 126, 127
definition of, 118
importance of to tracheal intuba-tion, 118–119
major causes of, 118
percentage of due to anesthesia, 119
morbidity and, deliberate hypotension as cause of, 102–103
Mucosa, engorged, of airway in parturi-ent, 119
Mucous blanket, description and func-tions of, 242–244, *243*
Muscle relaxants, use of in obstetric procedures, 120
Myocardium, contractility of, effects of anesthetics or adjuvants on, 137
depression of, as anesthetic com-plication, 148
oxygen balance in, *135*
oxygen consumption in, rate of under various circulatory conditions, *109*
oxygen demand in, determinants of, 136, 148
oxygen requirements of, factors governing, 108
oxygen supply of, major determinants of, 135

Parturients (*Continued*)
    tracheal intubation in, techniques
        for, 120–121
    types of personnel administering
        anesthesia for, 124(t)
    use of general anesthesia in, need for
        tracheal intubation with, 117–121
        results of without mandatory
            tracheal intubation, 125–126
Patient(s), care of, direction of in in-
        tensive care units, 277–301
    fragmentation of by multiple con-
        sultants, 283–284
    titrated, 282–283
        view of as responsibility of critical
            care medicine physicians, 279–
            291
    obstetric, number of given anesthesia,
        124
    surgical, bronchial hygiene and, 244–
        245
Peridural anesthesia, resurgence of use
    of, view of as threat to survival of
    spinal anesthesia, 16–17
Personnel, anesthesia. See *Anesthesia
    personnel.*
Phantom limb(s), painful sensations of,
    spinal anesthesia as cause of, 16
Physiology, maternal, importance of to
    tracheal intubation, 117–118
Plasma angiotensin II, rise in levels of
    during morphine-nitrous oxide
    anesthesia, 140
Preload, definition of, 137
Pregnancy, labor and, physiologic
    changes related to, 117–118
Pressure, arterial, monitoring of during
    deliberate hypotension, 99–100
Pulmonary disease, preoperative, IPPB
    therapy and, 246–247
Pulmonary system, functions of, 241
Puncture, lumbar. See *Lumbar puncture.*

Radial artery, catheter thrombectomy of,
    technique of, *263*
Regional anesthesia, administration of
    by nurse anesthetists, 225–229
        evidence supporting, 227
        view against, 231–235
    nurse anesthetists and, 223–237
Relaxants, muscle, use of in obstetric
    procedures, 120
Reproduction, anesthetic effects upon,
    45–70
Respiration, inadequacy of, as complica-
    tion of spinal anesthesia, 14–15
Respiratory tract, upper, infections of,
    anesthesia and, 74
    vascular tree and, as portals of entry
        and location for infection, 74

Safety, margin of, reduction of with
    deliberate hypotension, 111

Scopolamine, use of with morphine in
    coronary bypass operations, 150
Shock, common denominator of, 106
    signs of poor tissue perfusion with,
        106
Soda lime, ineffectiveness of as filter or
    bactericidal agent, 76–77
Spinal anesthesia, acceptance of, 6–17
    additional problems of, 14–15
    adhesive arachnoiditis due to, 12, *13*
    alternatives to, 7–8
    brain damage due to 9–10
    cauda equina syndrome as complica-
        tion of, 11–12
    choice of, patients as adversaries in,
        8–14
    effects of on regional circulation, 14
    epidural abscess and meningitis as
        complications of, 11
    epidural anesthesia and, physiologic
        responses to, 17
    exacerbation of antecedent neurologic
        disease by, 13–14
    failure of method for, 15–16
    headache due to, measure for pre-
        vention of, 10
    neurologic sequelae of, 6–7
        classification of, 9–10
    threat to survival of by resurgence
        of peridural anesthesia, 16–17
    unusual responses to, 15–16
Spinal cord, coverings of and, spinal
    anesthesia injuries localized to, 10–11
Splinter hemorrhage(s), as complication
    of arterial cannulation, 269
Stylets, contamination of during use, 80
Succinylcholine, nitrous oxide–oxygen
    and, use of during coronary bypass
    operations, 150
Surgeon(s), captain of the ship
        doctrine and, 3–5
    contributions of to intensive care,
        293–294
Surgery, advanced technology in, effects
        of on flammable anesthetics, 20–21
    anesthesia and, relationships between,
        3–4
    cardiac, morphine anesthesia and,
        benefits of, 149
        cardiovascular parameters during,
            140, *141*
    vessel, use of deliberate hypotension
        to facilitate, 96
Surgical practice, sound, fundamental
    tenets of, 95
Syndrome, cauda equina, as complica-
        tion of spinal anesthesia, 11–12
    signs and symptoms of, 11
    Mendelson's, use of oral antacids to
        reduce risk of in parturients, 119

Tachycardia, effects of, 98
    on myocardium, 148
    production of by hypotensive drugs,
        98